Pocketbook

From the publishers of the *Tarascon Pocket Pharmacopoeia*

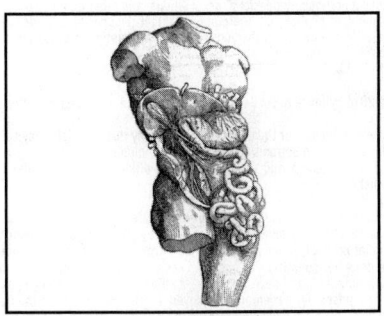

Eric Esrailian, MD, MPH
Co-Chief, Division of Digestive Diseases
Lincy Foundation Chair in Clinical Gastroenterology
Associate Clinical Professor of Medicine
David Geffen School of Medicine at UCLA
Los Angeles, CA
Website: http://gastro.ucla.edu

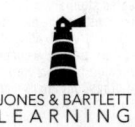

JONES & BARTLETT
LEARNING

World Headquarters
Jones & Bartlett Learning
5 Wall Street
Burlington, MA 01803
978-443-5000
info@jblearning.com
www.jblearning.com

Jones & Bartlett Learning books and products are available through most bookstores and online booksellers. To contact Jones & Bartlett Learning directly, call 800-832-0034, fax 978-443-8000, or visit our website, www.jblearning.com.

Substantial discounts on bulk quantities of Jones & Bartlett Learning publications are available to corporations, professional associations, and other qualified organizations. For details and specific discount information, contact the special sales department at Jones & Bartlett Learning via the above contact information or send an email to specialsales@jblearning.com.

Copyright © 2016 by Jones & Bartlett Learning, LLC, an Ascend Learning Company

All rights reserved. No part of the material protected by this copyright may be reproduced or utilized in any form, electronic or mechanical, including photocopying, recording, or by any information storage and retrieval system, without written permission from the copyright owner.

The content, statements, views, and opinions herein are the sole expression of the respective authors and not that of Jones & Bartlett Learning, LLC. Reference herein to any specific commercial product, process, or service by trade name, trademark, manufacturer, or otherwise does not constitute or imply its endorsement or recommendation by Jones & Bartlett Learning, LLC and such reference shall not be used for advertising or product endorsement purposes. All trademarks displayed are the trademarks of the parties noted herein. *Tarascon Gastroenterology Pocketbook* is an independent publication and has not been authorized, sponsored, or otherwise approved by the owners of the trademarks or service marks referenced in this product.

The authors, editor, and publisher have made every effort to provide accurate information. However, they are not responsible for errors, omissions, or for any outcomes related to the use of the contents of this book and take no responsibility for the use of the products and procedures described. Treatments and side effects described in this book may not be applicable to all people; likewise, some people may require a dose or experience a side effect that is not described herein. Drugs and medical devices are discussed that may have limited availability controlled by the Food and Drug Administration (FDA) for use only in a research study or clinical trial. Research, clinical practice, and government regulations often change the accepted standard in this field. When consideration is being given to use of any drug in the clinical setting, the health care provider or reader is responsible for determining FDA status of the drug, reading the package insert, and reviewing prescribing information for the most up-to-date recommendations on dose, precautions, and contraindications, and determining the appropriate usage for the product. This is especially important in the case of drugs that are new or seldom used.

NOTES

NOTES

NOTES

NOTES

NOTES

NOTES

Index

small intestinal bacterial overgrowth (SIBO), 28, 31, 88–89
small intestine, 96–97
SMV. *See* simeprevir
snare polypectomy, 163
SNRIs. *See* serotonin and norepinephrine reuptake inhibitors
sofosbuvir (SOF), 205–206
solid pseudopapillary neoplasms (SPNS), 133
somatic pain, 3
sorafenib, 270
splenic artery, 105
SPNS. *See* solid pseudopapillary neoplasms
spontaneous bacterial peritonitis (SBP), 252
sporadic vascular ectasia, 116
squamous cell carcinoma, 117
SSRIs. *See* selective serotonin reuptake inhibitors
Staphylococcus aureus, 158
steatohepatitis, 213
steatosis, 213
stenting/angioplasty of short venous stenosis, 212
steroids, 44
"stiff fundus," 14
stimulant laxative, 25*t*
stomach flu, 157
stool-based studies, 144
stool DNA, 144
stool osmotic gap, 30
stool softener/emollient, 25*t*
stricturing disease, 169
sub-mucosal epinephrine, 116*t*
superior mesenteric artery (SMA), 101, 103, 106
swallowed topical steroids, 11
symptomatic cholelithiasis, 140*t*, 141
symptomatic pseudocysts, 138
symptomatic therapy, 158

T

T2 hyperintense scar, 222
TACE. *See* transarterial chemoembolizations
TCAs. *See* tricyclic antidepressants
telaprevir, 205
tenofovir, 201
thiazolidinediones (TZDs), 243
thienopyridines, 310
third-degree burn, 42
third-line management, ascites, 252
thrombocytopenia, 114
thromboembolic disease, 296
thrombolytic therapy, 104
thrombosis, 103, 212
TIPS. *See* transjugular intrahepatic portosystemic shunt
TNM system, 128
traditional serrated adenomas, 162
transarterial chemoembolizations (TACE), 270
transjugular intrahepatic portosystemic shunt (TIPS), 111, 212, 261
Traveler's diarrhea, 30
tricyclic antidepressants (TCAs), 91
trientine, 215
Trousseau's syndrome, 127
tumor staging of esophageal cancer, 118
TZDs. *See* thiazolidinediones

U

UC. *See* ulcerative colitis
UDCA. *See* ursodeoxycholic acid
UGIB. *See* upper gastrointestinal bleeding
ulcerative colitis (UC), 153, 225
diagnosis, 166–167
differential diagnosis, 166
pathophysiology, 166
presentation, 165
treatment, 167

ulcers, 66, 110, 111
ultrasonography, 8
ultrasound, abdominal, 49
unconjugated hyperbilirubinemia, causes of, 195*t*
unifocal BD-IPMN, 132
upper area of abdomen, pain, 5*t*
upper esophageal foreign bodies, 36
upper gastrointestinal bleeding (UGIB)
differential diagnosis, 110
endoscopy, 110–111
gastropaedica, 110
post-endoscopy management, 111
pre-endoscopy management, 110
presentation, 109
upper gastrointestinal series, 51
ursodeoxycholic acid (UDCA), 227, 230
U.S. treatment algorithm, HBV, 202*f*

V

vague pain, 3
vascular access, 293
vascular malformations, 107
vasculitides, 107
venous drainage, 101
viral (rotavirus, adenovirus), 18
viral hepatitis, 209, 271
visceral pain, 3
vomiting, 7

W

Wegner's granulomatosis, 107
Whipple's disease, 28, 30, 31
widespread amyloid deposition, 74
Wilson's disease, 214–215, 245–246, 272

Z

Zenker diverticulum, 12

Index

pouchitis disease activity index (PDAI), 176
PPARG agonists. *See* peroxisome proliferator-activated receptor gamma agonists
PPIs. *See* proton pump inhibitors
pre-endoscopy management, 110
pre-pyloric feeding, 286
prednisone, 234
pregnancy, 19
  liver disease in. *See* liver disease, in pregnancy
preoperative embolization, 221
primary anal fissures. *See* anal fissures
primary biliary cirrhosis (PBC), 215, 216
  diagnosis, 230
  diagnostic algorithm for patients with, 231*f*
  differential diagnosis, 229
  pathophysiology, 229–230
  presentation, 229
  treatment, 230–231, 231*f*
primary sclerosing cholangitis (PSC), 216
  diagnosis, 226
  differential diagnosis, 226
  pathophysiology, 226
  presentation, 225–226
  treatment, 227
probiotics, 91, 176
prophylaxis, 176
proton pump inhibitors (PPIs), 11, 60
prucalopride, 25
pruritus, 264
PSC. *See* primary sclerosing cholangitis
pseudo-obstruction, 149
pseudocysts (PCs), 134
PTLD. *See* post-transplant lymphoproliferative disorders
PUD. *See* peptic ulcer disease

PVT. *See* portal vein thrombosis
pyogenic abscess, 223
pyrin, 75

R

radiation-induced colitis, 31
radiation therapy, 18
radiofrequency ablation, 270
radiologic studies for GI conditions. *See* GI conditions, radiologic studies for
randomized controlled trials, 66
Ranson's criteria, 136, 137*t*
RBV. *See* ribavirin
rectal foreign bodies, 39–40
recurrent pancreatitis, 135
recurrent pouchitis, 178
refeeding syndrome, 288
referred pain, 4
regurgitation, 17
renal insufficiency, 74
retroperitoneal hemorrhage, signs of, 135
revascularization, 105
ribavirin (RBV), 205–207
rifaximin, 178, 257
right lower quadrant (RLQ) ultrasound, 49
risk stratification tools, 110
RLQ ultrasound. *See* right lower quadrant ultrasound
rotavirus, 157
rumination process, 17
ruptured aortic aneurysm, 4
ruptured ectopic pregnancy, 4
RUQ ultrasound, 20

S

SBO. *See* small bowel obstruction
SBP. *See* spontaneous bacterial peritonitis
SCAD. *See* segmental colitis associated with diverticular disease
SCAs. *See* serous cystadenomas

SCID. *See* severe combined immunodeficiency
sclerosant injection, 111
sclerotherapy, 111
second-degree burn, 42
second-line management, ascites, 252
secretin stimulation test, 30
segmental colitis associated with diverticular disease (SCAD), 31
selective serotonin reuptake inhibitors (SSRIs), 91
self-expandable metal stents (SEMS), 120
sensitization, 85
serologic testing, 217
serotonin and norepinephrine reuptake inhibitors (SNRIs), 91
serous cystadenomas (SCAs), 133
serrated lesions, 162
serum lipase, 136
sessile serrated polyps, 162
severe acute pancreatitis, 135, 137
severe CDI
  presentation, 183–184
  treatment, 185
severe combined immunodeficiency (SCID), 94
severe-complicated CDI
  presentation, 184
  treatment, 185, 187
sharp and well localized, somatic pain, 3
SIBO. *See* small intestinal bacterial overgrowth
sigmoidoscopy, flexible, 101–102
simeprevir (SMV), 206–207
skin prick tests, 85
SMA. *See* superior mesenteric artery
small bowel foreign bodies, 37–38
small bowel imaging aids, 171
small bowel obstruction (SBO), 149

painless lower gastrointestinal bleeding, common causes of, 114*t*
palpable supraclavicular, 124
PAN. *See* polyarteritis nodosa
pancreas disease, 97
pancreatic cancer
 diagnosis, 128
 differential diagnosis, 127
 gastropaedica, 127
 presentation, 127
 prognosis, 129
 risk factors, 127–128
 staging, 128
 treatment, 129
pancreatic cystic neoplasms (PCNs), 131
pancreatic cysts
 differential diagnosis and treatment of different, 132–134
 gastropaedica, 131
pancreatic malignancies, 127
pancreatic necrosis, 137
pancreatic protocol, CT, 48–49
pancreatic pseudocysts, 138
pancreatitis
 diagnosis, 136
 differential diagnosis, 136
 gastropaedica, 135
 pathophysiology, 136
 presentation, 135
 treatment, 136–138
papain, 36
parenteral analgesia, 137
parenteral nutritional support
 complications, 295–296
 determine the composition of, 292–293
 gastropaedica, 291
 indications, 291–292
 infusions, 294
 monitoring, 294

nutritional needs and formulations, calculating, 292
parvovirus, 158
PAS. *See* pouchitis activity score
PAS stain. *See* periodic acid-Schiff stain
PBC. *See* primary biliary cirrhosis
PCNs. *See* pancreatic cystic neoplasms
PCOS. *See* polycystic ovarian syndrome
PCR. *See* polymerase chain reaction
PCs. *See* pseudocysts
PDAI. *See* pouchitis disease activity index
pegylated interferon (PEG), 206
 side effects of, 205
penicillamine, 215
peptic ulcer disease (PUD), 13, 65, 66
per-oral endoscopic myotomy (POEM), 11
percutaneous biopsy, 128
perforated duodenal ulcer, 4
perianal disease symptoms, 125
perinuclear antineutrophil cytoplasmic antibodies (p-ANCA), 166, 226
periodic acid-Schiff (PAS) stain, 211
perioperative chemotherapy, 125
peripheral leukocytosis, 183
periumbilical lymph nodes, 124
peroxisome proliferator-activated receptor gamma (PPARG) agonists, 243
persistent pseudocysts, 138
PET. *See* positron emission tomography
phenol, 42
plain radiographs, 35, 37, 39
plasma ammonia, 256

pleuritis, 74
PMNs. *See* polymorphonuclear leukocytes
POEM. *See* per-oral endoscopic myotomy
pollen food allergy syndrome, 83, 85
polyarteritis nodosa (PAN), 107
polycystic ovarian syndrome (PCOS), 239
polymerase chain reaction (PCR), 185
polymorphonuclear leukocytes (PMNs), 250
poorly localized pain, 3
porcelain gallbladder, 142
portal hypertension, 249, 260
portal vein thrombosis (PVT), 276
portal venous phase CT, 47
positron emission tomography (PET), 124
 esophageal cancer, 118–119
post-EGD proton pump inhibitor (PPI), 110
post-endoscopy management, 111
post-organ transplantation (HSCT/SOLID), 100
post-polypectomy bleed, 116
post-pyloric feeding, 286
post-transplant lymphoproliferative disorders (PTLD), 100
postoperative chemoradiation, 125
pouchitis
 cancer surveillance, 178
 diagnosis, 176
 differential diagnosis, 175
 pathophysiology, 175–176
 presentation, 175
 treatment, 176–178, 177*f*
pouchitis activity score (PAS), 176

Index

pathophysiology, 179–180
presentation, 179
treatment, 180–181, 181f
mid area of abdomen, pain, 5t
mild acute pancreatitis, 135
mild-to-moderate CDI
  presentation, 183
  treatment, 185
mild-to-moderate gallstone pancreatitis, patients with, 137
Mirizzi syndrome, 140t, 141
Model for End-Stage Liver Disease (MELD) score, 275
motility disorders, 19
MR enterography, 50
MRA. See magnetic resonance angiography
MRCP. See magnetic resonance cholangiopancreatography
mucinous cystic neoplasms (MCNS), 133
multifocal SB-IPMN, 133
multimodality treatment plan, 124
mutation
  analysis, 74
  HFE, 210
MVT. See mesenteric venous thrombosis

N

NAFLD. See nonalcoholic fatty liver disease
NASH. See nonalcoholic steatohepatitis
nasogastric tube (NGT), 102
  lavage, 110, 113
  placement, 111
National Polyp Study, 145
nausea and vomiting
  definitions, 17
  diagnosis, 20
  differential diagnosis, 18
  evaluation, 20
  pathophysiology, 17
  treatment, 21–22

negative pregnancy test, 92
negative upper endoscopy, 15
neuroendocrine tumors, 127
new-onset pouchitis, 176, 178
NHL. See Non-Hodgkin's lymphoma
NOMI. See non-occlusive mesenteric ischemia
non-gallstone gallbladder disease, 141
non-HBV/HCV hepatitis in clinical practice
  A1AT deficiency, 211
  AIH, 216–217
  ALD, 213–214
  BCS, 211–212
  cholestatic liver disease, 215–216
  differential diagnosis, 209
  DILI, 212–213
  gastropaedica, 209
  hepatitis A, 217–218
  HFE, 209–211
  NAFLD, 214
  Wilson's disease, 214–215
Non-Hodgkin's lymphoma (NHL), 99
non-occlusive mesenteric ischemia (NOMI), 103
nonalcoholic fatty liver disease (NAFLD), 214
  diagnosis, 240–242, 241f
  liver biopsy, 242
  natural history and cancer risks, 242
  pathophysiology, 239–240
  presentation, 240
  treatment, 242–243, 241f
nonalcoholic steatohepatitis (NASH), 214, 239, 275
nonmodifiable risk factors for gastric cancer, 123
nonsteroidal anti-inflammatory drug (NSAID), 109

norovirus, 157
NS. See nutcracker syndrome
NSAID. See nonsteroidal anti-inflammatory drug
nuclear scintigraphy, 115
nutcracker syndrome (NS), 106
nutritional requirements, calculation, 292
nutritional support, composition, 286

O

odynophagia, 34
Ogilvie syndrome, 149
  management of, 149
  pathophysiology of, 150
oligospermia/azoospermia, infertility with, 74
"onion skin" pattern, 226
oral agents, 201
oral allergy syndrome, 83, 85
oral antiviral therapy, 201–202
oral rehydration solutions (ORS), 302
oral/topical mesalamine, 178
oropharyngeal dysphagia, differential diagnosis of, 10t
ORS. See oral rehydration solutions
Osler-Weber-Rendu syndrome, 107
osmotic diarrhea, 28, 30
osmotic laxative, 25t
ovarian torsion, 4

P

p-ANCA. See perinuclear antineutrophil cytoplasmic antibodies
pain severity, 6
pain symptoms, characterization of, 5–7

Index

IPMNS. *See* intraductal papillary mucinous neoplasms
irritable bowel syndrome (IBS), 87, 299
   treatment for, 89–92, 90f
ischemic colitis, 101–102, 153
IV PPI. *See* intravenous proton pump inhibitor

J
jaundice, 7, 211

K
Kaposi's sarcoma (KS), 99, 100

L
L-ornithine-L-aspartate (LOLA), 257
labyrinthine disorders, 18
labyrinths, 17
lactulose, 256–257
laparoscopy, 151
large bowel obstruction (LBO), 149
large intestine, 96–97
laxatives, 91
LBO. *See* large bowel obstruction
LCHAD. *See* long-chain 3-hydroxyacyl-CoA dehydrogenase
LFTs. *See* liver function tests
LGIB. *See* lower gastrointestinal bleeding
liver
   with conventional contrast, MRI, 50
   with hepatobiliary contrast, MRI, 50
liver biopsy, 209, 210, 216, 225
   NAFLD, role of, 242
   PBC, 230
liver disease, 99, 296
   in pregnancy

acute fatty liver of pregnancy, 265–266
   HELLP syndrome, 264–265
   hyperemesis gravidarum, 263–264
   intrahepatic cholestasis of pregnancy, 264
liver function tests (LFTs), 213, 214, 230
liver injury, pattern of, 237
liver lesion, approach to patient
   abscesses, 223–224
   benign focal lesions, 220–223
   gastropaedica, 219
   malignant liver tumors, 220
liver panel abnormalities, 193
liver panel tests, 191, 192f
liver protocol, CT, 48
liver rupture, 265
liver transplantation (LT), 211, 270, 273
   gastropaedica, 275
   indications for, 275–276
   perioperative complications, 276–277
LOLA. *See* L-ornithine-L-aspartate
long-acting pegylated interferon alfa-2a, 201
long-chain 3-hydroxyacyl-CoA dehydrogenase (LCHAD), 265
lower area of abdomen, pain, 5t–6t
lower esophageal foreign bodies, 36–37
lower gastrointestinal bleeding (LGIB)
   diagnosis, 114–115
   differential diagnosis, 114
   gastropaedica, 113
   initial assessment, 113
   initial management, 113–114
   treatment, 115–116

LT. *See* liver transplantation
lubiprostone, 25
lung disease, 246
lye ingestions, 45
lymphocytic colitis, 179, 180

M
magnetic resonance angiography (MRA), 104
magnetic resonance cholangiopancreaticogram (MRCP), 216, 226
magnetic resonance cholangiopancreatography (MRCP), 49–50, 128, 139
magnetic resonance imaging (MRI)
   abdomen/pelvis, 50–51
   liver
      with conventional contrast, 50
      with hepatobiliary contrast, 50
maintenance therapy, 217
malignant liver tumors, 220
MCNS. *See* mucinous cystic neoplasms
mechanical obstruction, 19
median arcuate ligament syndrome, 105
MELD score. *See* Model for End-Stage Liver Disease score
Menetrier's disease, 28, 31
mercuric chloride, 42
mesenteric angiography, 114
mesenteric ischemia, 4
   treatment of, 104–105
mesenteric venous thrombosis (MVT), 103
metabolic disorders, 276
metastatic cancer, 120
metastatic tumors, 220
metoclopramide, 22
metronidazole, 178
microscopic colitis
   diagnosis, 180
   differential diagnosis, 179

Index

hepatitis C virus (HCV), 275
- definitions, 204
- extrahepatic disorders associated with, 204
- future of, 207
- history, 204
- transmission and susceptibility, 203
- treatments and caveats, 205–207
- virology and epidemiology, 203

hepatobiliary contrast, MRI liver with, 50
hepatobiliary iminodiacetic acid (HIDA) scan, 139
hepatocellular carcinoma (HCC), 220, 242
- diagnosis, 268
- differential diagnosis, 267–268
- pathophysiology, 268
- presentation, 267
- screening for, 202
- treatment, 268–270, 269t

hepatocellular injury, 193–194, 194t
hepatocyte-specific contrast agents, 223
hepatorenal syndrome (HRS)
- diagnosis, 260
- differential diagnosis, 259
- pathophysiology, 260
- presentation, 259
- treatment, 260–261, 261f

hepatotoxins, 271
HER2 oncogene, 125
hereditary hemochromatosis (HH), 209–211, 247–248
herpes simplex virus (HSV) esophagitis, 95
HG. *See* hyperemesis gravidarum
HH. *See* hereditary hemochromatosis
HIDA scan. *See* hepatobiliary iminodiacetic acid (HIDA) scan
high-resolution white light endoscopy (HR-WLE), 60

"high-risk stigmata" of malignant disease, 132
HIV. *See* human immunodeficiency virus
HLA genes. *See* human leukocyte antigen genes
HR-WLE. *See* high-resolution white light endoscopy
HRS. *See* hepatorenal syndrome
HSV. *See* herpes simplex virus esophagitis
human immunodeficiency virus (HIV), 94, 97, 99
- infections in, 95
human leukocyte antigen (HLA) genes, 78
humoral immune responses, 93, 217
hydrogen fluoride, 42
hyperemesis gravidarum (HG), 19, 263–264
hyperplastic polyps, 162

I

IBD. *See* inflammatory bowel disease
IBS. *See* irritable bowel syndrome
IBS-constipation predominant (IBS-C), 87, 88
IBS-diarrhea predominant (IBS-D), 87, 88
ICP. *See* intrahepatic cholestasis of pregnancy
IEL. *See* intraepithelial lymphocytes
IgE-mediated reactions, 83, 84
ileocolonoscopy, 171
IMA. *See* inferior mesenteric artery
imaging modalities, 171
immunodeficiency, 93–94
- acquired, 94–96

immunosuppressed patients, risk of GI malignancy in, 99–100
infectious diarrhea, 27
- diagnostic algorithm for, 98f
inferior mesenteric artery (IMA), 106–107
- pathology, 106
infertility, with oligospermia/azoospermia, 74
inflammatory bowel disease (IBD), 96, 153, 165, 166, 216, 225
inflammatory cytokines/endotoxins, 256
inflammatory disease, 169
inherited metabolic liver diseases
- alpha-1-antitrypsin deficiency, 246–247
- hereditary hemochromatosis, 247–248
- Wilson's disease, 245–246
injury
- causes of, 193–195
- patterns of, 193
- severity, 42
interferon-free therapies, 205
intestinal failure, 291–292
intestinal gas, 299
intestinal secretagogues, 91–92
intestinal strictures, 169
intestinal-type epithelium, 59
intraductal papillary mucinous neoplasms (IPMNS), 132–133
intraepithelial lymphocytes (IEL), 180
intrahepatic cholestasis, 195
intrahepatic cholestasis of pregnancy (ICP), 264
intravenous alimentation, 291
intravenous fluid resuscitation, 137
intravenous proton pump inhibitor (IV PPI), 43

gastroenteritis (*Cont.*)
  gastropaedica, 157
  presentation, 157
  treatment, 158–159
gastroesophageal junction (GEJ), 60
gastroesophageal reflux disease (GERD), 11, 300
  diagnosis, 55–56
  extraesophageal manifestations of, 57
  presentation, 55
  treatment, 56–58
gastrografin, 150
gastrointestinal (GI) disorders, 19, 299
gastrointestinal foreign bodies
  epidemiology, 33
  esophageal foreign bodies, 33–37
  gastric and small bowel foreign bodies, 37–38
  rectal foreign bodies, 39–40
gastropaedica, 93
GEJ. *See* gastroesophageal junction
genetic abnormalities, familial syndromes with, 128
GERD. *See* gastroesophageal reflux disease
GFD. *See* gluten-free diet
GGT. *See* gamma-glutamyl transpeptidase
GI conditions, radiologic studies for
  abdominal radiograph, 51
  abdominal ultrasound, 49
  CT enterography, 49
  CT liver protocol, 48
  CT pancreatic protocol, 48–49
  esophogram, 51
  MR enterography, 50
  MRCP, 49–50
  MRI abdomen/pelvis, 50–51

MRI liver
  with conventional contrast, 50
  with hepatobiliary contrast, 50
  noncontrast CT abdomen/pelvis, 49
  routine CT abdomen/pelvis with contrast, 47–48
  upper gastrointestinal series, 51
GI disorders. *See* gastrointestinal disorders
GI malignancy, in immunosuppressed patients, 99–100
GI mucosa, 95
Giardia, 158
gluten-free diet (GFD), 80
graft-versus-host disease (GVHD), 96
Grey Turner's sign, 135
guaiac-based fecal occult blood test (gFOBT), 144
guanylate cyclase agonist, 25*t*
GVHD. *See* graft-versus-host disease

H
HA. *See* hepatic adenoma
HAT. *See* hepatic artery thrombosis
HBcAg. *See* HBV core antigen
HBsAg. *See* HBV surface antigen
HBV. *See* hepatitis B virus
HBV core antibody (anti-HBc), 199
HBV core antigen (HBcAg), 199
HBV "e" antibody (anti-HBe), 200
HBV "e" antigen (HBeAg), 200
HBV serologic markers, 199*t*
HBV surface antibody (anti-HBs), 199
HBV surface antigen (HBsAg), 199

HCC. *See* hepatocellular carcinoma
HCV. *See* hepatitis C virus
HE. *See* hepatic encephalopathy
Helicobacter pylori infection, 111, 124
  diagnosis, 66–67
  differential diagnosis, 65
  pathophysiology, 65–66
  presentation, 65
  treatment, 67
  treatment failure, 67–68
Heller myotomy, 11
HELLP syndrome, 264–265
hematochezia, 109
hematopoietic stem cell, 96, 97
hemorrhoids
  diagnosis, 70
  differential diagnosis, 70
  pathophysiology, 69
  presentation, 69
  treatment, 70
hemostasis
  endoscopic treatments for, 116*t*
  maneuvers for lesions, 111
hemostatic clips, 116*t*
hepatic adenoma (HA), 221
hepatic artery thrombosis (HAT), 276
hepatic cysts, 221
hepatic encephalopathy (HE), 272
  diagnosis, 256
  pathophysiology, 255–256
  presentation, 255
  treatment, 256–257
hepatic synthetic function, tests of, 191
hepatitis A virus (HAV), 217–218
hepatitis B virus (HBV), 275
  diagnosis, 199–200, 199*t*
  evaluation, 200
  pathophysiology, 197
  presentation, 197–199
  treatment, 200–202, 201*t*, 202*f*

Index

Epstein-Barr virus (EBV) hepatitis, 209
eradication testing, 67–68
ERCP. *See* endoscopic retrograde cholangiopancreatography
esophageal cancer
 differential diagnosis, 118
 evaluation and staging, 118–119, 119f
 pathophysiology, 117, 118f
 presentation, 117
 treatment, 119–120
esophageal dysphagia, differential diagnosis of, 10t
esophageal foreign bodies, 33–37
esophageal/junctional, 95–96
 diseases, 96t
 varices, 111
esophageal manometry, 11
esophageal strictures, 45
esophagogastroduodenoscopy (EGD), 10, 30, 124, 307
esophagram, 10
esophagram, 51
EUS. *See* endoscopic ultrasound
EUS-FNA. *See* endoscopic ultrasound with fine-needle aspiration
exocrine tumors, 127
extrahepatic cholestasis, 194
extrahepatic disorders, associated with HCV, 204
extraintestinal manifestations of CD, 170

F

familial mediterranean fever (FMF)
 diagnosis, 75
 differential diagnosis, 74
 long-term complications, 74
 pathophysiology, 75
 presentation, 73–74

treatment, 76
fat, deposition in liver, 239
fecal elastase, 30
fecal immunochemical test (FIT), 144
fermentable oligosaccharides, disaccharides, monosaccharides and polyols (FODMAP) diet, 299, 301t
FHF. *See* fulminant hepatic failure
fiber, 91
fibrolamellar HCC, 268
fidaxomicin, 187
fine needle aspiration (FNA) biopsy, 219
first-degree burn, 42
first-line management, ascites, 250, 252
fistulizing disease symptoms, 169
5-HT4 agonist, 25t
5-HT3 antagonists, 22
5' nucleotidase, 191
flexible sigmoidoscopy, 101–102, 144–145, 162, 307
fluorouracil, 120
FMF. *See* familial mediterranean fever
FNA biopsy. *See* fine needle aspiration biopsy
focal nodular hyperplasia (FNH), 222–223
FODMAP diet. *See* fermentable oligosaccharides, disaccharides, monosaccharides and polyols diet
FOLFIRINOX, 130
food allergy, 83, 85
 treatment for, 85–86
 vs. food intolerance, 84t
food intolerance, food allergy vs., 84t
foodborne transmission, 217
forceps biopsy device, removal with, 163

Fukuoka guidelines, 132
fulminant hepatic failure (FHF), 276
 diagnosis, 272
 gastropaedica, 271
 pathophysiology and etiologies, 271–272
 presentation, 271
 treatment, 272–273
functional dyspepsia, 66
 management, 15

G

gadolinium-based hepatocyte-specific agents, 222
gallbladder adenocarcinoma, 142
gallbladder disease
 clinical features of, 140t
 gallstone disease, 141
 non-gallstone gallbladder disease, 141
 workup of, 139
gallbladder malignancy, 142
gallbladder polyps, 141
gallstone disease, 141
gallstone ileus, 140t, 141
gallstone pancreatitis, 140t, 141
gallstones, 135
gamma-glutamyl transpeptidase (GGT), 191, 240
gas-forming agents, 36
gastric cancer
 diagnosis, 124
 differential diagnosis, 124
 gastropaedica, 123
 pathophysiology, 123
 presentation, 123–124
 treatment, 124–125, 125t
gastric disease, 96
gastric emptying study, 20
gastric feeding, 286
gastric foreign bodies, 37–38
gastric lavage, 44
gastric varices, 111
gastroenteritis
 diagnosis, 158
 differential diagnosis, 157
 etiology, 157–158

Index

cytomegalovirus (CMV), 209
  esophagitis, 95

D

DAA. *See* direct acting antiviral
deamidated gliadin peptide (DGP), 78
defecatory disorders, 24
DGP. *See* deamidated gliadin peptide
diarrhea, 7, 93, 96, 288, 300, 302
  diagnosis, 29–30
  diagnostic for infectious, 97t
  pathophysiology, 27–28
  treatment, 30–31
dietary modification, 91
diffuse abdominal pain, 6
DILI. *See* drug-induced liver injury
direct acting antiviral (DAA), 205
disease severity, 170
diversion colitis, 31
diverticular bleed, 115–116
diverticulitis
  diagnosis, 154
  differential diagnosis, 153–154
  pathophysiology, 154
  presentation, 153
  treatment, 154–155
Doppler, abdominal ultrasound with, 49
dose-dependent pattern, injury in, 213
drooling, 34
drug-induced liver injury (DILI), 212–213
  diagnosis, 238
  differential diagnosis, 237
  pathophysiology, 238
  presentation, 237
  treatment, 238
dull pain, 3
duplex ultrasonography, 104
dyslipidemia, treatment of, 243
dyspepsia
  alarm signs associated with, 14
  definition, 13
  differential diagnosis, 13
  functional management, 15
  management, 14
  pathophysiology, 14
  refractory cases of, 15
dysphagia
  differential diagnosis, 118
  and motility disorders
    diagnostic tests, 10–11
    differential diagnosis, 10
  presentation, 9
  treatments, 11–12
dysplasia, 60, 62

E

EBL. *See* endoscopic rubber band ligation
EBV hepatitis. *See* Epstein-Barr virus hepatitis
EGD. *See* esophagogastroduodenoscopy
EGFR. *See* epidermal growth factor receptor
EIA. *See* enzyme immunoassay
electrolytes, 288
embolization, 105
emesis, 83
empiric antibiotics, 158
EMR. *See* endoscopic mucosal resection
endoscopic ablation, 62
endoscopic decompression and reduction, 151
endoscopic mucosal resection (EMR), 124, 163
endoscopic retrograde cholangiopancreatography (ERCP), 128, 139, 220, 226
endoscopic rubber band ligation (EBL), 111
endoscopic sphincterotomy, 137
endoscopic stent placement, 151
endoscopic treatment modalities, 115, 116t
endoscopic ultrasound (EUS), 124, 128
  esophageal cancer, 118
endoscopic ultrasound with fine-needle aspiration (EUS-FNA), 131
  cyst fluid analysis, 132t
endoscopy, 10, 36, 43, 95
  antibiotic prophylaxis in, 307–308
  antithrombotic agents in, 308–310
  indications for urgent, 307
  risk of bleeding and thromboembolic event, 309t
endovascular therapy, 104–105
energy requirements, determination, 292–293
Entamoeba histolytica, cysts of, 223
entecavir, 201
enteral feeding
  complications, 287–288
  continuous feeding *vs.* bolus feeding, 287
  contraindications, 285
  gastropaedica, 285
  indications, 285
  ineffective formulations and additives, 287
  nutritional requirements, 286
  pre- or post-pyloric feeding, 286
  value of, 286
enterography
  CT, 49
  MR, 50
environmental factors, PBC, 230
enzyme immunoassay (EIA), 185
eosinophilic esophagitis (EoE), 10, 11
epidermal growth factor receptor (EGFR), 268

cholangiocarcinoma, 142, 220
cholangiography, 225
choledochal cysts, 141
choledocholithiasis, 140t, 141
cholestatic injury, 194–195, 194t
cholestatic liver disease, 215–216, 275
cholestyramine, 91
chronic alcohol intake, 213
chronic antibiotic-responsive pouchitis, 178
chronic cholestatic liver diseases, 220
chronic constipation, 23, 24
  pharmacological treatment options for, 25t
chronic destructive arthritis, 74
chronic diarrhea, 30
chronic HBV infection, 198–199, 198t
chronic hepatitis B, treatment criteria for, 201t
chronic mesenteric ischemia (CMI), 103–105
chronic pancreatitis, 138
cirrhosis, 249
cisplatin, 120
Clostridium difficile infection (CDI)
  diagnosis, 185
  differential diagnosis, 184
  empiric antibiotic therapy for, 159
  pathophysiology, 184
  presentation, 183–184
  recurrent disease, 187
  risk factor for, 184
  symptoms of, 183
  treatment, 185–187, 186f
CMV. *See* cytomegalovirus
CNS. *See* central nervous system
coagulation techniques, 116t
coagulopathy, 114
  FHF, 273

colchicine, 76
collagenous colitis, 179, 180
colon cancer, 153
colon polyps
  diagnosis, 162
  differential diagnosis, 162
  gastropaedica, 161
  pathophysiology, 162
  presentation, 162
  treatment, 163
colonic angiodysplasia, 107
colonoscopy, 145, 162, 307
  diverticulitis, 154
  quality of, 145
colorectal cancer (CRC) screening
  algorithm for, 146f–147f
  colonoscopy, 145
  CT colonography, 144
  flexible sigmoidoscopy, 144–145
  gastropaedica, 143
  guidelines for, 145–147
  modalities for, 143
  screening strategies, 143
  stool-based studies, 144
compound heterozygotes, 209
computed tomography angiography (CTA), 104
computed tomography (CT) scans, 35, 47, 101, 128, 136, 150
  abdomen/pelvis
    with contrast, routine, 47–48
    with noncontrast, 49
  angiography, 115
  colonography, 144
  diverticulitis, 154
  enterography, 49
  esophageal cancer, 118
  imaging, 124
  liver protocol, 48
  pancreatic protocol, 48–49
condyloma, 71
  diagnosis, 72
  differential diagnosis, 72
  pathophysiology, 72

  presentation, 72
  treatment, 72
congenital anomalies, 291
conjugated hyperbilirubinemia, causes of, 195t
constipation, 302
  diagnosis, 24
  differential diagnosis, 24
  pathophysiology, 24
  presentation, 23
  treatment, 24–26
continuous feeding vs. bolus feeding, 287
contrast swallow studies, 35
conventional contrast, MRI liver with, 50
copper chelating agent, 215
CPENS. *See* cystic pancreatic endocrine neoplasms
cricopharyngeal bar, 12
Crohn's disease (CD), 153, 165
  diagnosis, 171
  differential diagnosis, 170
  pathophysiology, 170–171
  presentation, 169–170
  treatment, 172–173, 172f
cross-sectional imaging, 131
"cruise ship gastroenteritis," 157
Cryptosporidium, 158
CT scans. *See* computed tomography scans
Cullen's sign, 135
C282Y homozygotes, 209
cyclic vomiting syndrome, 19
cyst, types and characteristics, 131t
cystic pancreatic endocrine neoplasms (CPENS), 133–134
cystic tumors, 127
cysts, 221

Production Credits
Executive Editor: Nancy Anastasi Duffy
Editorial Assistant: Jade Freeman
Senior Production Editor: Daniel Stone
Digital Marketing Manager: Jennifer Sharp
Manufacturing and Inventory Control Supervisor: Amy Bacus
Rights and Photo Research Manager: Lauren Miller
Composition: diacriTech
Cover Image: Courtesy of the National Library of Medicine
Printer and Binding: Cenveo Publisher Services
Cover Printing: Cenveo Publisher Services

ISBN: 978-1-284-03855-2

6048

Printed in the United States of America
18 17 16 15 14   10 9 8 7 6 5 4 3 2 1

To Melina, Derek, and Andrew—you are the best part of me.

Tarascon Gastroenterology Pocketbook

Table of Contents

Contributor's List   xii
Abbreviations   xviii
Introduction   xxix

I APPROACH TO COMMON SYMPTOMS AND EMERGENCIES   1

1 Approach to Acute Abdominal Pain   3

- Overview   3
- Key Concepts   3
- Pathophysiology of Abdominal Pain   3
- Evaluation of Abdominal Pain   4
- Recognizing Potentially Emergent Conditions   4
- Characterize the Pain Symptoms   5
- Aggravating/Alleviating Factors   7
- Associated Symptoms   7
- Other Historical Elements   7
- Physical Findings   7
- Laboratory Testing   8
- Imaging   8
- References   8

2 Dysphagia and Motility Disorders   9

- Overview   9
- Presentation   9
- Differential Diagnosis   10
- Diagnostic Tests   10
- Treatments (Diagnosis-Specific)   11
- References   12

3 Dyspepsia   13

- Overview   13
- Definition   13
- Differential Diagnosis   13
- Pathophysiology of Functional Dyspepsia   14
- Alarm Signs Associated with Dyspepsia   14
- Management of Dyspepsia   14
- Functional Dyspepsia Management   15
- Refractory Cases of Dyspepsia   15
- References   15

4 Nausea and Vomiting   17

- Overview   17
- Definitions   17
- Pathophysiology   17
- Differential Diagnosis   18
- Evaluation   20
- Diagnosis   20
- Treatment   22
- References   22

5 Constipation   23

- Overview   23
- Presentation   23
- Differential Diagnosis   24
- Pathophysiology   24
- Diagnosis   24
- Treatment   24
- References   26

6 Diarrhea   27

- Overview   27
- Pathophysiology   27
- Diagnosis   29
- Treatment   30
- References   31

7 Gastrointestinal Foreign Bodies   33

- Overview   33
- Epidemiology   33
- Esophageal Foreign Bodies   33
- Gastric and Small Bowel Foreign Bodies   37
- Rectal Foreign Bodies   39
- References   40

8 Caustic Ingestions   41

- Overview   41
- Caustic Substances   41
- Clinical Presentation   42
- Acute WorkUp   42
- Endoscopy   43

	Treatment	43
	Long-Term Sequelae	45
	References	45
9	**Ordering Appropriate Radiologic Studies for GI Conditions**	**47**
	Overview	47
	Routine CT Abdomen/Pelvis with Contrast	47
	CT Liver Protocol	48
	CT Pancreatic Protocol	48
	CT Enterography	49
	Noncontrast CT Abdomen/Pelvis	49
	Abdominal Ultrasound	49
	MRCP	49
	MRI Liver with Hepatobiliary Contrast	50
	MRI Liver with Conventional Contrast	50
	MR Enterography	50
	MRI Abdomen/Pelvis	50
	Upper Gastrointestinal Series	51
	Esophogram	51
	Abdominal Radiograph	51
	References	51

II COMMON GASTRO-INTESTINAL DISORDERS   53

10	**The Diagnosis and Management of Gastroesophageal Reflux Disease (GERD)**	**55**
	Overview	55
	Presentation	55
	Diagnosis	55
	Treatment	56
	Approach to Extraesophageal Manifestations of GERD	57
	Treatment Approach to Unresponsive GERD	57
	References	58
11	**Barrett's Esophagus**	**59**
	Overview	59
	Presentation	59
	Pathophysiology	59
	Diagnosis	60
	Management/Treatment	60
	References	63
12	***Helicobacter Pylori* Infection**	**65**
	Overview	65
	Presentation	65

	Differential Diagnosis	65
	Pathophysiology	65
	Diagnosis	66
	Treatment	67
	Treatment Failure	67
	References	68
13	**Benign Anorectal Disorders (Hemorrhoids, Anal Fissure, Condyloma)**	**69**
	Overview	69
	Hemorrhoids	69
	Anal Fissures	70
	Condyloma	71
	References	72
14	**Familial Mediterranean Fever**	**73**
	Overview	73
	Presentation	73
	Differential Diagnosis	74
	Long-Term Complications	74
	Pathophysiology	75
	Diagnosis	75
	Treatment	76
	References	76
15	**Celiac Disease**	**77**
	Overview	77
	Presentation	77
	Differential Diagnosis	78
	Pathophysiology	78
	Diagnosis	78
	Treatment	80
	References	81
16	**Food Allergies**	**83**
	Overview	83
	Presentation	83
	Differential Diagnosis	85
	Pathophysiology	85
	Diagnosis	85
	Treatment	85
	References	86
17	**Irritable Bowel Syndrome and Small Intestinal Bacterial Overgrowth**	**87**
	Overview	87
	Presentation	87
	Differential Diagnosis	88
	Small Intestinal Bacterial Overgrowth	88
	Pathophysiology	89
	Diagnosis	89

Table of Contents

Treatment	89	
References	92	

18 Gastrointestinal Issues in the Immunocompromised Host — 93

- Overview — 93
- Primary Immunodeficiency — 93
- Acquired Immunodeficiency — 94
- Risk of GI Malignancy in Immunosuppressed Patients — 99
- References — 100

19 Vascular Disorders of the Gastrointestinal Tract — 101

- Overview — 101
- Blood Supply — 101
- Ischemic Colitis — 101
- Acute Mesenteric Ischemia (AMI) — 102
- Chronic Mesenteric Ischemia (CMI) — 103
- Celiac Artery Pathology — 105
- SMA Pathology — 106
- IMA Pathology — 106
- Vascular Malformations — 107
- References — 108

20 Upper GI Bleeding — 109

- Overview — 109
- Presentation — 109
- Differential Diagnosis — 110
- Pre-Endoscopy Management — 110
- Endoscopy — 110
- Post-Endoscopy Management — 111
- References — 112

21 Lower GI Bleeding — 113

- Overview — 113
- Initial Assessment — 113
- Initial Management — 113
- Differential Diagnosis — 114
- Diagnosis — 114
- Treatment — 115
- References — 116

22 Esophageal Cancer — 117

- Overview — 117
- Presentation — 117
- Pathophysiology — 117
- Differential Diagnosis in Patients with Dysphagia — 118
- Evaluation and Staging — 118
- Treatment — 118
- Consultations — 120
- References — 121

23 Gastric Cancer — 123

- Overview — 123
- Presentation — 123
- Differential Diagnosis — 124
- Pathophysiology — 124
- Diagnosis — 124
- Treatment — 124
- References — 126

24 Pancreatic Cancer — 127

- Overview — 127
- Presentation — 127
- Differential Diagnosis — 127
- Risk Factors — 127
- Diagnosis — 128
- Staging — 128
- Prognosis — 129
- Treatment — 129
- References — 130

25 Pancreatic Cysts — 131

- Overview — 131
- Differential Diagnosis and Treatment of Different PCNs — 132
- References — 134

26 Pancreatitis — 135

- Overview — 135
- Presentation — 135
- Differential Diagnosis — 136
- Pathophysiology — 136
- Diagnosis — 136
- Treatment — 136
- Reference — 138

27 Gallbladder Disease — 139

- Overview — 139
- Workup of Gallbladder Disease — 139
- Gallstone Disease — 141
- Non-Gallstone Gallbladder Disease — 141
- Gallbladder Malignancy — 142
- Reference — 142

28 Colorectal Cancer Screening — 143

- Overview — 143
- Screening Strategies — 143
- Guidelines for CRC Screening — 145
- References — 147

29 Bowel Obstruction — 149

- Overview — 149
- Presentation — 149
- Differential Diagnosis — 149

Table of Contents

Pathophysiology	150	
Diagnosis	150	
Treatment	151	
References	151	

30 Diverticulitis — 153

- Overview — 153
- Presentation — 153
- Differential Diagnosis — 153
- Pathophysiology — 154
- Diagnosis — 154
- Treatment — 154
- Reference — 155

31 Gastroenteritis — 157

- Overview — 157
- Presentation — 157
- Differential Diagnosis — 157
- Etiology — 157
- Diagnosis — 158
- Treatment — 158
- References — 160

32 Colon Polyps — 161

- Overview — 161
- Presentation — 162
- Differential Diagnosis — 162
- Pathophysiology — 162
- Diagnosis — 162
- Treatment — 163
- References — 163

33 Ulcerative Colitis — 165

- Overview — 165
- Presentation — 165
- Differential Diagnosis — 166
- Pathophysiology — 166
- Diagnosis — 166
- Treatment — 167
- References — 167

34 Crohn's Disease — 169

- Overview — 169
- Presentation — 169
- Differential Diagnosis — 170
- Pathophysiology — 170
- Diagnosis — 171
- Treatment — 172
- References — 173

35 Pouchitis — 175

- Overview — 175
- Presentation — 175
- Differential Diagnosis — 175
- Pathophysiology — 175
- Diagnosis — 176
- Treatment — 176
- Cancer Surveillance — 178
- References — 178

36 Microscopic Colitis — 179

- Overview — 179
- Presentation — 179
- Differential Diagnosis — 179
- Pathophysiology — 179
- Diagnosis — 180
- Treatment — 180
- References — 181

37 *Clostridium Difficile* Infection and Treatment — 183

- Overview — 183
- Presentation — 183
- Differential Diagnosis — 184
- Pathophysiology — 184
- Diagnosis — 185
- Treatment — 185
- References — 187

III HEPATOLOGY — 189

38 Approach to Abnormal Liver Tests — 191

- Overview — 191
- Liver Panel Tests — 191
- Patterns of Injury — 193
- Initial Approach — 193
- Causes of Injury — 193
- Abbreviations — 195
- Reference — 196

39 Hepatitis B Virus — 197

- Overview — 197
- Pathophysiology — 197
- Presentation — 197
- Diagnosis — 199
- Evaluation — 200
- Treatment — 200
- References — 202

40 Hepatitis C Infection — 203

- Overview — 203
- Virology and Epidemiology — 203
- Transmission and Susceptibility — 203

Table of Contents

Natural History	204	
Extrahepatic Disorders Associated with HCV	204	
Common Definitions to Know When Treating HCV	204	
Current Treatments and Caveats	205	
Future of HCV Therapy	207	
References	207	

41 How to Approach Non-HBV/HCV Hepatitis in Clinical Practice — 209

Overview	209
Differential Diagnosis	209
Hereditary Hemochromatosis (HFE)	209
Alpha-1 Antitrypsin (A1AT) Deficiency	211
Budd-Chiari Syndrome (BCS)	211
Drug-Induced Liver Injury (DILI)	212
Alcoholic Liver Disease (ALD)	213
Nonalcoholic Fatty Liver Disease (NAFLD)	214
Wilson's Disease	214
Cholestatic Liver Disease	215
Autoimmune Hepatitis (AIH)	216
Hepatitis A	217
References	218

42 Approach to the Patient with a Liver Lesion — 219

Overview	219
Malignant Liver Tumors	220
Benign Focal Lesions	220
Abscesses	223
References	224

43 Primary Sclerosing Cholangitis — 225

Overview	225
Presentation	225
Differential Diagnosis	226
Pathophysiology	226
Diagnosis	226
Treatment	227
References	227

44 Primary Biliary Cirrhosis — 229

Overview	229
Presentation	229
Differential Diagnosis	229
Pathophysiology	229
Diagnosis	230
Treatment	230
References	231

45 Autoimmune Hepatitis — 233

Overview	233
Presentation	233
Differential Diagnosis	233
Pathophysiology	233
Diagnosis	234
Treatment Indications	234
Treatment Regimens	234
References	236

46 Drug-Induced Liver Injury — 237

Overview	237
Presentation	237
Differential Diagnosis	237
Pathophysiology	238
Diagnosis	238
Treatment	238
References	238

47 Nonalcoholic Fatty Liver Disease — 239

Overview	239
Pathophysiology	239
Presentation	240
Diagnosis	240
Role of Liver Biopsy	242
Natural History and Cancer Risks	242
Treatment	242
References	243

48 Inherited Metabolic Liver Diseases — 245

Overview	245
Wilson's Disease	245
Alpha-1-Antitrypsin Deficiency	246
Hereditary Hemochromatosis (HH)	247
References	248

49 Ascites — 249

Overview	249
Presentation	249
Differential Diagnosis	249
Pathophysiology	249
Diagnosis	249
Treatment	250
References	253

50 Hepatic Encephalopathy — 255

- Overview — 255
- Presentation — 255
- Pathophysiology — 255
- Diagnosis — 256
- Treatment — 256
- References — 257

51 Hepatorenal Syndrome — 259

- Overview — 259
- Presentation — 259
- Differential Diagnosis — 259
- Pathophysiology — 260
- Diagnosis — 260
- Treatment — 260
- References — 262

52 Liver Disorders During Pregnancy — 263

- Overview — 263
- Hyperemesis Gravidarum — 263
- Intrahepatic Cholestasis of Pregnancy — 264
- HELLP Syndrome — 264
- Acute Fatty Liver of Pregnancy — 265
- Reference — 266

53 Hepatocellular Carcinoma — 267

- Overview — 267
- Presentation — 267
- Differential Diagnosis — 267
- Pathophysiology — 268
- Diagnosis — 268
- Treatment — 268
- References — 270

54 Fulminant Hepatic Failure — 271

- Overview — 271
- Presentation — 271
- Pathophysiology and Etiologies — 271
- Diagnosis — 272
- Treatment — 272
- References — 273

55 Liver Transplantation — 275

- Overview — 275
- Indications for Liver Transplantation — 275
- Perioperative Complications — 276
- Follow Up — 277
- References — 277

56 Alcoholic Hepatitis — 279

- Overview — 279
- Presentation — 279
- Differential Diagnosis — 279
- Pathophysiology — 279
- Diagnosis — 279
- Treatment — 280
- References — 280

IV NUTRITION — 283

57 Nutritional Support with Enteral Feeding — 285

- Overview — 285
- Indications — 285
- Contraindications to the Start of Enteral Feeding — 285
- Value of Enteral Nutrition — 286
- Pre- or Post-Pyloric Feeding — 286
- Nutritional Requirements — 286
- Formulations — 287
- Continuous versus Bolus Feeding — 287
- Complications — 287
- References — 288

58 Parenteral Nutritional Support — 291

- Overview — 291
- Indications — 291
- Calculating Nutritional Needs and Formulations — 292
- How to Determine the Composition of Parenteral Nutrition — 292
- Vascular Access — 293
- The Infusions — 294
- Monitoring and Follow Up — 294
- Complications — 295
- References — 296

59 Dietary Modifications for Gastrointestinal Symptoms — 299

- Overview — 299
- Gas/Bloating — 299
- GERD — 300
- Diarrhea — 300
- Constipation — 302
- References — 302

Table of Contents

V ENDOSCOPY GUIDELINES   305

60 Endoscopy Guidelines   307

Overview   307
Indications for Urgent Endoscopy   307
Antibiotic Prophylaxis in Endoscopy   307
Antithrombotic Agents in Endoscopy   308
References   310

Index   311

Contributor's List

Rini Abraham, MD, PharmD
Gastroenterology Fellow
NYU School of Medicine
New York, NY

Nikhil Agarwal, MD
Gastroenterologist
West Hollywood, CA

Vatche G. Agopian, MD
Assistant Professor of Surgery
Division of Liver Transplantation
David Geffen School of Medicine at UCLA
Los Angeles, CA

Michael J. Albertson, MD
Assistant Clinical Professor
Division of Digestive Diseases
David Geffen School of Medicine at UCLA
Los Angeles, CA

Christopher V. Almario, MD
Resident, Hospital of the University of Pennsylvania
Philadelphia, PA

Walid S. Ayoub, MD
Assistant Medical Director
Liver Transplant Program at Cedars Sinai Medical Center
Associate Professor of Medicine
UCLA
Los Angeles, CA

John Baber, MD
Gastroenterologist
Little Rock, AR

Simon W. Beaven, MD, PhD
Director, Metabolic Syndrome Program (COMET)
Division of Digestive Diseases & Pfleger Liver Institute
David Geffen School of Medicine at UCLA
Los Angeles, CA

Brigid Boland, MD
Gastroenterologist
UCSD Medical Center
San Diego, CA

Nirupama Bonthala, MD
Fellow, Keck School of Medicine of USC
Los Angeles, CA

Melinda Braskett, MD
Assistant Clinical Professor
David Geffen School of Medicine at UCLA
Los Angeles, CA

Moira E. Breslin, MD, MSC
Fellow Physician
Division of Allergy, Immunology, and Rheumatology
Department of Pediatrics
UCLA
Los Angeles, CA

Charles Brunicardi, MD
Moss Foundation Chair in Gastrointestinal and Personalized Surgery
Professor and Vice Chair Surgical Services
Chief of General Surgery
UCLA Santa Monica Medical Center
Department of Surgery
David Geffen School of Medicine at UCLA
Los Angeles, CA

Contributor's List

Joseph Chan, MD
Resident, Emergency Medicine
UCLA Emergency Medicine Center
Los Angeles, CA

Daniel D. Cho, MD
Assistant Clinical Professor
Division of Digestive Diseases
Department of Medicine
David Geffen School of Medicine at UCLA
Santa Monica/Redondo Beach, CA

Gina Choi, MD
Advanced Transplant Hepatology Fellow
Division of Gastroenterology at the
University of Pennsylvania
Philadelphia, PA

Jennifer M. Choi, MD
Associate Director, UCLA Center for
Inflammatory Bowel Diseases
Assistant Professor of Clinical Medicine
Division of Digestive Diseases
David Geffen School of Medicine at UCLA
Los Angeles, CA

Daniel Cole, MD, MPH
Associate Professor of Medicine
David Geffen School of Medicine at UCLA
Los Angeles, CA

Jeffrey L. Conklin, MD, FACG
Director, Center for Esophageal Disorders
and GI Motility Lab
Division of Digestive Diseases
David Geffen School of Medicine at UCLA
Los Angeles, CA

Lynn S. Connolly, MD, MSCR
Assistant Clinical Professor of Medicine
UCLA Division of Gastroenterology
Los Angeles, CA

Richelle J. Cooper, MD, MSHS
Professor, Emergency Medicine
UCLA Emergency Medicine Center
Los Angeles, CA

Sara E. Crager, MD
Chief Resident
UCLA Olive View Medical Center
Los Angeles, CA

Sheila E. Crowe, MD, FRCPC, FACP, FACG, AGAF
Professor of Medicine Director of
Research
Division of Gastroenterology
Department of Medicine
University of California, San Diego
La Jolla, CA

Hannah Do, MD
Los Angeles, CA

Timothy R. Donahue, MD
Assistant Professor of Surgery, and
Molecular & Medical Pharmacology
Director of the Core Surgery Residency
Program
Associate Director of the General Surgery
Residency Training Program
David Geffen School of Medicine at UCLA
Los Angeles, CA

Alexandra Drakaki, MD
Hematology Oncology
UCLA
Los Angeles, CA

Gareth S. Dulai, MD, MSHS
Chair, Gastroenterology SCPMG Downey
Assistant Clinical Professor of Medicine
UCLA
Los Angeles, CA

Parambir S. Dulai, MBBS
Fellow
Gastroenterology
University of California San Diego
San Diego, CA

Francisco A. Durazo, MD, FACP
Professor of Medicine and Surgery
Medical Director, Dumont-UCLA Liver Transplant Program
Digestive and Liver Diseases
David Geffen School of Medicine at UCLA
Los Angeles, CA

Mohamed El-Kabany, MD
Assistant Professor, Internal Medicine/Hepatology
David Geffen School of Medicine at UCLA
Pfleger Liver Institute
Los Angeles, CA

Mary Farid, DO
Assistant Clinical Professor
Division of Gastroenterology
UCLA
Los Angeles, CA

Dave Garg
Medical Student
David Geffen School of Medicine at UCLA
Los Angeles, CA

Terri Getzug, MD
Clinical Professor of Medicine
Division of Digestive Diseases
David Geffen School of Medicine at UCLA
Los Angeles, CA

Kevin Ghassemi, MD
Associate Director of Clinical Programs, Esophageal Center
Assistant Clinical Professor of Medicine
Division of Digestive Diseases
David Geffen School of Medicine at UCLA
Los Angeles, CA

Kourosh F. Ghassemi, MD
Interventional Gastroenterologist
Palo Alto Foundation Medical Group
Santa Cruz, CA

Christina Ha, MD
Clinical Assistant Professor
Center for Inflammatory Bowel Diseases
Division of Digestive Diseases
David Geffen School of Medicine at UCLA
Los Angeles, CA

Steven-Huy B. Han, MD, AGAF, FAASLD
Professor of Medicine and Surgery
Director, Hepatology Clinical Research Center
David Geffen School of Medicine at UCLA
Los Angeles, CA

Amy Lightner Hill, MD
Surgery Resident
Department of Surgery
UCLA
Los Angeles, CA

Darryl Hiyama, MD, FACS
Professor of Clinical Surgery
Division of General Surgery
David Geffen School of Medicine at UCLA
Los Angeles, CA

Andrew D. Ho, MD
Gastroenterology Fellow
Division of Digestive Diseases
David Geffen School of Medicine at UCLA
Los Angeles, CA

Nancee Jaffe, MS, RD
Registered Dietitian
Division of Digestive Diseases
UCLA
Los Angeles, CA

Contributor's List

Jeffery Kahn, MD
Associate Professor of Clinical Medicine
Transplant Hepatology
Keck School of Medicine at USC
Los Angeles, CA

Ciaran P. Kelly, MD
Professor of Medicine
Harvard Medical School
Director Gastroenterology Fellowship Training
Beth Israel Deaconess Medical Center
Boston, MA

Puja Khanna, MD
Clinical Instructor in Medicine, Rheumatology
UCLA Department of Medicine
Los Angeles, CA

Saro Khemichian, MD
Assistant Professor of Clinical Medicine
Transplant Hepatology
Keck School of Medicine at USC
Los Angeles, CA

Stephen Kim, MD
Clinical Instructor of Medicine
David Geffen School of Medicine at UCLA
Los Angeles, CA

Svetlana Kotova, MD
Division of Thoracic Surgery
David Geffen School of Medicine at UCLA
VA Greater Los Angeles Healthcare System
Los Angeles, CA

Peter F. Lawrence, MD
Chief of Vascular Surgery
Wiley Barker Chair in Vascular Surgery
Director Gonda Vascular Center
David Geffen School of Medicine at UCLA
Los Angeles, CA

Jay M. Lee, MD
Chief, Division of Thoracic Surgery
Surgical Director, Thoracic Oncology Program
Jonsson Comprehensive Cancer Center
Surgical Director, Center for Esophageal Disorders
Associate Professor of Surgery
David Geffen School of Medicine at UCLA
Los Angeles, CA

Anthony Lembo, MD
Associate Professor of Medicine
Harvard Medical School
Beth Israel Deaconess Medical Center
Boston, MA

Jeffrey R. Lewis, MD
Clinical Instructor, Division of Digestive Diseases
UCLA Medical Center
Los Angeles, CA

Anne Lin, MD
Assistant Professor of Surgery
Section of Colon and Rectal Surgery
David Geffen School of Medicine at UCLA
Los Angeles, CA

Mariela Macias, MD
Internist
San Diego, CA

Vignan Manne, MD
Resident, Internal Medicine
Akron General Medical Center
Akron, OH

Daniel J. A. Margolis, MD
Associate Professor of Radiology
Director, Virtual Colonography
David Geffen School of Medicine at UCLA
Los Angeles, CA

Contributor's List

Folasade P. May, MD, MPhil
Fellow in Gastroenterology
Division of Digestive Diseases
David Geffen School of Medicine at UCLA
Los Angeles, CA

Nelya Melnitchouk, MD
Colorectal Surgeon
Tufts Medical Center
Medford, MA

V. Raman Muthusamy, MD, FACG, FASGE
Director of Interventional Endoscopy
Clinical Professor of Medicine
David Geffen School of Medicine at UCLA
Los Angeles, CA

Nima Nassiri, BS
David Geffen School of Medicine at UCLA
Los Angeles, CA

Vivian Ng, MD
Resident
David Geffen School of Medicine at UCLA
Los Angeles, CA

Andrew H. Nguyen, MD
Fellow
UCLA Department of Surgery
Los Angeles, CA

Mark Ovsiowitz, MD
Assistant Clinical Professor of Medicine
Division of Digestive Diseases
David Geffen School of Medicine at UCLA
Los Angeles, CA

Vikas K. Pabby, MD, MPH
Clinical Instructor of Medicine
Division of Digestive Diseases
David Geffen School of Medicine at UCLA
Los Angeles, CA

Ishan Patel, MD
Clinical Research Fellow
Harvard Medical School
Gastroenterology Division
Beth Israel Deaconess Medical Center
Boston, MA

Michael A. Poles, MD, PhD
Associate Professor of Medicine,
Microbiology, and Pathology
Program Director of Gastroenterology
NYU School of Medicine
Section Chief of Gastroenterology
Manhattan Veteran's Hospital
New York, NY

Justin A. Reynolds, MD
Faculty Hepatologist
Center for Liver & Hepatobiliary Disease
St. Joseph's Hospital and Medical Center
Phoenix, AZ

Bennett E. Roth, MD
Professor of Clinical Medicine
David Geffen School of Medicine at UCLA
Los Angeles, CA

Steven J. Rottman, MD, FACEP
Professor, Emergency Medicine and
Community Health Sciences
David Geffen School of Medicine at UCLA
Fielding School of Public Health
UCLA
Los Angeles, CA

Bruce Allen Runyon, MD
Director of Hepatology, Santa Monica/UCLA
Clinical Professor of Medicine
David Geffen School of Medicine at UCLA
Santa Monica, CA

Contributor's List

Sammy Saab, MD, MPH, AGAF, FAASLD
Professor of Medicine and Surgery
Head, Outcomes Research in Hepatology
David Geffen School of Medicine at UCLA
Los Angeles, CA

Saeed Sadeghi, MD
Associate Clinical Professor of Medicine
Division of Hematology and Oncology
David Geffen School of Medicine at UCLA
Los Angeles, CA

Victor Sai, MD
Assistant Clinical Professor of Radiology
David Geffen School of Medicine at UCLA
Los Angeles, CA

Alireza Sedarat, MD
Interventional Endoscopy
Division of Digestive Diseases
David Geffen School of Medicine at UCLA and VA Greater Los Angeles Health Care System
Lost Angeles, CA

Rimma Shaposhnikov, MD
Assistant Clinical Professor
Division of Digestive Diseases
David Geffen School of Medicine at UCLA
Los Angeles, CA

Alan J. Sheinbaum, MD, FACG, AGAF
Associate Professor Medicine
David Geffen School of Medicine at UCLA
Los Angeles, CA

Vinay Sundaram, MD, MSC
Assistant Director of Hepatology
Cedars-Sinai Medical Center
Los Angeles, CA

Tram T. Tran, MD
Medical Director Liver Transplant
Director, Hepatology
Cedars Sinai Medical Center
Los Angeles, CA

Jorge H. Vargas, MD
Professor of Pediatrics
Division of Gastroenterology, Hepatology & Nutrition
David Geffen School of Medicine at UCLA
Los Angeles, CA

Michelle Vu, MD
Fellow, Gastroenterology
Ronald Reagan UCLA Medical Center
Los Angeles, CA

Zev Wainberg, MD
Co-Director GI Oncology Program
UCLA
Los Angeles, CA

Rabindra R. Watson, MD
Assistant Clinical Professor of Medicine
David Geffen School of Medicine at UCLA
Los Angeles, CA

James X. Wu, MD
General Surgery Resident
David Geffen School of Medicine at UCLA
Los Angeles, CA

James Yoo, MD
Chief, Division of Colon and Rectal Surgery
Tufts Medical Center
Boston MA

Christine Yu, MD
Quality Improvement fellow, Gastroenterology
UCLA
Los Angeles, CA

Kali Zhou, MD
Internal Medicine Resident
David Geffen School of Medicine at UCLA
Los Angeles, CA

NOTE: UCLA (University of California, Los Angeles)

Abbreviations

ORGANIZATIONS

AASLD	American Association for the Study of Liver Diseases
ACG	American College of Gastroenterology
ADA	American Dietetic Association
AGA	American Gastroenterological Association
AJCC	American Joint Committee on Cancer
APASL	Asian Pacific Association for the Study of the Liver
ASGE	American Society for Gastrointestinal Endoscopy
ASPEN	American Society for Parenteral and Enteral Nutrition
BCLC	Barcelona Clinic Liver Cancer
CDC	Center for Disease Control and Prevention
EASL	European Association for the Study of the Liver
ESPEN	European Society for Clinical Nutrition and Metabolism
ESPGHAN	European Society of Paediatric Gastroenterology, Hepatology, and Nutrition
ESPR	European Society of Paediatric Research
FDA	Food and Drug Administration
IDSA	Infectious Diseases Society of America
NCCN	National Comprehensive Cancer Network
NIAID	National Institute of Allergy and Infectious Diseases
NIH	National Institutes of Health
SHEA	Society for Healthcare Epidemiology of America
UCSF	University of California San Francisco
USPSTF	United States Preventive Service Task Force

MEASUREMENTS

cc	cubic centimeter
cm	centimeter
dL, dl	deciliter
Fr	franklin (electric charge)
g, gm	gram
IU	international unit
kcal	kilocalorie
kg	kilogram
L	liter
mcg	microgram
mEq	milliequivalent
mg	milligram

Abbreviations

mL, ml	milliliter
mm	millimeter
mmHg	millimeter of mercury
mosm	milliosmole
ng	nanogram
pg	picogram
U/L	unit per liter
µl	microliter
W	watt (electric charge)

GENERAL

5-FU	fluorouracil
5-HIAA	5-hydroxyindoleacetic acid
6MP	6-mercaptopurine
A1AT	alpha-1-antitrypsin
AA	abdominal aorta; amyloidosis
Ab	antibody
ACEI	angiotensin-converting enzyme inhibitor
ADR	adenoma detection rate
AFLP	acute fatty liver of pregnancy
AFP	alpha fetoprotein
AH	alcoholic hepatitis
AIDS	acquired immunodeficiency syndrome
AIH	autoimmune hepatitis
ALD	alcoholic liver disease
ALF	acute liver failure
ALKP, ALP	alkaline phosphatase
ALT	alanine aminotransferase
AMA	antimitochondrial antibody
AMI	acute mesenteric ischemia
ANA	antinuclear antibody (test)
ANCA	anti-neutrophil cytoplasmic antibody
anti-HBc	hepatitis B virus core antibody
anti-HBe	hepatitis B virus "e" antibody
anti-HBs	hepatitis B virus surface antibody
AP (or A/P)	anteroposterior
APACHE	Acute Physiology and Chronic Health Evaluation
APC	antigen-presenting cell
aPTT	activated partial thromboplastin time
ARB	angiotensin receptor blocker
ARDS	acute respiratory distress syndrome

Abbreviations

AS	aortic stenosis
ASA	aminosalicylic acid
ASMA	anti-smooth muscle antibody (test)
AST	aspartate aminotransferase
AT	ablative therapy
ATM	ataxia telangiectasia mutated
AXR	abdominal X-ray
AZA	azathioprine
BCS	Budd-Chiari syndrome
BD	branch duct
BE	Barrett's esophagus
BID	two times per day (*bis in die*)
BMI	body mass index
BNP	brain natriuretic peptide
BP	blood pressure
BRAT	banana, rice, applesauce, toast (diet)
BRCA	breast cancer
BRTO	balloon-occluded retrograde transvenous obliteration
BUN	blood urea nitrogen
Bx	biopsy
C	Celsius; cervical
C&M	C = circumferential length, M = maximal length (criteria)
C&S	culture and sensitivity (stool test)
Ca	calcium
CA	cancer
cAMP	cyclic adenosine monophosphate
CBC	complete blood count
CCK	cholecystokinin
CD	celiac disease; Crohn's disease
C. diff	*Clostridium difficile*
CDI	*Clostridium difficile* infection
CDKN	cyclic-dependent kinase inhibitor
CEA	carcinoembryonic antigen
CFTR	cystic fibrosis transmembrane (conductance) regulator
CHB	chronic hepatitis B
CHF	congestive heart failure
Cis	cisplatin
CK	creatinine kinase
CLO	*Campylobacter*-like organism
CMI	chronic mesenteric ischemia
CMP	comprehensive metabolic panel

Abbreviations

CMV	cytomegalovirus
CNS	central nervous system
CPEN	cystic pancreatic endocrine neoplasm
Cr	creatinine
CRC	colorectal cancer
CREST (syndrome)	calcinosis, Raynaud phenomenon, esophageal dysmotility, sclerodactyly, and telangiectasia
CRP	C-reactive protein
CSPY	colonoscopy
CT	computed tomography
CTA	computed tomography angiography
CTC	colonography
Cu	copper
CVID	common variable immunodeficiency
CXCR	CXC-chemokine receptor
CXR	chest X-ray
d	day
DAA	direct acting antiviral
DB	double-blind
DBE	double-balloon enteroscopy
DBPCFC	double-blind, placebo-controlled food challenge
DCD	donation (after) cardiac death
DEXA, DXA	dual-energy X-ray absorptiometry
DGP	deamidated gliadin peptide
DH	dermatitis herpetiformis
DIC	disseminated intravascular coagulation
DILI	drug-induced liver injury
DM	diabetes mellitus
DNA	deoxyribonucleic acid
DS	double strength
dsDNA	double-stranded DNA
EAC	esophageal adenocarcinoma
EBL	endoscopic (rubber) band ligation
EBV	Epstein-Barr virus
EF	ejection fraction
EGD	esophagogastroduodenoscopy
eGFR	estimated glomerular filtration rate
EGFR	epidermal growth factor receptor
EHEC	enterohemorrhagic *Escherichia coli*
EIA	enzyme immunoassay
EIEC	enteroinvasive *Escherichia coli*

EGD	esophagogastroduodenoscopy
EGJ	esophagogastric junction
EKG	electrocardiogram
ELISA	enzyme-linked immunosorbent assay
EM	electron microscopy
EMR	endoscopic mucosal resection
ENT	eyes, nose, throat (otolaryngology)
EoE	eosinophilic esophagitis
EOT	end of treatment
ER	endoplasmic reticulum
ERCP	endoscopic retrograde cholangiopancreatography
ESR	erythrocyte sedimentation rate
ESRD	end-stage renal disease
ETEC	enterotoxigenic *Escherichia coli*
EUS	endoscopic ultrasound
F	Fahrenheit; female
FAP	familial adenomatous polyposis
FB	foreign body
FDG	fluorodeoxyglucose
Fe	iron
FGID	functional gastrointestinal disorder
FHF	fulminant hepatic failure
FIT	fecal immunochemical test
FMF	familial Mediterranean fever
FMT	fecal microbiota transplantation
FNA	fine-needle aspiration
FNH	focal nodular hyperplasia
FODMAP	fermentable oligosaccharides, disaccharides, monosaccharides, and polyols
FOLFIRINOX	folinic acid, fluorouracil, irinotecan, and oxaliplatin
FSIG	flexible sigmoidoscopy
GABA	gamma-aminobutyric acid
GDH	glutamate dehydrogenase
GEJ	gastroesophageal junction
GERD	gastroesophageal reflux disease
GFD	gluten-free diet
gFOBT	guaiac-based fecal occult blood test
GFR	glomerular filtration rate
GGT	gamma-glutamyl transpeptidase
GI	gastrointestinal
GIST	gastrointestinal stromal tumor
GOO	gastric outlet obstruction

Abbreviations

G-tube	gastrostomy tube
GU	genitourinary
GVHD	graft-versus-host disease
HA	hepatic adenoma
HAART	highly active antiretroviral therapy
HAT	hepatic artery thrombosis
HAV	hepatitis A virus
HBc	hepatitis B virus core
HBcAg	hepatitis B virus core antigen
HBeAg	hepatitis B virus "e" antigen
HBs	hepatitis B virus surface
HBsAg	hepatitis B virus surface antigen
HBV	hepatitis B virus
HCC	hepatocellular carcinoma
HCV	hepatitis C virus
HCG	human chorionic gonadotropin
HCST	hematopoietic stem cell transplant
Hct	hematocrit
HDV	hepatitis D virus
HE	hepatic encephalopathy
HFE	hereditary hemochromatosis gene
HG	hyperemesis gravidarum
Hgb	hemoglobin
HGD	high-grade
HELLP	hemolysis, elevated liver enzymes, low platelets in pregnancy
HER2	human epidermal growth factor receptor 2
HH	hereditary hemochromatosis
HHT	hereditary hemorrhagic telangiectasia
HIDA	hepatobiliary iminodiacetic acid
HIV	human immunodeficiency virus
HLA	human leukocyte antigen
HNPCC	hereditary noncolorectal cancer polyposis syndrome
HP	*Helicobacter pylori*
HPLC	high-performance liquid chromatography
HPV	human papilloma virus
hr, H	hour
HR	heart rate; high-resolution
HRQOL	health-related quality of life
HRS	hepatorenal syndrome
HR-WLE	high-resolution white light endoscopy
HSCT	hematopoietic stem cell transplantation

HSV	herpes simplex virus
HTN	hypertension
HUS	hemolytic uremic syndrome
IBD	inflammatory bowel disease
IBS	irritable bowel syndrome
IBS-C	irritable bowel syndrome with constipation
IBS-D	irritable bowel syndrome with diarrhea
IBS-M	irritable bowel syndrome (mixed)
IBW	ideal body weight
ICP	intrahepatic cholestasis of pregnancy
ICU	intensive care unit
IEL	intraepithelial lymphocyte
IFN	interferon
IgA	immunoglobulin A
IgE	immunoglobulin E
IgG	immunoglobulin G
IgM	immunoglobulin M
IL	interleukin
IM	intestinal metaplasia
IMA	inferior mesenteric artery
INR	international normalized ratio
IPAA	ileal pouch-anal anastomosis
IPMN	intraductal papillary mucinous neoplasm
IV	intravenous
IVIG	intravenous immunoglobulin
K	potassium
KCl	potassium chloride
KS	Kaposi's sarcoma
KUB	kidney-ureter-bladder
LBO	large bowel obstruction
LC1	liver cytosol type 1
LCHAD	long-chain 3-hydroxyacyl-CoA dehydrogenase
LDH	lactate dehydrogenase
LES	lower esophageal sphincter
LFT	liver function test
LGD	low-grade
LGIB	lower gastrointestinal (GI) bleeding
LKM1	liver kidney microsome type 1
LN	lymph node
LOLA	L-ornithine-L-aspartate

Abbreviations

LR	lactated Ringer's (solution); liver resection
LRV	left renal vein
LSBE	low-segment Barrett's esophagus
LT	liver transplantation
M	male
MAC	*Mycobacterium avium* complex
MALT	mucosa-associated lymphoid tissue
MAP	mean arterial pressure
MCN	mucinous cystic neoplasm
MD	main duct; medical doctor
MEFV	familial Mediterranean fever gene
MELD	Model for End-Stage Liver Disease
MEN	multiple endocrine neoplasia
Mg	magnesium
min	minute
MR	magnetic resonance
MRCP	magnetic resonance cholangiopancreatography
MRA	magnetic resonance angiography
MRI	magnetic resonance imaging
MSM	men who have sex with men
MTX	methotrexate
MVT	mesenteric venous thrombosis
Na	sodium
NAFL	nonalcoholic fatty liver
NAFLD	nonalcoholic fatty liver disease
NAP-1	North American PFGE type 1 (*Clostridium difficile*)
NAS	NAFLD (nonalcoholic fatty liver disease) activity score
NASH	nonalcoholic steatohepatitis
NB	note well (*nota bene*)
NG	nasogastric
NGAL	neutrophil gelatinase-associated lipocalin
NGT	nasogastric tube
NH3	ammonia
NH4	ammonium
NHL	Non-Hodgkin's lymphoma
NL	normal
NOMI	non-occlusive mesenteric ischemia
NPO	nothing by mouth (*nil per os*)
NS	normal saline; nutcracker syndrome
NSAID	nonsteroidal anti-inflammatory drug

N&V	nausea and vomiting
OCP	oral contraceptive pill
O&P	ova and parasites (stool test)
ORS	oral rehydration solution
P	phosphorus
PAN	polyarteritis nodosa
pANCA	perinuclear antineutrophil cytoplasmic antibody
PAS	periodic acid-Schiff (stain); pouchitis activity score
PBC	primary biliary cirrhosis
PC	pseudocyst
PCN	pancreatic cystic neoplasm
PCOS	polycystic ovarian syndrome
PCR	polymerase chain reaction
PDAI	pouchitis disease activity index
PDT	photodynamic therapy
PEG	pegylated interferon; percutaneous endoscopic gastrostomy; polyethylene glycol
PET	positron emission tomography
PG	prostaglandin
PH	portal hypertension
PICC	peripherally inserted central catheter
PID	pelvic inflammatory disease
PMN	polymorphonuclear leukocyte
PO	by mouth (*per os*)
PO4	phosphate
POEM	per-oral endoscopic myotomy
PPARg	peroxisome proliferator-activated receptor gamma
PPD	purified protein derivative
PPI	proton pump inhibitor
PR	per rectum
PRBC	packed red blood cell
PRN	as needed (*pro re nata*)
PSC	primary sclerosing cholangitis
PT	prothrombin time
PTLD	post-transplant lymphoproliferative disorder
PTT	partial thromboplastin time
PUD	peptic ulcer disease
PVT	portal vein thrombosis
q	each/every (*quaque*)
QD	daily (*quaque die*)
QHS	every bedtime (*quaque hora somni*)

Abbreviations

QID	four times per day (*quater in die*)
QOL	quality of life
R	ratio
RBC	red blood cell
RBV	ribavirin
RFA	radiofrequency ablation
RLQ	right lower quadrant
RNA	ribonucleic acid
ROS	reactive oxygen species
RUQ	right upper quadrant
RVR	rapid viral response
SAA	serum amyloid A (protein)
SAAG	serum ascites albumin gradient
SB	side branch
SBO	small bowel obstruction
SBP	spontaneous bacterial peritonitis
SCA	serous cystadenoma
SCAD	segmental colitis associated with diverticular disease
SCFA	short-chain fatty acid
SCID	severe combined immunodeficiency
SCJ	squamocolumnar junction
SCN	serous cystadenoma
Se	selenium
sec	second
SEMS	self-expandable metal stent
seq	sequence
SGOT	serum glutamic oxaloacetic transaminase
SGPT	serum glutamic pyruvic transaminase
SIBO	small intestinal bacterial overgrowth
SIRS	systemic inflammatory response syndrome
SL	sublingual
SMA	smooth muscle antibody; superior mesenteric artery
SMV	simeprevir
SNRI	serotonin norepinephrine reuptake inhibitor
SOF	sofosbuvir
SPN	solid pseudopapillary neoplasm
SQ	subcutaneous
SSRI	selective serotonin re-uptake inhibitor
SVR	sustained viral response
TACE	transarterial chemoembolization
TAE	transarterial embolization

TB	total bilirubin, tuberculosis
TCA	tricyclic antidepressant
TE	treatment experienced
TH-1 and 2	T helper cells
TID	three times per day (*ter in die*)
TIPS	transjugular intrahepatic portosystemic shunt
TLF	toll-like receptor
TN	treatment naïve
TNF	tumor necrosis factor
TNM	tumor, (lymph) node, metastasis (cancer staging system)
TPMT	thiopurine methyltransferase
TPN	total parenteral nutrition
tRBC	tagged red blood cell (scan)
TS	transferrin saturation
TSH	thyroid-stimulating hormone
TTG	tissue transglutaminase
TTP	thrombotic thrombocytopenic purpura
TW	treatment week
TXT	taxotere
TZD	thiazolidinedione
UBT	urea breath test
UC	ulcerative colitis
UDCA	ursodeoxycholic acid
UGI	upper gastrointestinal
UGIB	upper gastrointestinal (GI) bleeding
ULN	upper limit of normal
US	ultrasound
U.S.	United States
UTI	urinary tract infection
VBG	venous blood gas
VIP	vasoactive intestinal (poly)peptide
vWD	von Willebrand disease
VZV	varicella zoster virus
WBC	white blood cell
WLE	white light endoscopy
XRT	X-ray (radiation) therapy
ZES	Zollinger-Ellison syndrome
Zn	zinc

Introduction

I first came across Tarascon's *Pharmacopoeia* as a medical student. Long before the days of smartphones and tablets, I was drawn to Tarascon's effort to provide a useful resource for clinicians in a simple, portable format. I am honored to have been able to put this work together with my outstanding co-authors and colleagues. It has truly been a team effort, and we know that this text can make a difference in daily practice. The practice of medicine is truly dynamic. Medical knowledge can now, thankfully, be accessed via innumerable sources. No one source can cover everything, but we have focused on the most relevant topics and strategies for patient care at this time.

I would like to thank the dedicated Tarascon team, including Nancy Duffy, Jade Freeman, Daniel Stone, and their colleagues, for their hard work, persistence, and passion towards creating and improving this book.

I often say that life is like chess—you must always think ahead. The field of medicine is no exception, and we are thrilled to have produced a tool for all practitioners and to enable…"thinking ahead."

Eric Esrailian, MD, MPH

PART I APPROACH TO COMMON SYMPTOMS AND EMERGENCIES

CHAPTER 1 ■ APPROACH TO ACUTE ABDOMINAL PAIN

Darryl Hiyama, MD

OVERVIEW

Abdominal pain is an extremely common presenting complaint for the gastroenterologist. From a diagnostic perspective, the potential causes of abdominal pain are numerous. Utilizing a sound and organized approach in evaluating patients with abdominal pain will prove invaluable to the clinician.

KEY CONCEPTS

- A need to understand the unique pathophysiology of abdominal pain.
- Early recognition of conditions requiring emergent treatment.
- A detailed history regarding the abdominal pain will often result in a "short list" of potential diagnoses.
- A focused physical examination often can complement historical information and dictate the timing and nature of needed interventions.
- Selective use of tests in evaluating abdominal pain is both time and cost-efficient.

PATHOPHYSIOLOGY OF ABDOMINAL PAIN

Visceral pain originates from the abdominal viscera in response to distension, muscular contraction, or ischemia. Because visceral innervation is by autonomic nerve fibers, the pain is typically **vague, dull, and poorly localized**. The perceived location of the pain tends to be referred to areas corresponding to the embryonic origin of the affected structure:

- Foregut to the upper abdomen (stomach, duodenum, liver, and pancreas)
- Midgut to the periumbilical region (small bowel, appendix, right colon, and proximal transverse colon)
- Hindgut to the lower abdomen (distal transverse colon, left colon, rectum, and genitourinary [GU] tract)

Somatic pain originates from stimulation of the parietal peritoneum in response to chemical, infectious, or other agents associated with inflammation. In contrast to visceral pain, somatic pain is **sharp and well localized**.

In essence, localized somatic pain represents a focal site of peritoneal inflammation. When somatic pain is generalized or diffuse (and accompanied by findings of diffuse abdominal tenderness), this is often a manifestation of generalized peritonitis.

Referred pain is in a distant location from its source as a result of the sharing of nerve roots between nonadjacent structures. Examples include scapular pain due to biliary colic, groin pain due to renal colic, and shoulder pain due to blood or infection irritating the diaphragm.

EVALUATION OF ABDOMINAL PAIN

The essential elements in the evaluation of abdominal pain include:

- Early recognition of potentially emergent conditions
- A thorough characterization of the pain (location, severity, character, onset, radiation, aggravating or alleviating factors, and associated symptoms)
- Vigilance for physical signs of shock, sepsis, abdominal distension, and localized or diffuse peritonitis
- Selective use of laboratory and imaging studies
- Initiating necessary treatment in a timely manner

RECOGNIZING POTENTIALLY EMERGENT CONDITIONS

Many conditions, such as mesenteric ischemia, or a perforated viscus, require expeditious diagnosis and treatment to prevent death or significant disability. In performing an evaluation, the clinician needs to be vigilant for symptoms or signs suggestive of these particular conditions ("if you aren't looking for it, you will never find it").

In general, two features characteristically mark this subset of abdominal conditions:

- Extreme pain
- Abrupt onset of the pain

Classic scenarios include:

- "Sudden tearing pain" (may be referred to the back), older male, history of hypertension, pulsatile abdominal mass = **ruptured aortic aneurysm**
- "Pain out of proportion to physical findings" = **acute mesenteric ischemia**
- "Sudden epigastric pain" = **perforated duodenal ulcer**
- "Sudden pelvic pain," woman of childbearing age = **ruptured ectopic pregnancy or ovarian torsion**

Chapter 1: Approach to Acute Abdominal Pain

CHARACTERIZE THE PAIN SYMPTOMS

LOCATION

The location of the pain—upper, mid (periumbilical), or lower areas of the abdomen—provides an important cue to possible causes. Vertical localization further helps focus upon likely causes (see **Table 1-1**).

Table 1-1 Possible Etiologies of Abdominal Pain by Location

	Right	Both	Left
Upper	Acute cholecystitis	Acute pancreatitis	Gastritis
	Biliary colic	Biliary colic	Splenic rupture or abscess
	Perforated duodenal ulcer	Perforated duodenal ulcer	
	Acute hepatitis	Myocardial ischemia	
	Congestive hepatomegaly	Lower lobe pneumonia	
		Herpes zoster	
	Choledocholithiasis		
	Acute cholangitis		
	Pyelonephritis		Pyelonephritis
Mid	Retrocecal appendicitis	Early appendicitis	
		Small bowel obstruction	
		Ruptured abdominal aortic aneurysm	
		Meckel's diverticulitis	
		Gastroenteritis	
Lower	Appendicitis	Acute cystitis	Sigmoid diverticulitis
	Cecal diverticulitis	Endometriosis	
	Meckel's diverticulitis	Ruptured aortic aneurysm	
		Acute colitis	Acute colitis
		Colonic ischemia	Colonic ischemia
	Incarcerated groin hernia		Incarcerated groin hernia

(Continues)

Table 1-1 Possible Etiologies of Abdominal Pain by Location (*Continued*)

	Right	Both	Left
Lower	Mesenteric adenitis		
	Psoas abscess		Psoas abscess
	Renal stone		Renal stone
	Inflammatory bowel disease	Inflammatory bowel disease	Inflammatory bowel disease
	Ruptured ectopic pregnancy		Ruptured ectopic pregnancy
	Torsion of gonad		Torsion of gonad
	Mittelschmerz		Mittelschmerz
	Abdominal wall hematoma	Abdominal wall hematoma	Abdominal wall hematoma
	Pelvic inflammatory disease	Pelvic inflammatory disease	Pelvic inflammatory disease

Diffuse abdominal pain may be caused by acute mesenteric ischemia, peritonitis of any cause, or medical conditions such as diabetic ketoacidosis, sickle cell crisis, and typhoid fever.

CHARACTER

The quality or character of the pain may also be telling.

- Sharp and constant: peritonitis
- Dull and constant: appendicitis, diverticulitis, biliary colic
- Sharp, comes in waves: renal stone, intestinal obstruction
- Dull, comes in waves: intestinal obstruction

ONSET

Sudden, abrupt, "woke me from sleep"

- Perforated ulcer
- Ruptured aneurysm
- Ruptured ectopic pregnancy
- Torsion of gonad
- Renal stone

SEVERITY

The perception of pain severity can vary between individuals. However, in general, more severe pain can be associated with the specific aforementioned conditions. Renal stones, biliary colic, and acute pancreatitis are also associated with severe pain.

RADIATION

- Right shoulder or scapula: biliary colic, acute cholecystitis
- Left shoulder or scapula: acute pancreatitis, splenic rupture

Chapter 1: Approach to Acute Abdominal Pain

- Flank: biliary colic, acute cholecystitis, acute pancreatitis, pyelonephritis
- Back: ruptured aortic aneurysm
- Groin: renal stone

AGGRAVATING/ALLEVIATING FACTORS

- Body movement worsens: peritonitis
- Leaning forward feels better: acute pancreatitis
- Antacids/proton pump inhibitor (PPI)/H2 blockers help: gastritis, peptic ulcer disease
- Vomiting helps: intestinal obstruction

ASSOCIATED SYMPTOMS

- Vomiting before pain: gastroenteritis
- Severe vomiting followed by upper abdominal or chest pain: Boerhaave syndrome
- Diarrhea: gastroenteritis, colitis, inflammatory bowel disease
- Jaundice: choledocholithiasis, cholangitis
- Bloody diarrhea: mesenteric ischemia, colonic ischemia, inflammatory bowel disease

OTHER HISTORICAL ELEMENTS

- Previous episodes of similar symptoms suggests chronic conditions, i.e., biliary colic
- Previous abdominal operations
- Significant medical conditions
- Current medications, especially immunosuppressive agents

PHYSICAL FINDINGS

Note: Elderly, pediatric patients, and those who are immunosuppressed may have very minimal physical findings despite bearing a serious intra-abdominal condition.

GENERAL APPEARANCE

- Quiet, lying still, or limited movement: diffuse peritonitis
- Doubled-over, writhing: renal stone, mesenteric ischemia (early)
- Pale, anxious, diaphoretic: shock, peritonitis, perforated viscus, ruptured aneurysm, ruptured ectopic pregnancy, ischemic bowel

ABDOMINAL EXAMINATION

Always approach with **patience and gentleness**:

- Shaking the bed or gurney yields abdominal pain: suggestive of peritoneal irritation. This is often a more accurate and reproducible test than involuntary guarding or rebound tenderness.
- Auscultate for the presence and quality of bowel sounds: absence is suggestive of ileus or peritonitis. High-pitched or rushing sounds suggestive of bowel obstruction.
- Inspect for surgical scars.
- Observe for abdominal distension: usually indicates a more serious condition such as intestinal obstruction, bowel ischemia, or ruptured aortic aneurysm.
- Examine for peritoneal signs. Always start *away* from the location of the pain and migrate back to the area of concern.
- Gentle percussion of the abdominal wall that elicits tenderness is often a gentler method of identifying the presence of peritonitis.
- Inspect for abdominal wall hernias at the umbilicus, any scars, inguinal and femoral regions.

LABORATORY TESTING

Note: For any patients with potentially emergent conditions, urgent resuscitation and early surgical consultation are more important than any testing or imaging.

- Routine blood tests (e.g., complete blood counts [CBC], basic metabolic panel) though routinely obtained, often yield nonspecific results.
- Directed blood tests ordered based upon the historical and physical findings, such as serum lipase to rule in acute pancreatitis or liver function tests to evaluate for liver or gallbladder conditions, are more useful.

IMAGING

- For patients who may have a perforated viscus and physical signs of diffuse peritonitis, an upright chest X-ray (CXR) to detect pneumoperitoneum is sufficient.
- Ultrasonography is the preferred study for evaluation of calculous biliary tract disease, ectopic pregnancy, and suspected appendicitis in children.
- Abdominal computerized tomography (CT) scan with oral and intravenous (IV) contrast is diagnostic in the great majority of cases of significant abdominal pain. This has largely supplanted plain and contrast radiography studies in the evaluation of acute abdominal pain.

REFERENCES

1. Silen W. Abdominal pain. In: Longo DL, Fauci AS, Kasper DL, Hauser SL, Jameson JL, J. Loscalzo J, eds. *Harrison's Principles of Internal Medicine*. 18th ed. New York: McGraw-Hill Professional; 2012.

CHAPTER 2 ■ DYSPHAGIA AND MOTILITY DISORDERS

Kevin A. Ghassemi, MD

OVERVIEW

- *Dysphagia* is the term used for difficulty with swallowing. It can mean that a bolus (food, liquid, and/or pills) does not pass down easily while traveling from the mouth to the stomach or that there is pain with swallowing (odynophagia).
- There are two general types of dysphagia based on anatomic location: oropharyngeal and esophageal.
- This chapter focuses on esophageal dysphagia, with reference to oropharyngeal dysphagia evaluation when appropriate.

PRESENTATION

- Presentation can depend on the cause of dysphagia and can help guide the evaluation.
- An immediate sensation of the bolus getting stuck in the throat, or coughing upon swallowing and/or true choking (the patient cannot breath), suggests an oropharyngeal cause. On the other hand, a sense of the bolus sticking a few seconds after swallowing is more likely to be esophageal in origin.
- Patient localization of where the bolus gets caught often does not correlate with the true location of the obstruction
- Dysphagia to solids alone, or that which *progresses* to both solids and liquids, usually is due to an anatomic obstruction. Dysphagia that begins in association with both solids and liquids may suggest a motility problem.
- A careful history should be performed to elucidate any potential contributory factors.
  - Symptoms suggestive of gastroesophageal reflux disease (GERD)
  - Medications
  - Prior surgeries (orthopedic, head and neck, esophageal) or neck trauma
  - History of radiation
  - History of autoimmune disorders
  - Concomitant allergic disorders

DIFFERENTIAL DIAGNOSIS

Table 2-1 Differential Diagnosis of Esophageal and Oropharyngeal Dysphagia

Esophageal		Oropharyngeal
Anatomic/Structural	Motility	
Peptic stricture	Achalasia	Head and neck tumors
Schatzki ring	Pseudoachalasia	Neurologic disease
Eosinophilic esophagitis	Scleroderma	Stroke
Anastomotic stricture		Trauma
Radiation-induced stricture		Autoimmune disorders
Caustic stricture		Cricopharyngeal bar
Malignancy		Cervical osteophyte
Diverticulum (including Zenker)		
Esophageal web		
Infection		
Candida		
Cytomegalovirus (CMV)		
Herpes simplex virus (HSV)		
Pill-induced esophagitis		
Vascular or other extrinsic compression		

DIAGNOSTIC TESTS

- Choice of test(s) should be guided by history.
- Endoscopy (esophagogastroduodenoscopy, or EGD) should be performed to evaluate for luminal narrowing, esophagitis, esophageal tumors, and for tumors of the cardia that may cause pseudoachalasia.
  - Typical endoscopic features of eosinophilic esophagitis (EoE) include concentric rings, linear furrows, and white exudates.
  - Biopsies should be taken from the proximal and distal esophagus. Presence of more than 15 eosinophils per high-power field in both locations suggests EoE while GERD typically causes increased eosinophils only in the distal esophagus.
  - Esophageal strictures should be biopsied to rule out a malignancy.
- Esophagram (barium swallow) can provide anatomic detail that may not be well appreciated by EGD.
  - Esophageal diverticula (particularly Zenker diverticulum)
  - Length of an esophageal stricture
  - Esophageal dilation and the classic "bird's beak" appearance in achalasia

Chapter 2: Dysphagia and Motility Disorders

- Esophageal manometry is the standard for assessing motility disorders.
  - In achalasia, there is impaired relaxation of the lower esophageal sphincter (LES) and absent peristalsis of the esophageal body.
  - In scleroderma, peristalsis usually is absent and the LES is hypotensive.
- Modified barium swallow study assesses oropharyngeal function, can identify aspiration, and can identify a cricopharyngeal bar.

TREATMENTS (DIAGNOSIS-SPECIFIC)

- EoE
  - Proton pump inhibitors (PPI) BID for 2–3 months should be tried first to rule out PPI-responsive esophageal eosinophilia.
  - Swallowed topical steroids (fluticasone 440 mcg BID or oral viscous budesonide 1 mg/2 ml BID) for 2–3 months are effective at inducing remission. Maintenance steroids (typically 50% of the initial dose) may be considered in severe cases or frequent relapses.
  - Six-food elimination diet (wheat, dairy, soy, nuts, eggs, seafood) is effective and is an accepted first-line therapy for EoE.
  - Dilation, with either balloon or wire-guided bougie, may be performed in cases of high-grade strictures and/or for immediate relief of symptoms. This does not treat the underlying inflammation.
- GERD
  - Peptic strictures and esophageal rings related to GERD can be dilated with balloon or bougie. Biopsy forceps may be used to disrupt a fibrous ring, either as a substitute for or in addition to dilation.
  - PPI should be used to reduce the risk of recurrent GERD-related complications.
- Achalasia
  - Heller myotomy (usually along with a Dor fundoplication) should be considered in all patients who are good operative candidates. The myotomy extends from several centimeters above the esophagogastric junction down to 3 cm along the lesser curvature of the stomach.
  - Pneumatic dilation (diameters of 30–40 mm) is an alternative to surgery. Patients with type I (no esophageal pressurization) or type III (spastic) achalasia are less likely to have success with this modality, as compared to type II (panesophageal pressurization).
  - Endoscopically directed injection of botulinum toxin into the LES should be considered in patients with a limited life expectancy or who are poor operative candidates. This has an effect duration of 6–12 months and may be repeated as needed.
  - Per-oral endoscopic myotomy (POEM) is a relatively new, but promising option for achalasia, which involves endoscopic dissection into the submucosal space and cutting of the LES and inner circular muscle of the esophagus and lesser curve of the proximal gastric body. It may be as effective as a Heller myotomy with either comparable or slightly higher rates of GERD postoperatively.

- Cricopharyngeal bar may be treated with an endoscopic or surgical myotomy.
- Zenker diverticulum may be treated by diverticulectomy or cricopharyngeal myotomy.

REFERENCES

1. Dellon ES, Gonsalves N, Hirano, I, Furuta GT, Liacouris CA, Katzka DA. ACG Clinical Guideline: evidence based approach to the diagnosis and management of esophageal eosinophilia and eosinophilic esophagitis (EoE). *Am J Gastroenterol*. 2013;108:679–92.
2. Kuo P, Holloway RH, Nguyen NQ. Current and future techniques in the evaluation of dysphagia. *J Gastroenterol Hepatol*. 2012;27:873–81.

CHAPTER 3 ■ DYSPEPSIA

Mary Farid, DO

OVERVIEW

- Dyspepsia is a common complaint encountered in clinical practice, accounting for ~ 20% of outpatient gastroenterology consultations.
- Dyspepsia is defined as chronic or recurrent pain or discomfort centered in the upper abdomen.
- Patients with dyspepsia who are over age 55 or who have alarm signs/symptoms should undergo prompt upper endoscopy.
- For all other patients, two treatment strategies are proposed, including (1) "test-and-treat" for *Helicobacter pylori* and (2) empiric trial of antisecretory therapy with a proton pump inhibitor (PPI).
- Functional dyspepsia (endoscopy-negative) accounts for the majority of cases.

DEFINITION

- Dyspepsia is defined as chronic or recurrent pain or discomfort centered in the upper abdomen. Discomfort is defined as a subjective negative feeling that is non-painful, and can incorporate a variety of symptoms including early satiety, nausea, bloating, or upper abdominal fullness.
- Patients presenting with predominant or frequent heartburn or acid regurgitation should be considered to have gastroesophageal reflux disease (GERD) until proven otherwise.

DIFFERENTIAL DIAGNOSIS

- Approximately 25% of patients with dyspepsia have an underlying organic cause.
- Peptic ulcer is responsible for approximately 10% of cases of dyspepsia.
- Other organic causes of dyspepsia include biliary pain, gastroparesis, nonsteroidal anti-inflammatory drugs (NSAIDs)/drug induced, pancreatic disorders, metabolic disturbances or systemic disorders (diabetes, thyroid disease, etc.).
- Less than 1% of cases are due to gastric malignancy.
- Functional dyspepsia accounts for approximately 75% and is by far the most common etiology.

PATHOPHYSIOLOGY OF FUNCTIONAL DYSPEPSIA

- Approximately 40% of patients with functional dyspepsia have delayed gastric emptying.
- There is evidence that the stomach, duodenum, and esophagus are hypersensitive to distention and this may lead to increased postprandial pain and belching.
- Impaired gastric accommodation ("stiff fundus") is also thought to play a role and is associated with early satiety.

ALARM SIGNS ASSOCIATED WITH DYSPEPSIA

Initial management of dyspepsia is largely dependent on the presence or absence of certain alarm signs and symptoms. These are: age over 55 years, weight loss, progressive dysphagia or odynophagia, recurrent vomiting, family history of upper gastrointestinal (GI) tract cancer, early satiety, evidence of GI bleeding or anemia, anorexia, palpable mass, or lymphadenopathy.

MANAGEMENT OF DYSPEPSIA

- Any patient above age 55 with new-onset dyspepsia should undergo prompt upper endoscopy to rule out underlying malignancy.
- Any patient with alarm signs or symptoms as listed should also undergo prompt upper endoscopy.
- In patients younger than 55 without alarm features, two main treatment strategies are recommended. The first is to test and treat for *H. pylori*, and the second is an empiric trial with a PPI.
- Testing and treating for *H. pylori* is most cost effective in high prevalence populations (recent immigrants from developing countries, populations where the prevalence of *H. pylori* exceeds 10%).
- The most accurate noninvasive method of testing for *H. pylori* is the stool antigen test or the urea breath test. If the patient will undergo endoscopy, biopsy for *H. pylori* should be done.
- The second strategy in younger patients without alarm signs is to begin an empiric trial of acid suppression for 4–8 weeks. PPI therapy has been shown to be more effective than H2 blockers in patients with dyspepsia.
- If either strategy fails to relieve symptoms, then the alternative strategy should be employed. In those patients who fail *both* test and treat and the empiric trial of acid suppression, the next step would be to perform an upper endoscopy.

Chapter 3: Dyspepsia

FUNCTIONAL DYSPEPSIA MANAGEMENT

- A negative upper endoscopy is required before a diagnosis of functional dyspepsia can be made.
- Some patients may not require treatment after they are given reassurance with a negative endoscopy.
- Lifestyle modifications should be employed, including avoiding high-fat meals, avoiding obvious food triggers, and eating smaller, more frequent meals throughout the day.
- Managing patients with functional dyspepsia who fail to respond to a 4–8 week course of PPI therapy can be challenging. They can be offered a trial of a low-dose tricyclic antidepressant or can be referred for cognitive behavioral therapy.

REFRACTORY CASES OF DYSPEPSIA

- In patients with resistant symptoms, it worth re-evaluating the diagnosis.
- Ultrasound can be obtained if the history is consistent with biliary colic.
- Although likely low yield, abdominal imaging to rule out chronic pancreatitis or small bowel pathology may be worth considering.
- Gastric emptying study may be considered.
- Re-evaluate the patient to see if they meet criteria for irritable bowel syndrome (IBS).
- Consider looking for rare metabolic or other causes of upper abdominal pain including thyroid disease, hypercalcemia, connective tissue disease, superior mesenteric artery (SMA) syndrome, or infiltrative disease.

REFERENCES

1. Talley NJ, Vakil N, Practice Parameters Committee of the American College of Gastroenterology. Guidelines for the management of dyspepsia. *Am J Gastroenterol.* 2005;100:2324–37.
2. Talley NJ, American Gastroenterological Association. American Gastroenterological Association medical position statement: evaluation of dyspepsia. *Gastroenterology* 2005;129:1753–55.

CHAPTER 4 ■ NAUSEA AND VOMITING

Rimma Shaposhnikov, MD

OVERVIEW

- Nausea and vomiting are common symptoms that can range from bothersome to disabling.
- The extensive list of underlying causes, with conditions beyond the gastrointestinal tract alone, presents a challenge for both diagnosis and treatment.

DEFINITIONS

- *Nausea* is a subjective unpleasant sensation in which one may vomit.
- *Vomiting* is a forceful expulsion of the gastric contents in retrograde fashion from the stomach, usually preceded by nausea. This is different from *retching*, which usually occurs in the absence of gastric evacuation, otherwise known as "dry heaves."
- *Regurgitation* is a passive flow of esophageal contents into the mouth, without abdominal or diaphragmatic muscular activity.
- *Rumination* is a process that occurs within minutes of eating or during eating through a voluntary increase in abdominal pressure. Regurgitated food is brought back to the mouth, with subsequent chewing and swallowing. It is not preceded by nausea.
- Symptoms of nausea and vomiting are defined as *chronic* if they persist for more than 1 month.

PATHOPHYSIOLOGY

- Etiologies causing acute nausea and vomiting affect separate anatomic regions via different receptors. Affected areas include area postrema, with activated dopamine receptors, as well as peripheral afferent pathways, which may stimulate the brainstem nuclei and activate serotonergic receptors.
- Cerebral cortex and labyrinths have also been implicated—with activation via histamine and muscarine cholinergic pathways.

DIFFERENTIAL DIAGNOSIS

- The differential diagnosis includes both pathologic and physiologic conditions encompassing disorders of the gut, peritoneum, as well as central nervous system (CNS), endocrine, and metabolic systems. In addition, medications, infections, and functional disorders need to be carefully assessed.
- Acute causes are generally related to side effects of medications recently prescribed, and infectious and iatrogenic causes, while other causes tend to be responsible for persistent symptoms.

MEDICATIONS/INFECTIOUS/IATROGENIC CAUSES

- Any medication recently prescribed should be assessed for possible adverse side effects. Most common drugs accounting for nausea and vomiting are chemotherapy drugs, which may cause acute (within 24 hours), delayed (after 1 day), and anticipatory nausea and vomiting. Acute reactions are usually mediated by serotonin, and respond better to a serotonin antagonist. Radiation therapy may cause symptoms with the highest occurrence after radiation of the upper abdomen.
- In addition, excess ethanol consumption and cannabinoid ingestion (suspect in young men with severe abdominal pain and relief of symptoms from excess hot showers), excessive consumption of vitamin A, and consumption of unripe akee fruit (Jamaican vomiting sickness) are rare causes and require meticulous history taking.

INFECTIOUS CAUSES

- Viral (rotavirus, adenovirus) causes tend to be self-limiting, and may be associated with diarrhea, fever, and myalgias. Bacterial gastroenteritis may occur within hours of toxin ingestion (*Staphylococcus aureus*, *Salmonella*, *Clostridium perfringens*, *Bacillus cereus*); other causes include otitis media, hepatitis, and meningitis, which can also present with acute onset of nausea and vomiting.
- Postoperative nausea and vomiting is affected by type of anesthetic use, duration, and type of surgery, and it is usually acute in presentation.

CNS CAUSES

- Common conditions include migraine headaches, seizure disorders, and any condition with increased intracranial pressure such as tumor, infarction, hemorrhage, abscess, and hydrocephalus. Labyrinthine disorders are often associated with vertigo (motion sickness, Meniere's disease)—activation via histamine and muscarine cholinergic pathway—and may therefore respond better to antihistamines and anticholinergics.
- Vomiting occurs in the morning before meals related to increased intracranial pressure; may be projectile and without preceding nausea.

Chapter 4: Nausea and Vomiting

May have severe headache, also worse in the morning. Presence of focal neurological deficits may occur.
- Psychiatric illnesses, including depression, anorexia nervosa, bulimia nervosa, psychogenic vomiting, anxiety, and emotional responses to particular smells, tastes, or unpleasant memories can also induce vomiting. May present with irregular or continuous vomiting.

ENDOCRINOLOGIC AND METABOLIC CAUSES

- Uremia, diabetic ketoacidosis, parathyroid and adrenal disorders, and hyperthyroidism can be elicited with history and laboratory evaluation.
- Pregnancy is the most common endocrine cause, and it should be considered in all women of childbearing age. Complicated conditions include: (1) hyperemesis gravidarum—intractable vomiting that may lead to electrolyte imbalance and (2) acute fatty liver of pregnancy, which presents in the 3rd trimester and may be complicated by liver failure, disseminated intravascular coagulation (DIC), and fetal/maternal death.

GASTROINTESTINAL DISORDERS

- Acute processes such as peptic ulcer disease, acute pancreatitis, cholecystitis, and appendicitis will lead to acute presentation of nausea and vomiting.
- Biliary colic and cholecystitis (suspect with right upper quadrant [RUQ] pain, radiation to right shoulder blade), pancreatitis (epigastric pain radiating to the back, worse pain with eating), and peptic ulcer disease are more common causes. Dyspepsia, gastroesophageal reflux disease (GERD), and irritable bowel syndrome may cause symptoms as well.
- Mechanical obstruction such as gastric outlet obstruction (GOO) is characterized as intermittent vomiting, delayed by at least an hour after eating, lack of bile, and absence of pain. Small bowel obstruction, on the other hand, presents as acute, painful episodes, associated with bilious vomiting, and improvement of pain after vomiting. Symptoms may be acute or chronic.
- Motility disorders such as gastroparesis should be suspected with systemic diseases such as diabetes mellitus, scleroderma, systemic lupus erythematosus, and amyloidosis—emesis may have putrid odor due to stagnation and inability to move the food out into the small bowel. Early satiety and postprandial fullness are additional complaints.

FUNCTIONAL CAUSES

- Cyclic vomiting syndrome: presents as acute episodes of nausea and vomiting, followed by asymptomatic periods. Often seen in children and females, with some association with personal or family history of migraines.

- Functional nausea and vomiting, according to Rome III criteria, is characterized by absence of criteria for any major disease and absence of abnormalities on labs or studies; it is, therefore, a diagnosis of exclusion.

EVALUATION (SEE FIGURE 4-1)

- The American Gastroenterological Association (AGA) guidelines recommend a three-step approach. The goal is to first recognize and correct any associated consequences of nausea and vomiting, namely fluid loss, electrolyte imbalance. The second step is to identify the underlying etiology and provide appropriate therapy. The third step is to provide empiric therapy to treat the symptoms if no cause is found.
- Physical exam: a complete physical exam may provide clues. Patient should be evaluated for signs of dehydration, orthostatic vital signs, skin turgor, mucous membranes. General examination should be performed, with particular emphasis on signs associated with self-induced vomiting such as parotid enlargement, loss of dental enamel, calluses on dorsal surfaces of the fingers, and lanugo hair.
- Abdominal exam: succession splash may identify gastric outlet obstruction, bowel sounds—increased in obstruction and diminished in ileus; tenderness in RUQ may help with biliary colic.
- Neurological exam should be considered.

DIAGNOSIS

- Laboratory tests may be helpful depending on the etiology. Due to the myriad possible diseases, the recommendation is to check for signs of dehydration with comprehensive metabolic panel (CMP), complete blood count (CBC), and human chorionic gonadotropin (HCG) test to rule out pregnancy, all of which should be part of an acute evaluation. Additional tests such as thyroid-stimulating hormone (TSH), amylase, lipase, and erythrocyte sedimentation rate (ESR) may be needed depending on history.
- Imaging tests such as supine and upright abdominal films should be ordered if an acute episode of small bowel obstruction is suspected. Additional imaging such as MRI/CT of head is recommended if CNS etiology is suspected and workup is warranted. RUQ ultrasound is beneficial with the diagnosis of biliary etiology; esophagogastroduodenoscopy (EGD) will evaluate for mucosal lesions such as ulcers. A gastric emptying study may reveal gastroparesis, but it is less helpful in an acute illness.

Chapter 4: Nausea and Vomiting

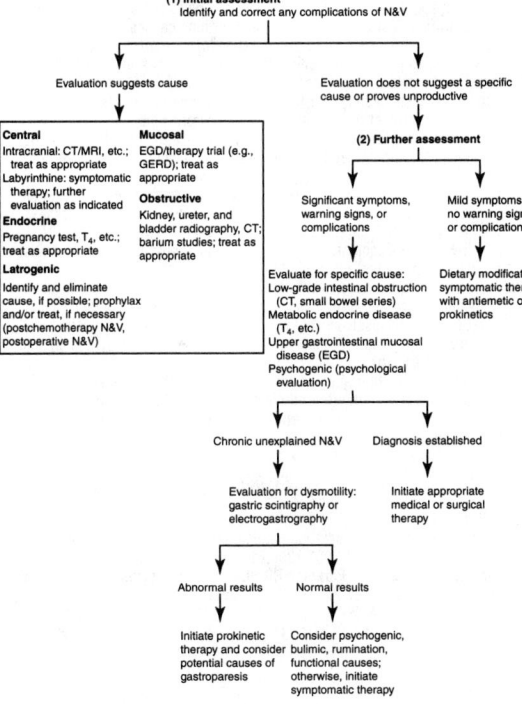

Figure 4-1 Initial assessment: Identify and correct any complications of N & V.

Adapted from Quigley EM, Hasler WL, Parkman HP. AGA technical review on nausea and vomiting. *Gastroenterol.* 2001;120:263–86. With permission from Elsevier.

TREATMENT

- First and foremost, the goal is to correct electrolyte and fluid imbalance. Second step is to offer targeted therapy if the cause or pathophysiology is identified. Motion sickness and labyrinthine causes are treated with histamine H1 and muscarinic/cholinergic M1 receptor antagonists such as scopolamine transdermal patch; antihistamines include meclizine and diphenhydramine. Acute symptoms related to chemotherapy will respond to use of serotonergic 5-HT3 receptor antagonists.
- Empiric treatment may be initiated if no culprit is located to help with the presenting symptoms. Due to limited data on the efficacy of the medications, suggested therapies that have been noted in the literature are listed as follows:
  - Phenothiazines, prochlorperazine, and promethazine are available rectally, orally, and parenterally and may work in motion sickness, vertigo, postchemotherapy, and postoperative symptoms.
  - 5-HT3 antagonists—such as ondansetron, cannabinoids, benzodiazepines, corticosteroids, butyrophenones (droperidol, haloperidol)—have been shown to work in anticipatory and acute chemotherapy-related nausea, as well as postoperative nausea.
  - Benzamides, such as metoclopramide, exert prokinetic effect and are used for gastroparesis but have unfavorable extrapyramidal side effects such as tardive dyskinesia.
  - Alternative therapies such as acupuncture may work for postoperative patients and chemotherapy patients. Ginger, 250 mg before meals, may work, and pyridoxine (vitamin B6) may be used for early pregnancy.

REFERENCES

1. Talley NJ, American Gastrointestinal Association. American Gastroenterological Association medical position statement: nausea and vomiting. *Gastroenterol.* 2001;120:261–3.
2. Quigley EM, Hasler WL, Parkman HP. AGA technical review on nausea and vomiting. *Gastroenterol.* 2001;120:263–86.
3. Scorza K, Williams A, Phillips JD, Shaw J. Evaluation of nausea and vomiting. *Am Fam Physician.* 2007;76(1):76–84

CHAPTER 5 ■ CONSTIPATION

Anthony Lembo, MD

OVERVIEW

- Constipation is defined as unsatisfactory defecation characterized by infrequent stools, difficult stool passage, or both. Difficult stool passage includes straining, a sense of difficulty passing stool, incomplete evacuation, hard/lumpy stools, prolonged time to pass stool, or the need for manual maneuvers to pass stool.
- Constipation is a common complaint, is reported to be present in approximately 12–19% of the general population, and is particularly prevalent in women and the elderly.
- Invasive diagnostic testing such as colonoscopy is only necessary when alarm features are present such as new onset in the elderly, rectal bleeding, weight loss, or family history of colorectal cancer.
- Chronic constipation can be associated with significant negative impact on quality of life.

PRESENTATION

- Most individuals experience intermittent and mild constipation at some time in their lives, rarely require medical consultation, and generally respond to changes in diet or mild laxatives. When constipation is chronic, more severe, and does not respond to simple dietary changes and mild laxatives, some of these individuals seek consultation.
- Infrequent stools (i.e., less than three bowel movements per week) are often present; however, patients also frequently complain of difficulty evacuating their bowels, excessive straining, and incomplete emptying of their rectum. Bloating and abdominal discomfort are also commonly present.
- The presence of unexplained rectal bleeding, severe constipation, new onset of constipation in the elderly, excessive weight loss, and family history of colorectal cancer could be a sign of an organic cause for constipation and further evaluation of the colon may be necessary.

DIFFERENTIAL DIAGNOSIS

- While chronic constipation is most often functional (i.e., idiopathic) secondary causes to consider include a number of medications (iron, narcotics, antidepressants, calcium channel blockers, antacids, etc.). Likewise, anatomical (neoplasm, diverticular disease, prolapse, etc.), neurological (spinal lesions, autonomic neuropathy, Parkinson's disease, etc.), and metabolic/endocrine (diabetes, Addison's, hypercalcemia, etc.) abnormalities should be considered.

PATHOPHYSIOLOGY

- Frequently multifactorial. The three main categories of functional constipation include slow transit constipation, normal transit constipation, and defecatory disorders.
- Defecatory disorders (i.e., pelvic floor dyssynergia) are secondary to incomplete relaxation of the anal sphincter and pelvic floor muscles or inadequate pressure in the rectum during defecation.

DIAGNOSIS

- The diagnosis is made clinically based on symptoms, a detailed physical examination (including a digital rectal examination), and by excluding secondary causes of constipation.
- The Rome III Criteria for diagnosing functional constipation include two or more of the following symptoms: fewer than three bowel movements per week or during at least 25% of defecations, lumpy or hard stools, sensation of incomplete evacuation, sensation of anorectal obstruction or blockage, manual maneuvers to facilitate defecation. Loose stools should be rarely present without the use of laxatives.
  - If symptoms persist despite medical management, further evaluation of pelvic floor function (e.g., anorectal motility/balloon expulsion) and colonic motility could be considered.

TREATMENT (SEE TABLE 5-1)

- If a secondary cause is identified, eliminating the offending medication or treating the underlying medical condition may relieve constipation.
- Counsel on dedicating regular time (preferably the morning) for bowel function, elevating the feet 6–12 inches while defecating, avoiding excessive straining.
- Advocate for simple lifestyle changes such as increasing dietary fiber and drinking adequate water.

Chapter 5: Constipation

Table 5-1 Pharmacological Treatment Options for Chronic Constipation

Medication	Maximal Recommended Dose	Comments
Bulk laxative		
Psyllium	Titrate up to 20 g	Natural soluble
Methylcellulose	Titrate up to 20 g	Semisynthetic cellulose
Polycarbophil	Titrate up to 20 g	Synthetic
Osmotic laxative		
Magnesium based products	dosage varies	Draws water into the lumen
Lactulose	15–30 ml once or twice a day	Poorly absorbed sugar (disaccharide—galactose and fructose)
Polyethylene glycol	17–36 g once or twice a day	Organic polymers that are poorly absorbed and not metabolized by colonic bacteria
Stimulant laxative		
Anthraquinones	325 mg (or 5 ml) daily	Increase contractions in the intestines and promote secretions
Cascara sagrada	187 mg daily	
Senna	5–10 mg every night	
Castor oil	5–10 mg every night	
Bisacodyl	5–10 mg every night	
Sodium picosulfate	5–10 mg every night	
Stool softener/ emollient		
Docusate sodium	100 mg twice a day	Ionic detergents soften stool
Mineral oil	5–15 ml orally every night	
Chloride channel agonist		
Lubiprostone	24 mcg twice a day	Increases fluid in the lumen
Guanylate cyclase agonist		
Linaclotide	145 mcg once a day	Increases fluid in the lumen
5-HT4 agonist		
Prucalopride	2 mg twice a day	Increases motility

- Empiric treatment with fiber and laxatives can increase bowel frequency and improve some symptoms of constipation.
- Prescription therapies like lubiprostone, a chloride channel activator, and linaclotide, a guanylate cyclase-C agonist, increase fluid in the lumen of the intestine, increase intestinal transit, and improve bowel function. Prucalopride, a 5-HT4 agonist, is available in Europe and several other countries but not currently in the United States.

- Anorectal biofeedback for sphincter retraining is the treatment of choice for defecatory disorder or pelvic floor dysfunction.
- Surgery to remove a portion or the entire colon is rarely indicated and generally reserved only for patients with severe slow transit constipation without small bowel dysmotility or pelvic floor dysfunction.

REFERENCES

1. Lembo AJ, Camilleri M. Chronic constipation. *N Engl J Med*. 2003; 349:1360–68.
2. Lacy BE, Lovenick JM, Crowell M. Chronic constipation: new diagnostic and treatment approaches. *Therap Adv Gastroenterol*. 2012;5(4):233–247.

CHAPTER 6 ■ DIARRHEA

Vikas K. Pabby, MD, MPH

OVERVIEW

- Diarrhea is defined as a stool weight of more than 200 grams per 24 hours in a person consuming a Western diet.
- Diarrhea can be classified in several ways, and based on:
  o Duration of symptoms: acute (≤ 4 weeks' duration) versus chronic (> 4 weeks' duration). Chronic diarrhea further classifies into watery, fatty, or inflammatory.
  o Cause of diarrhea: infectious, inflammatory, malabsorption, secretory, osmotic, functional.
  o Stool osmolality: osmotic versus secretory.

PATHOPHYSIOLOGY

INFECTIOUS DIARRHEA

Generally acute but some organisms can cause chronic symptoms:

- Acute invasive: causes include *Salmonella* (contaminated eggs, poultry, meat, unpasteurized milk or juice, cheese, raw fruits and vegetables), *Shigella* (contaminated food and water), enteroinvasive *Escherichia coli* (EIEC), *Yersinia* (from contaminated milk and pork products), and *Campylobacter* (undercooked poultry, unpasteurized milk, contaminated water).
- Acute watery diarrhea: *Rotavirus* (young children), *Norovirus* (older children and adults, associated with cruise ships), enterotoxigenic *Escherichia coli* (ETEC; traveler's diarrhea), and *Vibrio cholera* (produces rice water diarrhea), which stimulates cAMP-mediated chloride secretion.
- Preformed toxin: *Bacillus cereus* (fried rice) and *Staphylococcus aureus* (salads and bakery products). These organisms generally cause diarrhea within 6 hours of ingestion.
- Preformed spores: *Clostridium perfringens* (poultry and beef).
- Acute bloody diarrhea: enterohemorrhagic *Escherichia coli* (EHEC) or *E. coli* O157:H7 (undercooked hamburger meat, associated with hemolytic uremic syndrome—HUS), *Shigella*, EIEC, *Yersinia*, *Campylobacter*.
- Antibiotic associated: *Clostridium difficile*, which produces a cytotoxin.
- Acute to chronic symptoms: *Giardia*, *Amebae*, *Cryptosporidium*, *Cyclospora*, and *Isospora*.

INFLAMMATORY

- Inflammatory bowel disease (IBD), microscopic colitis
- Ischemic: colonic ischemic, mesenteric ischemia
- Medication induced: due to drugs such as nonsteroidal anti-inflammatory drugs (NSAIDs), isotretinoin, ipilimumab
- Radiation induced
- Diversion colitis
- Segmental colitis associated with diverticular disease (SCAD)

MALABSORPTION

- Whipple's disease: a rare, systemic disease caused by *Tropheryma whipplei*. Extraintestinal manifestations include signs of malabsorption with potential involvement of the neurologic, cardiovascular, pulmonary, ophthalmologic, and musculoskeletal systems.
- Menetrier's disease: a rare, acquired disorder causing gastric rugae to enlarge, forming giant folds in the stomach.
- Celiac disease or gluten sensitive enteropathy.
- Chronic pancreatitis.

SECRETORY

This type of diarrhea occurs due to toxins or tumors producing excessive mucosal secretion. Apart from infectious causes, which include *Staphylococcus*, *Escherichia coli*, and *Vibrio cholerae*, causes of secretory diarrhea include bile acid–induced diarrhea, long-standing diabetes mellitus, and neuroendocrine tumors, including VIPoma, Zollinger-Ellison syndrome (ZES), medullary carcinoma of the thyroid, and carcinoid tumors.

OSMOTIC

This type of diarrhea occurs due to poorly absorbed osmotic substances that are present in the stool.

- Small intestinal bacterial overgrowth (SIBO): risk factors include scleroderma, small bowel diverticula, gastric or small bowel surgeries, chronic pancreatitis, Crohn's disease of the terminal ileum, and proton pump inhibitor (PPI) use.
- Lactose intolerance.
- Intake of polyethylene glycol (PEG), sugar, sorbitol, and lactulose.

FUNCTIONAL

Diarrhea-predominant irritable bowel syndrome (IBS-D)

Chapter 6: Diarrhea

DIAGNOSIS (SEE FIGURE 6-1)

- For acute diarrhea based on the clinical suspicion, stool studies should be sent for stool culture, *C. difficile* enzyme immunoassay (EIA), ova and parasites, *Giardia* antigen testing if possible exposure, and *E. histolytica* fecal antigen assay. In immunocompromised patients, *Cryptosporidium*, *Cyclospora*, and *Isospora* testing may be indicated.
- If there is a history of IBD, a disease flare should be ruled out with inflammatory biomarkers (C-reactive protein [CRP], fecal lactoferrin, fecal calprotectin) or endoscopic evaluation. *C. difficile* or cytomegalovirus infection should be ruled out.
- Endoscopic evaluation with biopsies for pathological examination and virology. Besides *C. difficile* infection, pseudomembranes can also be seen in *E. coli* colitis, ischemic colitis, and chemical colitis. In IBD, crypt

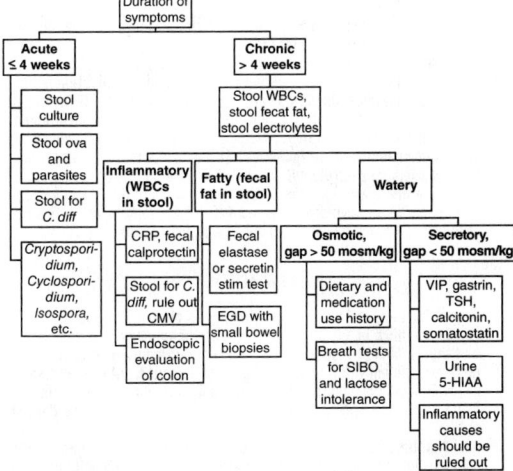

Figure 6-1 Recommended diagnostic approach to treating diarrhea.

CRP = C-reactive protein; CMV = cytomegalovirus; EGD = esophagogastroduodenoscopy; SIBO = small intestinal bacterial overgrowth; VIP = vasoactive intestinal peptide; TSH = thyroid-stimulating hormone; 5-HIAA = 5-hydroxyindoleacetic acid.

distortion with branching or budding, basal plasmacytosis, and paneth cell metaplasia are seen.
- Esophagogastroduodenoscopy (EGD) should be considered in those with malabsorptive disorders. The differential diagnosis of villous blunting on small bowel biopsy includes celiac disease, *Giardia* infection, and common variable immune deficiency (CVID). Whipple's disease will show periodic acid-Schiff positive, acid-fast bacillus negative duodenal biopsies. Menetrier's disease will show crypt elongation and dilation with foveolar hyperplasia on gastric biopsy.
- In chronic diarrhea associated with anemia, a tissue transglutaminase (tTG) antibody IgA and/or IgG should be checked.
- Fecal elastase or secretin stimulation test should be ordered in suspected chronic pancreatitis.
- Stool osmotic gap is used to differentiate between osmotic and secretory diarrhea. This is calculated by obtaining the difference between normal gut lumen osmolality (290 mosm/kg) and the calculated stool osmolality, which is equal to $2 \times (Na + K)$.
  - Osmotic diarrhea: gap > 50 mosm/kg. In carbohydrate malabsorption, the stool pH will be less than 5.3.
  - Secretory diarrhea: gap < 50 mosm/kg.
- For osmotic diarrhea, a detailed dietary history and a medication history for use of laxatives should be taken. Breath tests for SIBO (hydrogen and methane breath testing following oral glucose or lactulose ingestion) and lactose intolerance (hydrogen breath testing following consumption of lactose) are indicated. The gold standard of diagnosing SIBO is a jejunal aspirate/culture, but it is infrequently done.
- For secretory diarrhea, check vasointestinal peptide (VIP), gastrin, calcitonin, 5-hydroxindoleacetic acid (5-HIAA), somatostatin, thyroid-stimulating hormone (TSH), and chromogranin A levels.

TREATMENT

- Acute diarrhea: oral rehydration therapy as opposed to sports drinks, which are high in glucose, "BRAT" diet (bananas, rice, applesauce, and toast). Milk products should be avoided in adults due to transient lactase deficiency during acute diarrheal episodes. Infants and small children should be continued on breastmilk, formula, or cow's milk.
- Avoid antibiotics with suspected *E. coli* O157:H7: may increase the risk of HUS.
- Avoid antimotility agents such as loperamide and diphenoxylate/atropine in patients with bloody diarrhea or suspected inflammatory diarrhea. Otherwise, use in low doses to slow down bowel movement frequency without causing constipation.
- Traveler's diarrhea: prophylaxis is with bismuth subsalicylate. Treatment is with fluoroquinolones, azithromycin, or rifaximin.

- SIBO: rifaximin, metronidazole, amoxicillin/clavulanate, or fluoroquinolones for 7–14 days.
- Radiation-induced colitis: short-chain fatty acid (SCFA) enemas, endoscopic argon plasma coagulation, and hyperbaric oxygen therapy are used.
- SCAD: 5-aminosalicylic acid (5-ASA) orally or topically.
- Diversion colitis: SCFA enemas or 5-ASA enemas.
- Whipple's disease: Penicillin G and streptomycin or a third-generation cephalosporin followed by trimethoprim/sulfamethoxazole for at least 1 year to decrease the risk of relapse.
- Menetrier's disease: PPI, histamine-2 receptor antagonists, octreotide, and cetuximab have been used. Gastrectomy is used for those patients who are refractory to medical therapy.

REFERENCES

1. Binder HJ. Causes of chronic diarrhea. *N Engl J Med*. 2006;355:236–9.
2. Ryan ET, Madoff LC, Ferraro MJ. Case records of the Massachusetts General Hospital. Case 20-2011. A 30-year-old man with diarrhea after a trip to the Dominican Republic. *N Engl J Med*. 2011;364(26):2536–41.
3. Thielman NM, Guerrant RL. Clinical practice: acute infectious diarrhea. *N Engl J Med*. 2004 Jan 1;350(1):38–47.
4. Sandhu DK, Surawicz C. Update on chronic diarrhea: a run-through for the clinician. *Curr Gastroenterol Rep*. 2012;14(5):421–7.
5. Schiller LR. Definitions, pathophysiology, and evaluation of chronic diarrhoea. *Best Pract Res Clin Gastroenterol*. 2012;26(5):551–62.
6. Pagès C, Gornet JM, Monsel G, et al. Ipilimumab-induced acute severe colitis treated by infliximab. *Melanoma Res*. 2013;23(3):227–30.

CHAPTER 7 ■ GASTROINTESTINAL FOREIGN BODIES

Joseph Chan, MD and Richelle J. Cooper, MD, MSHS

OVERVIEW

- Gastrointestinal foreign bodies can be broadly divided into three main categories by location: esophageal, gastric/intestinal, and rectal.
- Esophageal foreign bodies can further be functionally divided into upper and lower esophageal.
- Although children make up the largest subset of patients with gastrointestinal foreign bodies (> 80%), this chapter focuses on adults.
- The importance of this topic lies mainly in the potentially disastrous complication of perforation of the gastrointestinal tract. The focus of diagnosis and management is risk stratifying those who will need emergent intervention versus conservative management.

EPIDEMIOLOGY

- In adults, predisposing factors include patients who have dentures (edentulous), esophageal disease, psychiatric illness, or who are incarcerated.
- The most common foreign bodies (FB) in adults are impacted meat, bones, toothpicks, dentures, and oral piercings. The most dangerous objects are packets of illicit drugs, disc batteries, multiple magnets, and sharp objects (bones/toothpicks/razors).
- Up to 80–90% of FBs will pass through the gastrointestinal tract uneventfully. 10–20% will require endoscopic removal and only 1% will require surgery.
- Early endoscopy is required for cases with the potential for toxicity, altered anatomy (including prior surgery), sharp foreign bodies, and esophageal impactions that do not resolve spontaneously. Emergent surgery is indicated for perforation or for cases that are refractory to endoscopy.

ESOPHAGEAL FOREIGN BODIES

- Sharp objects (such as fish bones) often become impaled in the posterior oropharynx or in the upper/cervical esophagus (above the thoracic inlet or clavicular level on plain radiograph).

- Food impactions, the most common lower esophageal FB in adults, will usually be lodged at either the level of the aortic arch or lower esophageal sphincter (two to four vertebral bodies superior to the gastric bubble on plain film).
- Esophageal FBs have a high probability of associated preexisting esophageal pathology (> 75%) including anatomic or functional abnormalities such as vascular rings, esophageal diverticula, strictures, masses, webs, achalasia, or diffuse esophageal spasm. In general, complications are rare (2%), but severe.
- Any FB, including meat, can cause esophageal rupture if it induces enough repeated vomiting. Objects impacted longer than 24 hours have a higher risk of mucosal erosion, thus urgent gastroenterology (GI) consultation and removal within 12 hours is the expected standard.
- Button batteries are a high-risk subset of FB. They are extremely corrosive if impacted in the esophagus and result in high risk of perforation due to liquefaction necrosis; erosion into nearby structures can lead to esophagotracheal or esophagoaortic fistulas. Immediate GI consultation is required as esophageal button batteries universally need to be removed emergently within 2 hours.

PRESENTATION

- Odynophagia is the most common symptom of obstruction, but patients can also experience dysphagia, neck pain, substernal pain, vomiting, and wheezing. Patients are usually able to accurately pinpoint the location of their FB.
- Drooling is a sign of high-grade obstruction, and an indication for urgent endoscopy to prevent aspiration. Shortness of breath is uncommon unless the FB is so large it impinges on the trachea. Late sequelae from perforation may present with symptoms of mediastinitis; erosion into vasculature may be heralded by a small bleed followed by massive hemorrhage.
- The exam is usually normal unless perforation has already occurred, in which case there may be subcutaneous emphysema or signs of infection.

DIAGNOSIS

- FBs in the posterior oropharynx (such as fish bones) not seen initially can sometimes be directly visualized after stimulating the patient's gag reflex with a tongue depressor, thus elevating the soft palate, revealing the previously hidden FB. FBs in the upper esophagus may be visualized by video laryngoscopy at bedside.
- In general, imaging is not indicated in most patients with symptomatic esophageal food impaction diagnosed by history and physical—additional radiation from imaging will not preclude their need for management with endoscopy whether the diagnostic testing is definitive or not.

Chapter 7: Gastrointestinal Foreign Bodies

- Plain radiographs (chest anterior-posterior [AP] and cervical [C]-spine AP/lateral) aid in the diagnosis in approximately 50% of patients.
  - Most helpful in children who swallow radiopaque objects, such as coins or batteries, and are unable to relate symptoms to the examiner.
  - Fish bones are detected on plain radiographs only 25% of the time.
  - Plastic foreign bodies are usually not visible.
  - Plain radiographs are not indicated if meat or other soft food bolus is known to be impacted in the esophagus as these are radiolucent.
- Computed tomography (CT) scans with three-dimensional reconstruction (for potentially radiolucent objects such as fish bones) or endoscopy are the recommended primary diagnostic tool if plain radiographs are negative.
- Contrast swallow studies (such as barium or gastrografin esophagrams or barium-soaked contrast cotton balls) are not recommended. They are of low diagnostic yield and complicate definitive treatment with endoscopy as they may hide a foreign body or mucosal injury and also risk aspiration.

MANAGEMENT

- The most emergent but uncommon complication related to upper esophageal FB is airway compromise—airway is always the first priority in any patient's management. Anyone with difficulty managing their secretions is at risk for aspiration/airway compromise and needs urgent intervention.
- The consulting service for definitive management will largely depend on the location of the FB.
  - FBs in the upper/cervical esophagus are usually managed by emergency physicians or otolaryngologists (ENT).
  - FBs below the clavicles (lower esophagus) are managed by GI with endoscopy.
  - If at any time (including upon presentation) the patient has evidence of perforation, either by imaging or by clinical findings consistent with mediastinitis or peritonitis (as manifested by severe chest or abdominal pain, ill appearance, subcutaneous emphysema, significant hematemesis or hematochezia, abdominal rebound or guarding, or signs of shock), the appropriate place for removal of the FB is in the operating room by a surgeon. After immediately consulting general surgery, one should obtain adequate IV access, resuscitate with crystalloid boluses and/or vasopressors as needed, administer broad-spectrum antibiotics (such as piperacillin-tazobactam to cover Gram-negative enterics and anaerobes), withhold oral food and fluids from the patient (NPO), and manage the airway as needed.

Upper Esophageal Foreign Bodies

- If the FB can be visualized directly or on video laryngoscopy, an experienced physician can attempt removal with Magill forceps at bedside.
- Expectant management is often successful (overall > 95%); ideal patients are those seen within 24 hours of ingestion of a radiographically "safe" object, such as a coin.
- With suspected fish bones in particular, if neither plain radiographs nor CT scan reveal any fish bones, and the patient has persistent mild symptoms but is well appearing, it is reasonable to have the patient return to the emergency department in 24 hours for a recheck rather than moving straight to endoscopy. A mucosal scratch alone can cause symptoms mimicking impaction even in the absence of a FB, but should resolve in < 24 hours because the mucosa heals rapidly. Acid-blocking medication (H2 blocker or PPI—proton pump inhibitor) is recommended.

Lower Esophageal Foreign Bodies

- Lower esophageal food impactions require GI consultation for treatment of the acute presentation and identification of any underlying pathology.
- Medical management, although frequently suggested, is of no proven benefit, may cause harm, and should not delay needed consultation or intervention.
  - Glucagon, although it is thought to potentially decrease smooth muscle tone of the lower esophageal sphincter, is not routinely recommended. No good quality randomized controlled trials prove efficacy, and it commonly induces vomiting—which can increase the risk of rupture as well as aspiration. Its use should be avoided.
  - Other medications, including nitroglycerin and nifedipine (thought to work similarly to glucagon—although even less effective than unproven glucagon) are also not recommended due to lack of efficacy data.
  - Gas-forming agents (carbonated drinks) have not been shown to be effective.
  - Papain (or other proteolytic enzymes) should *never* be used for food impaction, due to risk of mucosal erosion, perforation, and hypernatremia.
- With meat or soft food impactions, if the patient only has minor symptoms, a trial of expectant management for 12 hours is reasonable.
- Endoscopy is the preferred strategy for removal if necessary. During endoscopy, if removal is difficult, the impaction may also safely be resolved by pushing the meat into the stomach with minimal pressure.
- Sharp objects (such as bones, safety pins, hat pins, razor blades, toothpicks, and nails) impacted in the esophagus should be removed endoscopically—or in the operating room if the endoscopist is unsuccessful or deems it unsafe.
- All patients who have spontaneous clearing of a FB should have a trial of oral intake prior to discharge and be put on a soft diet. Due to the high

incidence of underlying pathology (> 75%), all patients with esophageal FB (most often food impaction) need a referral to a gastroenterologist for endoscopic evaluation.
- Any patient treated conservatively with expectant management and discharged from the emergency department tolerating oral intake should be instructed to return for shortness of breath, pain (chest or abdominal), persistent vomiting, hematemesis, bloody or black stool, or any difficulty swallowing their own secretions.

GASTRIC AND SMALL BOWEL FOREIGN BODIES

Once foreign bodies pass the esophagus, they will usually pass through the rest of the gastrointestinal tract within a few days uneventfully, surprisingly often even if they are sharp FBs. If impaction, perforation, or obstruction does occur, the FB is usually lodged at either the gastric outlet or the ileocecal valve.

PRESENTATION

- Patient symptoms range from asymptomatic to vague abdominal pain, obstruction, or peritonitis from perforation.
- The physical exam should be normal unless there is a large bezoar, small bowel obstruction, or perforation.
- A subset of adult patients have secondary gain with ingestion of foreign bodies for the intent of hiding illicit drugs. If the packet contains toxic substances such as cocaine, rupture can result in rapid deterioration and death. *Body packing* involves a premeditated act of previously prepared packets, and should be differentiated from *body stuffing*, which is usually done in haste when facing imminent police search—because the latter is more likely to have toxic consequences because of poor packaging.
- Other important historical features are known ingestion of magnets (which have a much higher likelihood of complications), medical implants (dental, esophageal, biliary) that can migrate, as well as a history of habits leading to bezoar formation.

DIAGNOSIS

Plain radiographs are often diagnostic. Even when suspicion is low, they can identify foreign bodies as the source of symptoms. Plain radiography is 90% sensitive for body packers, but often negative in body stuffers (including ingestion of crack vials). If plain radiographs are negative, consider CT scan (contrast may not be necessary with the current generation of CT scanners) or contrast swallow study.

MANAGEMENT

- The vast majority of patients with FBs that have successfully navigated the esophagus into the stomach or small bowel will do well with expectant management. However, a select group of objects require more urgent evaluation.

- Any patient known to have ingested two or more magnets will almost always require removal by either GI or surgery because of the high incidence of complications due to pressure necrosis from bowel wall caught between the two objects.
- GI should be consulted about sharp objects in the stomach because even if they pass the pylorus, they may perforate the small intestine. However, the incidence of sharp objects (even razor blades) perforating the gastrointestinal tract once already in the stomach varies widely from none to 25% depending on the case study—so the decision will need to be made on a case-by-case basis.
- Intervention should be considered for objects larger than 2 cm (difficulty passing the pylorus), objects longer than 5–6 cm (difficulty passing the duodenal sweep), or any object that has not passed through the stomach after 72 hours.
- In the case of body packers or stuffers, regardless of the patient's legal situation, the physician should only intervene if medically reasonable to prevent injury from the ingested object or substance. Patients should be admitted to the hospital for observation until passage of all material. Passage can be facilitated with polyethylene glycol (PEG) solution and/or laxatives. If signs of intestinal obstruction or drug toxicity occur, immediate removal by surgery is warranted (endoscopic removal is not recommended secondary to the risk of rupture).
- Intact button batteries that reach the stomach, unlike the esophagus, do not necessitate immediate removal unless they later fail to progress or the patient develops pain.
- If expectant management is chosen, patients with FBs expected to pass uneventfully (small, blunt objects) should be advised that most likely the object will pass unnoticed in their stool but to return if they develop symptoms of obstruction (pain, vomiting, obstipation). For objects that are higher risk (button batteries or objects that are sharp/irregularly shaped/large) and for whom expectant management is still deemed acceptable by the consulting service, the patient should return for serial radiographs taken 24 hours apart until the object passes. Intervention should be performed if there is no progression on interval radiographs indicating impaction, or sooner if the patient develops symptoms of bowel obstruction or perforation. In the case of magnets, if the number ingested is uncertain, the patient should be more closely followed with repeat imaging to detect failure of progression through the GI tract. Delayed passage might imply the presence of multiple magnets as set of plain radiographs at one point in time is unreliable in being able to differentiate a single magnet versus multiple.

Chapter 7: Gastrointestinal Foreign Bodies

RECTAL FOREIGN BODIES

Result from retrograde introduction due to sexual practices (most commonly) and also in patients with psychiatric disorders (one-third of cases).

PRESENTATION

- Patients are often hesitant to give accurate histories—making early diagnosis crucial because complications are higher with a delayed diagnosis. It is not uncommon for these patients to present after a complication, such as obstruction or perforation, has already occurred. It is of utmost importance to have a high index of suspicion and perform a thorough physical exam. One should also remember to ask about abuse or assault.
- In the absence of physical exam findings concerning for complications such as obstruction or perforation, the digital rectal exam should universally be performed unless the object is potentially sharp.

DIAGNOSIS

- Plain radiographs are diagnostic in over half of patients with rectal foreign bodies and are also useful in detecting secondary findings of perforation, such as free air. If those are unrevealing, contrast studies can be helpful (water-soluble contrast and gentle pressure should be utilized if there is concern for perforation). CT scan is usually not required in the workup (but is extremely useful for detecting complications such as perforation).
- If the object(s) is not among the majority that are found with direct palpation, the physician should progress to anoscopy, or rigid sigmoidoscopy, with sedation if required.

MANAGEMENT

- Transanal removal in the emergency department is successful in the majority of patients (60–75%), with the remaining being managed in the operating room (either transanal removal facilitated by general anesthesia or laparotomy). Avoid removing objects with a high risk of complications (sharp edges or high risk of dangerous breakage such as light bulbs).
- Initial attempts with digital extraction are often successful and can be aided by ring forceps combined with an anoscope or vaginal speculum. Passing one or more Foley catheters beyond the foreign body and proximally inflating air through the catheter, after filling the balloon, can break the vacuum seal that is oftentimes formed by the object within

the rectum. Vacuum devices to grasp the FB are other adjuncts that have been successfully used.
- If there is any doubt about integrity of the anorectal mucosa, the object should be removed in the operating room.
- After removal of the FB, assess the amount of injury to the rectum. If there is evidence of increased tenderness or rectal bleeding, post-removal sigmoidoscopy may identify mucosal injury, and plain radiographs may reveal free air, indicating perforation. Hospitalization is usually unnecessary unless a significant rectal laceration or perforation is found. If perforation is diagnosed, one should administer appropriate antibiotics to treat secondary bacterial peritonitis and obtain a surgical consultation.
- If transanal removal in the emergency department is successful without evidence of complication on exam or by symptoms, the patient should at a minimum be observed for several hours. Patients should be told to return if they develop fevers, worsening pain, or bleeding.

REFERENCES

1. American Society for Gastrointestinal Endoscopy (ASGE) Standards of Practice Committee, Ikenberry SO, Jue TL, Anderson MA, et al. Management of ingested foreign bodies and food impactions. *Gastrointest Endosc.* 2011;73(6):1085–91.
2. Crockett SD, Sperry SL, Miller CB, Shaheen NJ, Dellon ES. Emergency care of esophageal foreign body impactions: timing, treatment modalities, and resource utilization. *Dis Esophagus.* 2013;26(2):105–12.
3. Ambe P, Weber SA, Schauer M, Knoefel WT. Swallowed foreign bodies in adults. *Dtsch Arztebl Int.* 2012;109(5):869–75.
4. Arora S, Galich P. Myth: glucagon is an effective first-line therapy for esophageal foreign body impaction. *CJEM* 2009;11(2):169–171.
5. Pinto A, Muzi C, Gagliardi N, et al. Role of imaging in the assessment of impacted foreign bodies in the hypopharynx and cervical esophagus. *Semin Ultrasound CT MR.* 2012;33(5):463–70.
6. Goldberg JE, Steele SR. Rectal foreign bodies. *Surg Clin North Am.* 2010;90(1):173–84.
7. Cologne KG, Ault GT. Rectal foreign bodies: what is the current standard? *Clin Colon Rectal Surg.* 2010;23(4):214–8.

CHAPTER 8 ■ CAUSTIC INGESTIONS

Sara E. Crager, MD and Steven J. Rottman, MD, FACEP

OVERVIEW

- Most caustic ingestions occur in children under age 6 years and are of small volume.
- Adolescent and adult ingestions tend to be more severe due to higher frequency of intentional, large-volume ingestions.

CAUSTIC SUBSTANCES (SEE TABLE 8-1)

Primarily acid or alkali; pH < 2 or > 12.5 generally results in severe tissue damage, but less extreme pH can also cause serious injury. Determine pH with litmus paper or from substance's material safety data sheet (http://www.msdsonline.com).

- Acid
  - Bitter taste and pain with ingestion often results in smaller ingested volumes.
  - Causes coagulation necrosis: thrombosis of underlying mucosal blood vessels and formation of an eschar.
  - Lower viscosity commonly causes stomach and duodenal injuries.
- Alkali
  - Usually odorless and tasteless; can result in larger ingested volumes.

Table 8-1 Common Caustic Substances*

Acid	Alkali
Rust remover	Oven cleaner
Toilet bowl cleaner[†]	Drain opener
Soldering flux	Hair relaxers
Metal cleaner	Swimming pool cleaners
Automotive battery liquid	Dishwashing detergent
Photography products	Laundry detergent
Cement cleaner	Bleach[‡]

*Industrial strength cleaners generally have higher concentrations of caustic substances
[†]Most fatalities due to drain and toilet bowl cleaners
[‡]Significant injury extremely rare with household bleach (5% NaClO)
Data from Ferry GD. Caustic ingestion. In: Robert MD, Wyllie JS, Hyams MD (eds), *Pediatric Gastrointestinal Disease: Pathphysiology, Diagnosis, Management*. Philadelphia: WB Saunders; 1993.

- Causes liquefactive necrosis: mucosal inflammation, sloughing and ulceration, transmural damage over 3–4 days.
- Higher viscosity and gastric pH neutralization causes esophageal injuries.

CAUSTIC AGENTS WITH HIGH RISK OF SYSTEMIC TOXICITY

- Hydrogen fluoride
  - Found in rust remover and metal cleaners. Even small quantities can cause fatal arrhythmias due to severe hypocalcemia, hypomagnesemia, and hyperkalemia.
- Zinc chloride
  - Found in soldering flux. Can cause pancreatitis, pancreatic insufficiency, and renal failure.
- Mercuric chloride
  - Found in some skin-lightening products. Can cause renal failure.
- Phenol (carbolic acid)
  - Found in no-lye hair relaxer, disinfectants and antiseptics, lubricating oils. Can cause renal failure, dysrhythmias, seizures, and coma.

CLINICAL PRESENTATION

- Initial signs/symptoms do not reliably predict extent of injury.
- Symptoms: oropharyngeal, retrosternal, or epigastric pain, as well as dysphagia/odynophagia, drooling, feeding refusal, vomiting, and hematemesis.
- Complications: esophageal/gastric perforation, mediastinitis, peritonitis, respiratory distress, renal failure, disseminated intravascular coagulation (DIC), and shock.

INJURY SEVERITY

- First-degree burn: superficial mucosal damage with focal or diffuse erythema, edema, and hemorrhage
- Second-degree burn: mucosal and submucosal damage with ulcerations, exudates, and vesicle formation
- Third-degree burn: transmural damage with deep ulcers, black discoloration, and possible perforation

ACUTE WORKUP

Complete blood count (CBC), Chem-10, venous blood gas (VBG), liver function tests (LFTs), DIC panel, type/screen, aspirin/acetaminophen levels, electrocardiogram (EKG) (for suspected concurrent toxic ingestion), and upright chest X-ray (CXR). Use water-soluble contrast agents if contrast study indicated; barium studies not reliable for evaluating acute injury.

ENDOSCOPY

Upper endoscopy indicated in most patients during the first 24–48 hours after ingestion in order to assess injury severity, determine prognosis, and guide therapy (see Figure 8-1).

INJURY SEVERITY GRADING SCALE BY ENDOSCOPY

Grade 0	Normal
Grade 1	Mucosal edema and hyperemia
Grade 2A	Superficial ulcers, bleeding, exudates
Grade 2B	Deep focal or circumferential ulcers
Grade 3A	Focal necrosis
Grade 3B	Extensive necrosis

- *Grades 1 and 2A*: excellent prognosis without significant risk of acute morbidity or subsequent stricture formation.
- *Grades 2B and 3A*: development of strictures in over 70% of cases.
- *Grade 3B*: 65% early mortality rate; most require esophageal resection.

CONTRAINDICATIONS TO ENDOSCOPY

- Presentation suggestive of perforation; obtain emergent surgical consultation.
- Hemodynamic instability, severe respiratory distress, or severe oropharyngeal or glottic edema/necrosis.

TREATMENT (SEE FIGURE 8-1)

- Manage all caustic ingestions in consultation with Poison Control: 1-800-222-1222.
- Secure airway early if any indication of airway compromise. May require surgical airway if evidence of epiglottic/laryngeal injury.
- Treat hypotension and hemorrhage as required; keep NPO.
- Third-generation cephalosporins for patients with third-degree burns or if suspected perforation; antibiotics controversial in second-degree burns.
- Intravenous proton pump inhibitor (IV PPI) suggested to prevent stress ulcer development.
- Admit to intensive care unit (ICU) if endoscopic findings of injury grade 2B or higher, or ingestions with high risk of systemic toxicity.

CONTRAINDICATED IN THE MANAGEMENT OF CAUSTIC INGESTIONS

- *Emetics*: cause re-exposure of esophagus to caustic substance.
- *Neutralizing agents*: questionable efficacy, cause exothermic reaction with thermal injury. Milk/water dilution can cause emesis.

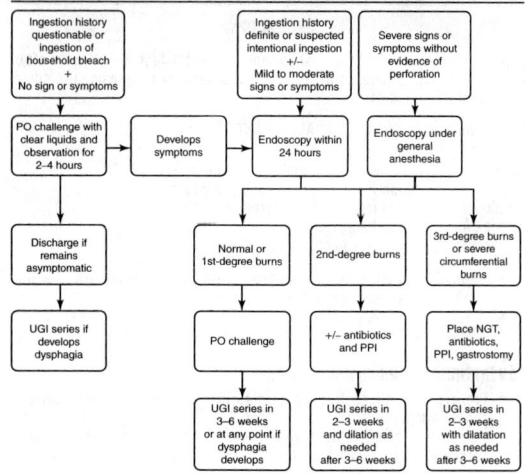

Figure 8-1 Management of caustic ingestions.

NGT = nasogastric tube; PO = oral; UGI = upper gastrointestinal.
Data from Ferry GD. Caustic ingestion. In: Robert MD, Wyllie JS, Hyams MD (eds), *Pediatric Gastrointestinal Disease: Pathophysiology, Diagnosis, Management*. Philadelphia: WB Saunders; 1993.

- *NGT placement*: blind placement of a nasogastric tube (NGT) risks creating a false passage; if needed, place NGT at time of endoscopy.
- *Gastric lavage*: no benefit, retching increases risk of perforation and aspiration. Possible exception: large-volume liquid acid ingestions; discuss with Poison Control.
- *Activated charcoal*: poor adsorption; interferes with endoscopy.
- *Steroids*: previously thought to prevent stricture formation; current consensus is that steroids do not improve outcomes and may cause harm.

LONG-TERM SEQUELAE

- Esophageal strictures are associated with esophageal squamous cell carcinomas. Majority who do develop strictures become symptomatic within 2 months; in cases of severe burns symptoms may manifest in as little as 3 weeks.
- Strictures are treated with esophageal dilations. Early dilation not recommended due to the high risk of perforation; defer dilation until 3–6 weeks after initial injury.
- Development of early satiety and postprandial emesis months to years after initial injury suggests pyloric stenosis with gastric outlet obstruction (usually acid-induced injury).
- Lye ingestions (e.g., drain cleaner, oven cleaner, hair relaxers) confer 1000-fold increased risk of developing esophageal squamous cell carcinoma; endoscopic surveillance should begin ~15 years after lye ingestion.

REFERENCES

1. Kay M, Wyllie R. Caustic ingestions in children. *Curr Op Pediatri.* 2009;21:651–4.
2. Salzman M, O'Malley R. Updates on the evaluation and management of caustic exposures. *Emerg Med Clin N Am.* 2007;25:459–76.
3. Pelclova D, Navratil T. Do corticosteroids prevent oesophageal stricture after corrosive ingestion? *Toxicol Rev.* 2005;24:125–9.

CHAPTER 9 ■ ORDERING APPROPRIATE RADIOLOGIC STUDIES FOR GI CONDITIONS

Victor Sai, MD and Daniel J. A. Margolis, MD

OVERVIEW

- When in doubt, order intravenous (IV) contrast-enhanced studies (oral contrast will be administered per radiologist discretion but IV contrast must be ordered by the referring physician).
- Computed tomography (CT) is the workhorse of abdominal imaging; magnetic resonance imaging (MRI) is more suited for problem solving and generally less helpful for acute conditions and workup of unknown diagnoses. (MRI is not better than CT in abdominal imaging but occasionally may be complementary.)
- Always describe the symptoms and clinical question to help the radiologist select the most appropriate protocol and provide the best interpretation.
- If unsure about what to order, consult a radiologist! Inappropriate ordering leads to delay in diagnosis and added burden on the patient and medical system.
- Order with *and without* contrast if no prior imaging. This allows for detection of hemorrhage and discrimination of complex cysts from hypovascular lesions.

ROUTINE CT ABDOMEN/PELVIS WITH CONTRAST

(Portal venous phase CT)

- [BEST] Abdominal pain of unknown etiology (see **Figure 9-1**)
- [BEST] Suspected small/large bowel obstruction, volvulus, bowel ischemia
- [BEST] Suspected inflammation (appendicitis, diverticulitis, colitis), abscess, perforation, hemorrhage
  - NB: Enteric contrast is highly recommended if perforation or fluid collection is suspected, but not for obstruction.
- [BEST] Suspected neoplasms, staging, and follow-up: gastrointestinal (GI) tract malignancies (hepatocellular carcinoma [HCC] and pancreatic malignancies are covered in more detail later in this chapter), lymphadenopathy, metastases
- [EXCELLENT] Suspected acute/chronic cholecystitis and choledocholithiasis or biliary obstruction, especially for complications thereof

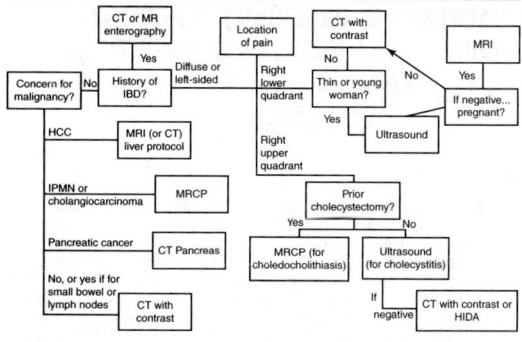

Figure 9-1 Algorithm for abdominal pain imaging.

CT = computed tomography; HCC = hepatocellular carcinoma; HIDA = hepatobiliary scan; IBD = inflammatory bowel disease; IPMN = intraductal papillary mucinous neoplasm; MRCP = magnetic resonance cholangiopancreatography; MRI = magnetic resonance imaging

- NB: best test for cholecystitis: biliary scintigraphy or ultrasound
- NB: best test for ducts = magnetic resonance cholangiopancreatography (MRCP) or endoscopic retrograde cholangiopancreatography (ERCP)

CT LIVER PROTOCOL

(CT anterior/posterior [A/P] with contrast + arterial images timed to liver + delayed images)

- [BEST] Liver transplant workup, follow-up after liver transplant
- [EXCELLENT] Suspected HCC, cholangiocarcinoma, and workup of nonspecific liver lesion (best test = MRI Liver Protocol)
- [EXCELLENT] Follow-up after treatment of HCC, cholangiocarcinoma

CT PANCREATIC PROTOCOL

(CT A/P with contrast + arterial images timed to pancreas + delayed images)

- [BEST] Suspected pancreatic adenocarcinoma (e.g., new onset diabetes mellitus, depression, and weight loss) and pancreatic neuroendocrine tumors, including insulinomas, gastrinomas, glucagonomas
- [BEST] Painless jaundice

Chapter 9: Ordering Appropriate Radiologic Studies

- [NOT NECESSARY] Follow-up after resection of pancreatic lesion or pancreatitis (CT A/P will suffice.)

CT ENTEROGRAPHY

(CT A/P with IV contrast + nonabsorbable water-density enteric contrast)

- [BEST] Suspected (new diagnosis) inflammatory bowel disease (IBD)
- [EXCELLENT] Presumed IBD flare (best test = MR enterography to assess peristalsis and to avoid repeated radiation) or suspected complications of IBD, including strictures, fistulas, abscesses. (However, a routine CT A/P will usually suffice.)

NONCONTRAST CT ABDOMEN/PELVIS

- [GOOD] Suspected inflammation, obstruction, perforation, fluid collection in patients with renal dysfunction (eGFR < 45 or serum Cr > 1.8)
  - NB: For suspected perforation or fluid collection, in the absence of IV contrast, enteric contrast is highly recommended. It is not necessary for obstruction.
- [GOOD] Painful hematuria and evaluation of known renal/ureteral stones
  - NB: CT with contrast is far superior for nearly all other abdominal indications.
- [POOR] Suspected solid organ neoplasms or evaluation of ischemia

ABDOMINAL ULTRASOUND

- [BEST] Suspected gallbladder disease (gallstones and cholecystitis), biliary obstruction
- [BEST] Abdominal ultrasound with Doppler: evaluation of hepatic vasculature
  - NB: Best way to show portal venous flow direction, MRI being less reliable
- [BEST FIRST TEST] Limited right lower quadrant (RLQ) ultrasound: if suspect acute appendicitis in pregnant patients, children, or thin females of childbearing age
- [EXCELLENT] Suspected cirrhosis or hepatomegaly/splenomegaly
  - NB: liver protocol CT or MRI is better in known liver disease.
- [GOOD] Suspected HCC
- [NOT USEFUL] Suspected bowel pathology

MRCP

(Magnetic resonance cholangiopancreatography = fluid-sensitive MRI to examine biliary system and pancreatic duct)

- [BEST] Suspected choledocholithiasis, evaluate unknown cause of biliary obstruction.

- [BEST] Workup of cystic pancreatic neoplasm, evaluate unknown cause of pancreatic ductal obstruction.
- NB: Also order MRI with IV contrast to evaluate pancreatic parenchyma (i.e., solid component of pancreatic cystic neoplasm).

MRI LIVER WITH HEPATOBILIARY CONTRAST

(Noncontrast + arterial, portal venous, and delayed magnetic resonance images timed to liver using hepatobiliary-specific contrast agent such as gadoxetate disodium)

- [BEST] Suspected IICC, cholangiocarcinoma, and workup of nonspecific liver lesion (including to distinguish malignant lesions from focal nodular hyperplasia [FNH], hepatic adenoma).
- [BEST] Follow-up of HCC and cholangiocarcinoma after treatment.
- NB: In presumed hepatic hemangioma, MRI liver with an extracellular agent is preferred.

MRI LIVER WITH CONVENTIONAL CONTRAST

(Noncontrast + arterial, portal venous, and delayed MRI timed to liver using extracellular contrast such as gadopentetate dimeglumine)

- [BEST] Suspected hepatic hemangioma.
- NB: Unless specified the radiologist will choose the appropriate MR contrast agent (hepatobiliary vs. extracellular) to answer the clinical question.

MR ENTEROGRAPHY

(MRI A/P with extracellular IV contrast and nonabsorbable enteric contrast)

- [BEST] Known IBD (Crohn's disease or ulcerative colitis [UC]) and workup of presumed flare (better than CT due to lack of radiation and added advantage of functional peristalsis images)
- [EXCELLENT] Suspected complications of IBD, including strictures, fistulas, abscesses
  - NB: CT is preferable if urgent.

MRI ABDOMEN/PELVIS

- [BEST] Suspected appendicitis in pregnant woman
  - NB: IV contrast is generally avoided in pregnancy.
- [GOOD] Evaluation of acute intra-abdominal pathology in patients with iodinated contrast allergy

UPPER GASTROINTESTINAL SERIES

(Fluoroscopic study with enteric contrast targeting the esophagus, stomach, and duodenum)

- [BEST] Suspected anastomotic leak after proximal GI tract surgery
- [BEST] Functional abnormality of the stomach (e.g., delayed emptying)
- [GOOD] Upper GI series with small bowel follow through: evaluation of small bowel filling defects, strictures, fistulas, and intraluminal transit
- [FAIR] Evaluation of abdominal pain of unknown etiology, vomiting
  - NB: endoscopy is superior for mucosal abnormalities, especially as they are now generally detected earlier, and CT or MRI is better for mural abnormalities as only the lumen is seen with fluoroscopy.

ESOPHOGRAM

(Fluoroscopic study with enteric contrast targeting the esophagus only)

- [BEST] Suspected anastomotic leak after esophageal surgery
- [BEST] Evaluation of dysphagia, suspected esophageal motility disorder
  - [BEST] NB: If achalasia is suspected, the technique is modified to avoid gas granules.
- Evaluation of gastric fundoplication or other gastroesophageal surgical interventions
- [GOOD] Evaluation of underlying esophageal lesions

ABDOMINAL RADIOGRAPH

(Kidney-ureter-bladder = "KUB")

- [BEST] Confirm tube position, evaluate presence of foreign bodies
- [EXCELLENT] Follow-up of known enteric obstruction or ileus
- [GOOD] Suspected bowel obstruction or ileus or intraperitoneal free air
  - NB: Best test = CT
- [POOR] Evaluation of nonspecific acute intra-abdominal pathology

REFERENCES

1. American College of Radiology Appropriateness Criteria. Available at: http://www.acr.org/Quality-Safety/Appropriateness-Criteria.

- NB: best test = CT with contrast as MRI has poorer spatial resolution and is more fraught with motion artifact compared to CT.

PART II COMMON GASTROINTESTINAL DISORDERS

…

CHAPTER 10 ■ THE DIAGNOSIS AND MANAGEMENT OF GASTROESOPHAGEAL REFLUX DISEASE (GERD)

Jeffrey L. Conklin, MD, FACG

OVERVIEW

- Gastroesophageal reflux disease (GERD) is one of the most frequent reasons why patients see both primary care physicians and gastroenterologists.
- The Montreal consensus defined GERD as the presence of bothersome symptoms or complications when gastric contents reflux into the esophagus.
- GERD may have both esophageal and extraesophageal symptoms.
- The diagnosis can usually be made, and treatment can be initiated, without endoscopy in low-risk patients.

PRESENTATION

- Esophageal symptoms of GERD include heartburn, regurgitation, chest pain, and dysphagia.
- Esophageal complications of GERD include esophagitis, esophageal ulcer, stricture, Barrett's esophagus, and adenocarcinoma.
- The consequences of extraesophageal reflux are sinusitis, cough, laryngitis, asthma, and pulmonary fibrosis.

DIAGNOSIS

- For patients who present with typical symptoms of heartburn and/or regurgitation and no "alarm" symptoms (chest pain, dysphagia, odynophagia, vomiting, hematemesis, melena, or anemia), the presumptive diagnosis of GERD can be made by a treatment trial with a proton pump inhibitor (PPI).
- Endoscopy is not needed when the patient has typical symptoms of GERD, is low risk, and responds to a PPI treatment trial. It is part of the evaluation when a PPI trial fails, and it is necessary to rule out esophageal complications of GERD in patients with alarm symptoms. It is also warranted to screen patients at high-risk of Barrett's esophagus. Finally, endoscopy should be performed after PPI treatment of patients

with erosive or ulcerative esophagitis to rule out an underlying Barrett's esophagus or neoplasm.
- Patients suspected of having noncardiac chest pain due to GERD must have cardiac chest pain ruled out.
- Ambulatory intraesophageal pH testing is used when the patient is unresponsive to PPI treatment, and endoscopy does not identify signs of esophageal inflammation. It is used when a patient with previous, objectively diagnosed GERD (erosive esophagitis or previous positive pH testing) is not responding to PPI therapy. Finally, pH testing is used when a patient has GERD symptoms after surgical treatment.
- Barium X-rays are of no value in the diagnosis of GERD.

TREATMENT

- Lifestyle modifications like weight loss, avoiding eating 2–3 hours before bed, and elevation of the head of the bed are first-line therapies for GERD. Avoidance of things thought to trigger GERD (alcohol; chocolate; nicotine; carbonated beverages; fatty, spicy, or citrus foods) is of questionable benefit, unless a specific food causes symptoms.
- Eight weeks of treatment with a PPI is the recommended initial pharmacological therapy for patients with symptoms of GERD or erosive esophagitis. The PPI should be taken once a day, *before* the first meal of the day. Those who respond partially might benefit from changing the PPI, adding another dose of PPI prior to the evening meal, or an H2-antagonist before bed. Patients who do not respond to PPIs should be sent for diagnostic evaluation.
- Maintenance therapy is instituted if GERD symptoms recur after the PPI is stopped, or if the patient has complications of GERD like erosive or ulcerative esophagitis, esophageal stricture, or Barrett's esophagus. Patients with uncomplicated GERD can often be managed using intermittent or on-demand PPI therapy, or with H2-antagonists.
- Baclofen is a GABA-B receptor agonist that blocks transient lower esophageal sphincter relaxation. It is efficacious as a GERD treatment, but frequently causes unacceptable somnolence. It is not used as first-line therapy, but may be added when symptoms are not adequately controlled by PPIs.
- The use of prokinetic agents as treatment for GERD is dubious. Data regarding the efficacy of metoclopramide as treatment for GERD are scant, and it has potential neurologic side effects. Domperidone is not available in the US, there are essentially no data demonstrating its efficacy in the treatment of GERD, and it increases the risk of cardiac death from ventricular arrhythmia. Prucalopride is not available in the US and is essentially unstudied for this purpose.
- Surgery is an accepted and effective long-term therapy for GERD. Current approaches include laparoscopic fundoplication or a ring of

magnetic beads placed at the esophagogastric junction, called the Linx. In the obese patient, consideration may be given to doing a gastric bypass. The preoperative evaluation includes ambulatory pH monitoring for patients who do not have erosive esophagitis, and esophageal manometry to rule out severe esophageal motor abnormalities like achalasia or aperistalsis resembling what is seen in scleroderma. In general, patients who do not improve when taking a PPI are not good candidates for surgery.
- The efficacies of endoscopic therapies like transoral incisionless fundoplication and radiofrequency treatments are still unclear, and are not recommended.

APPROACH TO EXTRAESOPHAGEAL MANIFESTATIONS OF GERD

- Include: chronic cough, asthma, laryngitis.
- For patients who present with extraesophageal *and* typical GERD symptoms (heartburn and/or regurgitation), an 8-week PPI trial is initiated. Those who fail this trial should stop the PPI, and be referred to evaluate head and neck, pulmonary, and allergic causes of symptoms.
- For patients who present with extraesophageal symptoms only, ambulatory pH testing of therapy should be considered prior to treatment with a PPI. If the pH study is negative, head and neck, pulmonary, and allergy evaluations should be considered.
- Doing impedance/pH testing on therapy has been touted as a way to diagnose extraesophageal symptoms caused by non-acid reflux. Recent studies call the usefulness of impedance testing into question.
- Diagnosis of reflux laryngitis should not be made solely by laryngoscopic findings.
- Anti-reflux surgery should not be done for extraesophageal symptoms that do not respond to PPI therapy.

TREATMENT APPROACH TO UNRESPONSIVE GERD

- The first thing to do if the patient is not responding to a PPI is make sure the drug is being taken appropriately. Are doses being missed? Is it being taken before meals? Taking the PPI correctly often improves treatment response. Sometimes doubling the dose of PPI or switching to a different PPI is useful. Adding baclofen can sometimes be beneficial.
- If symptoms of GERD remain refractory after optimizing therapy, endoscopy should be done to rule out other causes of symptoms like eosinophilic esophagitis, esophageal infections, an inlet patch, or erosive esophagitis not responsive to the therapy.
- If the endoscopy is normal, ambulatory intraesophageal pH testing is done to determine the amount and extent of esophageal acid exposure

and to determine the association between symptoms and reflux events. The study is done after stopping the PPI for 7 days. Many authors advocate using impedance/pH testing in this situation to determine if non-acid reflux is causing symptoms.

REFERENCES

1. Vakil N, van Vanten SV, Kahrilas P, Dent J, Jones R. The Montreal definition and classification of gastroesophageal reflux disease: a global evidence-based consensus. *Am J Gastroenterol*. 2006;101:1900–20.
2. Katz PO, Gerson LB, Vela MF. Guidelines for the diagnosis and management of gastroesophageal reflux disease. *Am J Gastroenterol*. 2013;108:308–28.

CHAPTER 11 ■ BARRETT'S ESOPHAGUS

Kourosh F. Ghassemi, MD and V. Raman Muthusamy, MD, FACG, FASGE

OVERVIEW

- Barrett's esophagus (BE) is defined as a condition in which metaplastic columnar epithelium replaces the stratified squamous epithelium that normally lines the tubular esophagus.
- The presence of intestinal-type epithelium (intestinal metaplasia, IM) in the columnar-lined esophagus predisposes to esophageal adenocarcinoma (EAC).
- The prevalence of BE is 1–2% in large population-based studies. Over 40% of these individuals are asymptomatic (no reflux symptoms).
- In patients with chronic gastroesophageal reflux disease (GERD) undergoing upper endoscopy, long-segment BE (≥ 3 cm) is present in 3–5% and short-segment BE (< 3 cm) in up to 10–15%.
- BE is predominantly a disease of middle-aged to older white men, and it is uncommon in black and Asian populations. The male-to-female ratio is 2:1. Obesity, especially abdominal fat distribution, is a risk factor while aspirin/nonsteroidal anti-inflammatory drugs (NSAIDs) use may be protective.
- Although the risk of EAC is up to 30-fold higher in patients with BE compared with the general population, the absolute risk remains low. The incidence of EAC in patients with BE is estimated to be between 0.12–0.5% per year, but increases to 6–10% per year when high-grade dysplasia is present.

PRESENTATION

BE is asymptomatic, although most patients diagnosed with the condition are initially seen for GERD. In those with GERD, erosive esophagitis and possibly peptic strictures confer an increased risk for BE.

PATHOPHYSIOLOGY

- The precise sequence of events remains to be determined. The prevailing hypothesis suggests that chronic reflux of gastric contents, primarily acid, and the ensuing inflammation damages the squamous epithelium, exposing pluripotent stem cells and stimulating their differentiation into intestinal-type columnar cells.

- The metaplastic epithelium is likely a protective mechanism in response to tissue injury, but it also predisposes to neoplasia.

DIAGNOSIS

- The diagnosis is definitively made by endoscopy with biopsies. One must identify both the squamocolumnar junction (SCJ) and the gastroesophageal junction (GEJ) to document that the tubular esophagus is lined by columnar epithelium. The GEJ is defined as the most proximal extent of the gastric folds.
- In the United States, diagnosis requires biopsies from the columnar-lined esophagus to show histologic evidence of intestinal metaplasia.
- The Prague C+M criteria—circumferential extent and maximal extent of IM above the GEJ—shows good intra-observer variability for reporting the extent of BE, especially for low-segment Barrett's esophagus (LSBE).
- Premalignant genetic changes in BE epithelium causes morphologic changes recognized by pathologists as dysplasia. Dysplasia is categorized as low-grade (LGD) or high-grade (HGD). Due to variable interobserver agreement for LGD and HGD, at least two expert pathologists should review histology prior to diagnosis.
- The American Gastroenterological Association (AGA) recommends limiting screening patients for the presence of BE to those who have multiple risks for acquiring the condition: age 50 years or older, male, white race, chronic GERD, hiatal hernia, increased body mass index (BMI)/intra-abdominal body fat distribution.

MANAGEMENT/TREATMENT (SEE FIGURE 11-1)

- Three components of managing BE include treatment of associated GERD, endoscopic surveillance for dysplasia, and treatment of dysplasia.
- Treatment of GERD in patients with BE is similar to those without this condition. An important difference is that proton pump inhibitors (PPIs) are used as initial therapy rather than a "step up" approach. Although observational data suggest PPIs can reduce progression of BE to HGD/EAC, this concept has not been established in prospective clinical trials. Fundoplication appears no more effective in preventing EAC than medical therapy.
- Visible yet subtle changes of dysplasia using high-resolution white light endoscopy (HR-WLE) are seen in most cases. Endoscopic surveillance in BE should consist of careful inspection and biopsy of any visible abnormalities, mucosal resection (for treatment and staging) of any nodular areas within the BE segment, and four quadrant random biopsies using established protocols (such as the Seattle protocol). Techniques (such

Chapter 11: Barrett's Esophagus

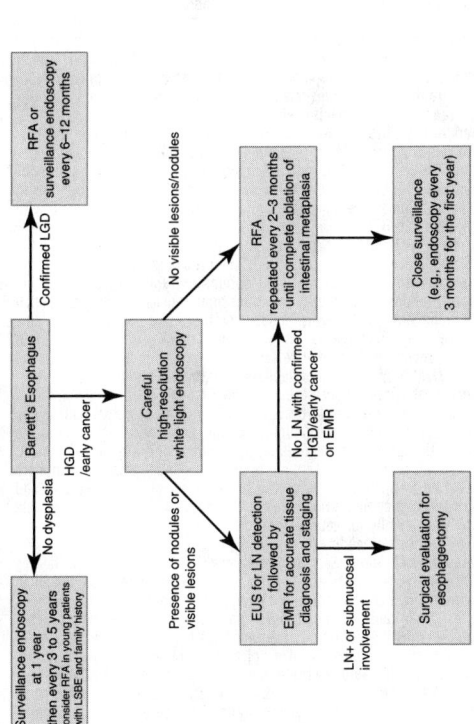

Figure 11-1 Treatment algorithm for patients with Barrett's Esophagus (BE).
HGD = high grade dysplasia; LGD = low grade dysplasia; LSBE = long-segment Barrett's esophagus; RFA = Radiofrequency ablation therapy.

as chromoendoscopy, narrow band imaging, endosonography, and confocal endomicroscopy) to enhance dysplasia for targeted biopsies in BE are available, yet none has provided a clear benefit to justify routine clinical use.
- Some experimental and epidemiologic evidence supports an inverse association of progression to EAC in patients with BE taking aspirin or NSAIDs. Further data are needed, but low-dose aspirin in patients with concurrent cardiovascular risks (such as male, over 50 years old) may be a reasonable approach to chemoprevention.
- There are insufficient data for efficacy of cancer prevention in patients with nondysplastic BE to recommend endoscopic therapy, and endoscopic surveillance is currently recommended every 3–5 years for non-dysplastic BE. Endoscopic treatment can be considered in patients with a family history of esophageal cancer or who are under age 50 with long-segment BE.
- For those with LGD confirmed by two pathologists, endoscopic therapy or surveillance endoscopy every 6–12 months is recommended.
- In those with HGD, the treatment options are endoscopic eradication therapy (endoscopic ablation or endoscopic mucosal resection [EMR]) or esophagectomy. Typically, endoscopic therapy is preferred, with surgery reserved for those failing endoscopic therapy or those desiring a single procedure. Surveillance for HGD is generally avoided given the high risk of progression and available treatment options.
- The risk of lymph node metastases in BE with HGD or intramucosal carcinoma is estimated to be 1–2%, allowing for effective endoscopic therapy in these patients. Esophagectomy, however, removes all of the neoplastic epithelium, regional lymph nodes, and any occult cancer. However, it carries a mortality of up to 5% (in older patients with more advanced EAC), as well as prolonged hospitalization (~2 weeks), and postoperative complication rates of 30–50%. It remains a reasonable option, especially for younger and otherwise fit patients who desire a single curative procedure.
- Endoscopic ablation uses radiofrequency (RFA), photodynamic therapy (PDT), or cryotherapy to ablate the abnormal epithelium. In a nonacidic environment, the ablated mucosa heals with growth of neosquamous epithelium. Albeit rare, ablated BE can heal with neosquamous epithelium overlying metaplastic tissue, and the "buried" BE can progress to EAC. Complete eradication of dysplasia can be achieved in over 90% of patients using ablative therapies. Given the available evidence, currently RFA is the preferred modality for ablation in BE. Recurrence rates of 30% for IM and 10% for dysplasia can be seen after ablative therapies, thus adherence to a rigorous endoscopic surveillance protocol is essential in the post-ablation period.
- EMR involves resection of a large segment of mucosa down to the submucosa, providing specimens for histology and staging. It can be combined with ablative therapies for eradication of BE in patients with

visible lesions. In BE with early EAC, excellent outcomes have been achieved (98% 5-year survival), but recurrent/metachronous rates of up to 12% have been reported, highlighting the need for ongoing surveillance following therapy.

REFERENCES

1. Spechler SJ, Sharma P, Souza RF, et al. American Gastroenterological Association technical review on the management of Barrett's esophagus. *Gastroenterology.* 2011;140(3):e18–52.
2. Spechler SJ, Souza RF. Barrett's esophagus. In Feldman M, Friedman LS, Brandt LJ, eds., *Sleisenger and Fordtran's Gastrointestinal and Liver Disease*, 9th ed. Philadelphia: Saunders; 2010.

CHAPTER 12 ■ *HELICOBACTER PYLORI* INFECTION

Daniel Cole, MD, MPH

OVERVIEW

- Until 1980, peptic ulcer disease (PUD) was thought to be caused by stress, aspirin, and nonsteroidal anti-inflammatory drugs (NSAIDs). The vast majority of non-NSAID related ulcers are now thought to be secondary to *Helicobacter pylori* (HP) infection.
- Marshall and Warren first recognized that the HP bacterium was in fact the cause of PUD. It was subsequently recognized that it was also a common cause of chronic gastritis, gastric adenocarcinoma, and mucosa-associated lymphoid tissue (MALT) lymphoma.

PRESENTATION

The HP infection causes symptoms depending on the extent and duration of disease. It is the most common cause of PUD—both gastric and duodenal—besides NSAIDs. The complications of bleeding, gastric outlet obstruction, and perforation can be attributed to HP. However, HP is also associated with the development of gastric cancer and gastric MALT lymphoma. Nonspecific abdominal pain usually does not respond to treatment of HP if the cause is multifactorial.

DIFFERENTIAL DIAGNOSIS

Functional abdominal pain/dyspepsia, NSAID-induced PUD, gastric cancer, pancreatic cancer, gallbladder disease, gastroesophageal reflux disease (GERD)

PATHOPHYSIOLOGY

BACTERIOLOGY

HP is a spiral-shaped, Gram-negative bacterium. Urease production is vital to its survival. This is clinically important because it forms the basis for many diagnostic tests. Urease, along with bacterial motility, allows HP to survive in the hostile, acidic gastric environment.

EPIDEMIOLOGY

HP is the most common chronic bacterial infection in humans. It has been demonstrated worldwide and in all ages possibly infecting as much as 50% of the world's population. It is usually acquired at an early age in underdeveloped countries, and it persists indefinitely. In more developed countries, it is acquired at a later age. The infection is more prevalent in African American and Latino patients. Factors such as housing density, number of siblings, lack of running water, income, and level of education have all been associated with the rate of development of HP. The bacteria can be cultured from vomitus and stool, and it is more likely to be spread within a family during periods of illness.

ULCERS

HP is one of the most common causes of peptic ulcer disease—both gastric and duodenal. The other common cause is NSAID use. It is still important to document the cause of the ulcer and testing should be done. Biopsy should be done at the time of endoscopy if PUD is detected. When ulcers are present in the absence of HP, PUD has a worse prognosis and is more difficult to cure. When HP is not treated, the recurrence rate of ulcers is > 80% in the first year. When treated successfully, the recurrence is < 5%.

FUNCTIONAL DYSPEPSIA

Randomized controlled trials have failed to show a clear relationship between treatment of HP infection and resolution of functional abdominal pain. While infection may cause various minor alterations in gastric motility, there is no evidence that these minor changes are associated with abdominal pain.

DIAGNOSIS

WHEN TO TEST

The American College of Gastroenterology (ACG) guidelines include the following recommendations:

1. Testing for HP should be performed only if the clinician plans to offer treatment for positive results.
2. Testing is indicated in patients with gastric MALT lymphoma, active peptic ulcer disease, or prior history of peptic ulcer disease.

WHICH TEST TO USE

- The test-and-treat strategy for HP is a very acceptable management technique. Treat all positive tests in symptomatic patients under age 55—assuming there are no alarm features including bleeding, anemia, weight loss, dysphagia, vomiting, or family history of gastric cancer. Multiple factors determine which test to perform. Financial considerations should be included in the decision making.

- If the patient has never been treated before, then the most convenient test is serologic testing. This test maintains high sensitivity but low specificity. However, if the patient is going to have an endoscopy, then a biopsy for (*Campylobacter*)-like organism (CLO) testing can be performed. Antral biopsy for histopathology remains the gold standard for this diagnosis.
- Other accurate noninvasive tests include stool antigen testing and the urea breath test (UBT), which are both very accurate. If the patient has previously been treated for HP, then the serology is of no value because it may remain positive for years—even after successful treatment. Therefore, stool antigen, UBT, or biopsy is needed.

TREATMENT

The most common treatment regimen is "triple therapy," which includes two antibiotics and a proton pump inhibitor (PPI). A combination of amoxicillin, 1 g twice daily; clarithromycin, 500 mg twice daily; and a full-strength PPI twice daily for 10 to 14 days is used as a first-line regimen. In patients who are allergic to penicillin, metronidazole, 500 mg twice daily, can replace the amoxicillin with no significant reduction in effectiveness.

TREATMENT FAILURE

- There is great variability worldwide in HP susceptibility to individual antibiotics. Approximately 20% of patients will fail the initial treatment of HP. It is recommended that repeat treatment be started with an alternative antibiotic regimen plus twice daily PPI therapy. This approach will result in ~70% success rate for previously resistant patients. If the patient was initially treated with amoxicillin and clarithromycin, then tetracycline, 500 mg twice daily, and metronidazole, 500 mg twice daily, should be substituted. Regardless of the new antibiotic regimen used, it is suggested that bismuth subcitrate caplets, 240 mg twice daily, be added for "quadruple therapy."
- There have been many newer antibiotic regimens proposed including those using levofloxacin, rifabutin, and moxifloxacin in various combinations with the standard antibiotics of tetracycline, amoxicillin, and metronidazole. These options should probably be reserved for multiple treatment failures, and an infectious diseases specialist should be consulted.

ERADICATION TESTING

Because of widespread resistance, it is recommended that all patients have eradication testing. As previously mentioned, serology is not useful because it will remain positive even if treatment is successful. Stool antigen or UBT should be performed about 4 to 6 weeks after treatment is completed.

PPI therapy may give a false-negative result and should be stopped at least a week before eradication testing. Antibiotics for treatment of other conditions can also give a false-negative result and should be stopped 3 to 4 weeks prior to eradication testing.

REFERENCES

1. Garza-Gonzalez E, Perez-Perez GI, Maldonado-Garza HJ. A review of Helicobacter pylori diagnosis, treatment, and methods to detect eradication. *World J Gastro*. 2014;20(6):1438–49.
2. Federico A, Gravina AG, Miranda A. Eradication of *Hellcobacter pylori* infection: which regimen first? *World J of Gastro*. 2014;20(3):665–72.

CHAPTER 13 ■ BENIGN ANORECTAL DISORDERS (HEMORRHOIDS, ANAL FISSURE, CONDYLOMA)

Amy Lightner Hill, MD and Anne Lin, MD, MSHS

OVERVIEW

- Hemorrhoids are one of the most common indications for visits to gastroenterologists and colorectal surgeons.
- Most patients with hemorrhoids and anal fissures will have resolution of symptoms with conservative management.
- Patients with condylomas are at increased risk of anogenital cancers.

HEMORRHOIDS

- Hemorrhoids are highly vascularized cushions of thick submucosa in the left lateral, right anterior, and right posterior quadrants of the anal canal.
- Hemorrhoids may be internal (proximal to the dentate line) or external (distal to the dentate line) and are insensate or sensate, respectively.
- Internal hemorrhoids are graded by the degree of prolapse:
  - 1st degree: no prolapse
  - 2nd degree: prolapse with spontaneous reduction
  - 3rd degree: prolapse requiring digital reduction
  - 4th degree: prolapsed, cannot be reduced

PRESENTATION OF HEMORRHOIDS

- Hemorrhoids are present equally among men and women with a prevalence of 4%—peaking between the ages of 45 and 65 years.
- Patients with external hemorrhoids typically complain of perianal itching and burning. When a patient has a thrombosed external hemorrhoid, they present with a painful, hard perianal nodule.
- Patients with internal hemorrhoids typically present with painless bleeding from the rectum that is worse with straining or bowel movements. When hemorrhoids prolapse, patients may also experience leakage of stool contents.

DIFFERENTIAL DIAGNOSIS OF HEMORRHOIDS

Skin tags, anal fissures, rectal prolapse, condylomas, perianal Crohn's disease, or anal cancer may be mistaken for hemorrhoids. When an age-appropriate patient presents with bleeding or anemia, it is important to rule out a more serious condition (i.e., malignancy) with endoscopy.

PATHOPHYSIOLOGY OF HEMORRHOIDS

The etiology is unknown, but hemorrhoids are associated with advancing age, diarrhea, pregnancy, pelvic tumors, prolonged sitting, straining, and chronic constipation.

DIAGNOSIS OF HEMORRHOIDS

Diagnosis is made by physical exam including digital examination and anoscopy.

TREATMENT OF HEMORRHOIDS

- Conservative: most patients will have resolution of symptoms with dietary modification (fiber supplements), hydration, and sitz baths alone.
- Office-based procedures: second- and third-degree internal hemorrhoids generally require intervention with an office-based procedure including rubber band ligation (treating one to two cushions at a time) or injection sclerotherapy.
- Surgical: fourth-degree internal hemorrhoids, or combined internal/external hemorrhoids, often require excisional hemorrhoidectomy.
- For patients who present with a thrombosed external hemorrhoid, excision and drainage of thrombus is recommended only if within 72 hours of symptom onset.

ANAL FISSURES

- Tear in the anoderm distal to the dentate line, most commonly located in the posterior midline. Next most common location is anterior midline.
- By definition, an acute anal fissure heals within 6 weeks with conservative therapy, whereas a chronic anal fissure may require more aggressive intervention to heal.
- Primary anal fissures are due to local trauma and secondary anal fissures are due to underlying medical conditions, such as Crohn's disease or malignancy.

PRESENTATION OF ANAL FISSURES

- Patients complain of tearing pain with bowel movements, occasional blood on toilet paper or stool, and occasional pruritus.

- Fissures are most commonly located in the posterior midline. If the fissure is lateral, it is most likely a secondary fissure and the patient should be evaluated for associated medical conditions including Crohn's disease, tuberculosis, sarcoidosis, malignancy such as squamous cell carcinoma and leukemia, and communicable diseases such as HIV infection, syphilis, and chlamydia.

DIFFERENTIAL DIAGNOSIS OF ANAL FISSURES

Perianal ulcers or sores, anorectal fistulas, and hemorrhoids

PATHOPHYSIOLOGY OF ANAL FISSURES

Anal fissures are the result of stretching the anal mucosa past its capacity, causing a tear. This tear causes the exposed underlying internal sphincter to spasm, pulling the edges of the fissure apart—further impeding wound healing. Decreased blood flow to the posterior midline causing relative ischemia may also contribute to anal fissures.

DIAGNOSIS OF ANAL FISSURES

- The diagnosis is definitively made by physical exam demonstrating a superficial tear in the anoderm. Chronic anal fissures often appear hypertrophied with a skin tag at the distal end.
- Most patients will not be able to tolerate a digital rectal exam or anoscopy due to pain.

TREATMENT OF PRIMARY ANAL FISSURES

- Conservative: most patients will have resolution of symptoms with local wound care (sitz baths) and relief of constipation (fiber supplements).
- Medical: topical diltiazem 2% cream or gel applied three times a day to the perianal area for 8 weeks may be effective in approximately 70% of patients. Patients with recurrent symptoms can be treated with a second course. Botox injections may be used if conservative management is ineffective. Temporary fecal incontinence may be noted.
- Surgical: lateral internal sphincterotomy is effective in 95% of patients when medical management fails. Risk of fecal incontinence is less than 10%.

CONDYLOMA

- Condyloma acuminatum is caused by human papillomavirus (HPV).
- Condylomas are related to sexual activity and are more common in immunosuppressed individuals—such as HIV patients.
- Patients with condylomas are at increased risk of anogenital cancers.

PRESENTATION OF CONDYLOMA

- Symptoms include pruritus, bleeding, burning, tenderness, vaginal discharge (women), or pain.
- Large exophytic condylomas can be obstructive, interfering with defecation and intercourse.

DIFFERENTIAL DIAGNOSIS OF CONDYLOMA

Skin tags, molluscum, squamous cell carcinoma, and vulvar lesions in females

PATHOPHYSIOLOGY OF CONDYLOMA

HPV, a common sexually transmitted disease

DIAGNOSIS OF CONDYLOMA

- Physical exam shows skin-colored or pink lesions ranging from smooth, flattened papules to a verrucous, papilliform appearance.
- Extent of involvement can be documented by anoscopy.

TREATMENT OF CONDYLOMA

- Treatment options depend on size and location of lesions and may include chemical (trichloroacetic acid, 5-fluorouracil/epinephrine gel, or podophyllin) or physical destruction (liquid nitrogen, laser therapy), immunologic therapy (imiquimod, interferon alpha), or surgical excision (for large warts). Imiquimod 5% cream may be used after excision.
- Following treatment, timely follow-up and continued surveillance are important to detect recurrence.

REFERENCES

1. Townsend, CM. Common benign anal disorders. In: Townsend CM, Beauchamp D, Evers BM, Mattox, KL, eds. *Sabiston Textbook of Surgery*, 18th ed. Philadelphia: Elsevier; 2013.
2. Bleday R, Breen E. Treatment of hemorrhoids. Available at: http://www.uptodate.com/contents/treatment-of-hemorrhoids. Updated: Oct 16, 2013.

CHAPTER 14 ■ FAMILIAL MEDITERRANEAN FEVER

Terri Getzug, MD

OVERVIEW

- Familial Mediterranean fever (FMF) is an autosomal recessive systemic autoinflammatory disorder characterized by recurrent episodes of fever accompanied by peritonitis, pleuritis, and arthritis or erysipelas-like erythema.
- FMF is the most common periodic fever syndrome—affecting more than 10,000 patients worldwide.
- The disease is most prevalent in populations of the Mediterranean basin: Turks, Armenians, Arabs, non-Ashkenazi Jews, Greeks, and Italians. It can be seen less commonly in others such as Ashkenazi Jews, Japanese, Chinese, Europeans, and South Americans.
- The diagnosis is made clinically; however, genetic testing for mutations of the MEFV (Mediterranean fever) gene can help make the diagnosis in more challenging situations. In general, a careful history and familiarity with FMF will make the diagnosis.

PRESENTATION

- The majority of affected individuals present before 10 years of age and 90% before age 20.
- A typical FMF attack lasts approximately 24 to 72 hours with the frequency of episodes varying from once weekly to several times a year. In between attacks, patients are generally well.
- Fever is a feature of every acute attack, and, rarely, can be the only manifestation of FMF.
- Painful abdominal attacks, which mimic acute peritonitis both by history and physical examination, are the most common presentation, occurring in 95% of patients. Symptoms resulting from ileus are frequent.
- Arthritis is the second most common manifestation of FMF and is usually monoarticular or oligoarticular with the knee, ankle, hip, and elbow being most commonly affected. The attacks, usually of short duration (up to 1 week), start abruptly with no prodrome. These usually resolve completely.

- Pleuritis, most commonly unilateral and occasionally associated with a transient pleural effusion, is another frequent manifestation of FMF.
- A more rare erysipeloid skin lesion reminiscent of cellulitis may occur unilaterally on the extensor surface of the lower leg, ankle, or dorsum of the foot. It is tender, raised, and well demarcated and can be 10 to 35 cm^2 in area. It resolves spontaneously and does not need antibiotics.
- Other acute manifestations of FMF include pericarditis, orchitis, and recurrent aseptic meningitis.
- FMF has also been associated with different vasculitides, including protracted febrile myalgia, Henoch-Schonlein purpura, and polyarteritis nodosa.

DIFFERENTIAL DIAGNOSIS

Other disease processes can be confused with FMF but can be excluded based on historical features, laboratory testing, and imaging. Some of these include acute surgical emergencies (appendicitis, cholecystitis, small bowel obstruction, perforated peptic ulcer, mesenteric ischemia), pancreatitis, hereditary angioedema, mastocytosis, juvenile rheumatoid arthritis, systemic lupus erythematosus and vasculitis, acute intermittent porphyria, pneumonia, intestinal migraines, and other rare, hereditary periodic fever syndromes.

LONG-TERM COMPLICATIONS

- Secondary amyloidosis (AA) with associated renal failure is the major source of mortality in untreated patients with FMF. Renal insufficiency can begin subtly but progress to frank nephrotic syndrome and end-stage renal disease requiring dialysis or renal transplantation. Widespread amyloid deposition can also affect the gastrointestinal tract (resulting in malabsorption and intestinal pseudoobstruction), as well as the liver, spleen, and thyroid.
- Certain ethnic groups (Turkish, North African Jewish, and Armenians from Yerevan—the capital of Armenia) are more predisposed to develop renal amyloidosis. Mutation analysis has revealed a high association with M694V homozygosity, severe disease, and the development of amyloidosis.
- Recurrent attacks of peritonitis may lead to unnecessary operations, and small bowel obstruction from adhesions may occur.
- Infertility with oligospermia/azoospermia in men or due to recurrent peritoneal inflammation leading to abdominal and ovarian adhesions in women may also complicate untreated FMF.
- Chronic destructive arthritis involving the hips and knees, sacroiliitis, and spondyloarthritis, are rare (0.4–5%) but can result in the need for joint replacement or immunosuppressant therapy.

PATHOPHYSIOLOGY

- The FMF gene, MEFV, located on the short arm of chromosome 16, encodes for a protein named pyrin, which is expressed only in circulating neutrophils and acts as a regulator of inflammation. Pyrin is an important mediator in the innate immune system.
- The neutrophil appears to be the effector of the inflammatory response at the serosal surfaces but the exact mechanism is still unknown. Deficiency of a C5a inhibitor and/or interleukin 8 (IL-8) may also be involved in the production of an FMF attack.
- Over 50 disease-associated mutations in MEFV have been identified, and patients with clinical FMF have either one or no mutations.
- The five most common mutations (M694V, M694I, V726A, E148Q, and M680I) are responsible for more than 85% of FMF patients in the Middle Eastern region and are associated with variable degrees of disease severity, risk of severe arthritis, and amyloidosis.

DIAGNOSIS

- The diagnosis of FMF is based primarily on clinical factors. Because FMF is an episodic disease, the patient's history of intermittent fever associated with serositis lasting 1 to 3 days, ethnic background, family history, and physical exam findings are critical to make the proper diagnosis.
- Laboratory testing during an acute attack will reveal a nonspecific increase in acute phase reactants such as leukocytosis with neutrophils, C-reactive protein, erythrocyte sedimentation rate, fibrinogen, and serum amyloid protein (SAA). Markers of inflammation will generally revert to normal between attacks—which may be a distinguishing feature between FMF and other diagnoses.
- Joint aspiration during attacks usually reveals a sterile pyogenic synovial effusion.
- Otherwise unexplained proteinuria in between attacks raises the question of amyloidosis and warrants further testing.
- Targeted genetic testing for the most prevalent MEFV mutations is reserved for atypical cases as it is not diagnostic unless two mutations are present or if no mutations are present. If targeted mutation testing is negative or reveals only one mutation, a therapeutic trial of colchicine may be given. If the diagnosis is still uncertain, full gene sequencing of the MEFV gene may be performed.

TREATMENT

- Colchicine is the treatment of choice for both children and adults with FMF worldwide.
- Goals of treatment are to prevent the painful attacks and the development of amyloidosis. Daily, lifelong administration of colchicine is required.
- Adult dosing is 1.2–2.4 mg/day whereas children usually start at 0.3–1.2 mg/day.
- Response rates to colchicine are over 90%. Most patients will have complete suppression of attacks or marked reduction in attack frequency and severity.
- Side effects to colchicine are unusual but may include diarrhea, abdominal cramps, and rare neuromyopathy and bone marrow suppression—all responsive to dose reduction.
- Unresponsiveness to colchicine may be due to noncompliance, drug interactions affecting metabolism, possible lack of efficacy of one formulation over another, or in 5–10% of cases true colchicine resistance.
- Off-label treatment trials and case reports with other agents such as the anti-interleukin-1 targeting drugs anakinra, canakinumab, and rilonacept show some promise for the treatment of resistant FMF but are in need of formal clinical trials. It is also unclear as to whether or not they would prevent amyloidosis.
- Colchicine is generally felt to be safe during pregnancy and breastfeeding. Some recommend holding colchicine for 2 to 3 months prior to conception and the first trimester depending on the clinical situation. There is no consensus on the need for amniocentesis.

REFERENCES

1. Zadeh N, Getzug T, Grody WW. Diagnosis and management of familial Mediterranean fever: integrating medical genetics in a dedicated interdisciplinary clinic. *Genet Med*. 2011;13(3):263–9.
2. Ben-Chetrit E, Touitou I. Familial Mediterranean fever in the world. *Arthritis Rheum* 2009;61(10):1447–53.

CHAPTER 15 ■ CELIAC DISEASE

Brigid Boland, MD, and Sheila E. Crowe, MD, FRCPC, FACP, FACG, AGAF

OVERVIEW

- Celiac disease (CD) refers to a chronic small intestine immune-mediated enteropathy that is driven by exposure to dietary gluten in genetically predisposed individuals. Destruction of the small intestinal villi leads to chronic malabsorption with reduction in absorptive area and diminished absorption of critical nutrients and vitamins.
- CD affects approximately 1% of the US population; however, only a small proportion of the cases of celiac disease have been diagnosed in the United States.
- CD is 4 times more prevalent than it was 50 years ago for reasons that are not entirely clear.
- First-degree relatives of individuals with celiac disease have an increased risk of celiac disease and should be tested for this condition if they develop clinical features of celiac disease.
- CD is an autoimmune disorder that is associated with many other autoimmune diseases, including microscopic colitis, Type 1 diabetes, and autoimmune thyroid disease.
- If a patient has common gastrointestinal (GI) symptoms, other autoimmune disorders, or presentations of malabsorption, consider CD!

PRESENTATION

- Historically, classic celiac disease presented at a young age with failure to thrive, diarrhea, protuberant abdomen, and weight loss; however, this is no longer the most frequent presentation.
- Typically, so-called atypical or nonclassical celiac disease presents with a variety of nonspecific gastrointestinal symptoms such as diarrhea, altered bowel habits, bloating, abdominal pain, and even nongastrointestinal symptoms.
- CD frequently presents with extra-intestinal manifestations including dermatitis herpetiformis (DH), iron-deficiency anemia, fat-soluble vitamin deficiencies, osteoporosis, microscopic colitis, other autoimmune diseases, and/or elevated transaminases.
- CD may present as dermatitis herpetiformis, a blistering pruritic skin rash on extensor surfaces often without digestive symptoms in spite of enteropathy.

DIFFERENTIAL DIAGNOSIS

Irritable bowel syndrome, functional dyspepsia and other functional GI disorders, small intestinal bacterial overgrowth, Crohn's disease, ulcerative colitis, peptic ulcer disease, microscopic colitis, non-celiac gluten sensitivity, chronic infections such as giardiasis

PATHOPHYSIOLOGY

- Celiac disease is an immune-mediated process driven by gluten exposure in genetically susceptible individuals. Cereal prolamines, like gluten, that are derived from wheat, rye, and barley are the antigens that cause an immune response involving T lymphocytes.
- For poorly understood reasons, some individuals develop a defect in the intestinal epithelium that allows undigested polypeptides, like α-gliadin, to cross into the lamina propria. In genetically susceptible individuals, tissue transglutaminase, a celiac auto-antigen, deamidates α-gliadin and thereby enhances its affinity for binding to HLA-DQ2 and DQ8 molecules on antigen-presenting cells (APCs). Such APC gluten peptides activate CD4 T cells that in turn activate the innate immune system and adaptive immune response, leading to production of autoantibodies and T cell—mediated inflammation. The end result is an inflammatory destruction of the small intestinal villi.
- To develop celiac disease, an individual must have certain human leukocyte antigen (HLA) genes that encode for antigen-presenting cell surface markers that are able to bind to α-gliadin and activate CD4 T cells. Individuals who possess certain HLA haplotypes DQ2 and DQ8 are at risk for celiac disease. HLA DQ2 and DQ8 are common in the population and are required but not sufficient for developing CD.

DIAGNOSIS (SEE FIGURE 15-1)

- Ultimately, diagnosis of celiac depends on history, physical examination, serology, and duodenal biopsies with characteristic changes associated with celiac disease.
- The first step in evaluating for celiac disease is serologic testing in the setting of ongoing gluten ingestion. The recommended screening test is tissue transglutaminase immunoglobulin A (TTG IgA), which has an overall sensitivity and specificity of 90% with higher titers associated with greater specificity.
- Deamidated gliadin peptide (DGP) is another serologic test for celiac disease that can be used to confirm diagnosis or monitor therapy but does not replace TTG IgA as the primary screening tool due to lower sensitivity.

Chapter 15: Celiac Disease

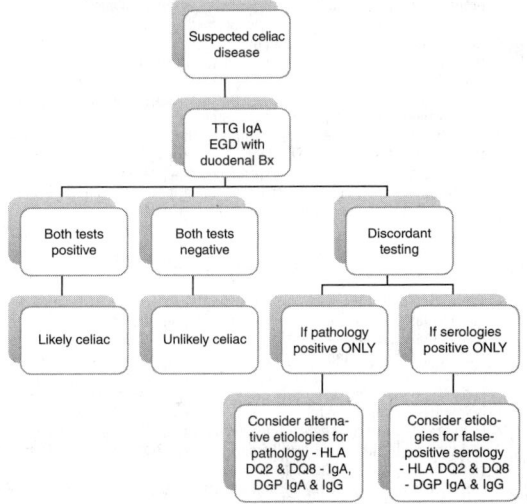

Figure 15-1 Algorithm for diagnosis of suspected celiac disease.

Bx = biopsy; DGP = deaminated gliadin peptide; HLA = human leukocyte antigen; IgA = immunoglobulin A; IgG = immunoglobulin G; TTG = Tissue transglutaminase
Source: Data from Rubio-Tapia A, Hill ID, Kelly CP, et al. ACG: Clinical guidelines: diagnosis and management of celiac disease. *Am J Gastro.* 2013;108:656–76.

- In patients with IgA deficiency, TTG IgA may be undetectable in the setting of celiac disease. DGP IgG, which is more commonly available than TTG IgG, should be checked in this situation. However, TTG IgA performance in the setting of IgA insufficiency is the same as in those with normal serum IgA levels.
- If suspicion for CD is high, endoscopy and duodenal biopsies are recommended even in the setting of negative serologies (5–16% will have negative serologies, an average false-negative rate of 1 in 10 cases of suspected CD).
- Confirmation of the diagnosis requires endoscopy with duodenal biopsies that show characteristic findings of CD, including villous atrophy, crypt hyperplasia, and lymphocytic infiltrate including the epithelium (intraepithelial lymphocytes) at the villous tips and in the lamina

propria. Endoscopic findings of duodenal fissuring or scalloping may be present in CD but are not necessary for the diagnosis.
- At a minimum, four biopsies from distal duodenum and one biopsy from the duodenal bulb should be obtained to ensure adequate tissue for diagnosis.
- While a clinical response to a gluten-free diet may support diagnosis of CD, it cannot distinguish non-celiac gluten sensitivity and CD.
- In the setting of dermatitis herpetiformis, the diagnosis of CD can be made with a characteristic skin biopsy.
- Genetic testing for HLA DQ2 and DQ8 should not be used for diagnosis of CD, but its high negative predictive value may help rule out celiac disease in certain instances.

TREATMENT

- The only treatment at present is a gluten-free diet (GFD), including avoidance of food containing wheat, rye, and barley. There are no medications currently available to protect the intestine from gluten-mediated damage. Adherence to a GFD is associated with improved symptoms and avoidance of complications. After diagnosis, patient consultation and follow-up with a registered dietitian familiar with CD is strongly recommended.
- Evaluate for nutritional deficiencies, including iron, folate, vitamin B12, and vitamin D, that could result from malabsorption and any deficiencies or insufficiencies should be treated.
- Consider dual-energy X-ray absorptiometry (DEXA) scan to evaluate for osteoporosis with standard follow-up for abnormal scans.
- After initiation of GFD, monitoring the patient entails confirmation of laboratory abnormalities, including CD serologies returning to normal. After normalization of lab tests, annual serologic tests are often advised.
- If symptoms relapse or persist, recommend review for continued gluten ingestion including medications, and re-evaluation of the diagnosis (review original biopsies), also consider possible coexisting conditions (persistent lactose intolerance, small intestinal bacterial overgrowth [SIBO], functional gastrointestinal disorders [FGID] including irritable bowel syndrome [IBS]) and, potentially, repeat endoscopy with biopsies. Refractory CD that does not respond to GFD is quite rare but is associated with a poor prognosis. Infrequently, patients will require steroids and immune modulators.
- Risks associated with untreated CD include osteoporosis, nutritional deficiencies, infertility, and, less frequently, enteropathy-associated T-cell lymphoma.

REFERENCES

1. Green PH, Cellier C. Celiac disease. *N Engl J Med*. 2010;357:1731–43.
2. Rostom A, Murray JA, Kagnoff MF. AGA Institute technical review on the diagnosis and management of celiac disease. *Gastro*. 2006; 131:1981–2002.
3. Rubio-Tapia A, Hill ID, Kelly CP, et al. ACG Clinical Guidelines: diagnosis and management of celiac disease. *Am J Gastro*. 2013;108(5):656–76.
4. Crowe, SE. In the clinic: celiac disease. *Ann Internal Med*. 2011;154(9):ITC5–14.

CHAPTER 16 ■ FOOD ALLERGIES

Moira E. Breslin, MD, MSc and Melinda Braskett, MD

OVERVIEW

Food allergy describes immune-mediated adverse reactions due to foods.

- "Classic" food allergy is characterized by IgE-mediated immediate hypersensitivity reactions to an ingested food protein.
- 90% of food allergies are due to one of the following eight major allergens: milk, egg, fish, crustacean shellfish, tree nuts, wheat, peanut, and soybean.
- Classic food allergies affect up to ~4–5% of adults and are more prevalent in children. The incidence of self-reported food allergy is significantly higher than physician-diagnosed food allergy. Accordingly, food intolerance reactions are much more common than hypersensitivity reactions (see **Table 16-1**).
- Pollen food allergy syndrome, or oral allergy syndrome, is the most common food allergy in adults and occurs in individuals with concomitant pollen allergy. Highly conserved domains on food proteins cross-react with receptors for pollen proteins and result in oropharyngeal urticaria. These proteins are extremely susceptible to proteolysis, and thus reactions are generally self-limited and do not cause systemic symptoms.
- Non-IgE-mediated reactions will be described elsewhere.

PRESENTATION

IgE-mediated reactions are rapid with reproducible objective findings.

- Classic food allergy reactions are reproducible adverse reactions with pathognomonic clinical features including a short timeline with rapid progression. Most have urticarial or angioedema manifestations. Emesis is much more common than diarrhea, although both occur. Involvement of the upper or lower airway inflammation can be life threatening with accompanying arrhythmia, hypotension, and syncope.
- The onset of symptoms occurs within minutes after ingestion and may take up to 2 hours to evolve. The peak of the adverse reactions generally lasts about 30 minutes. The exception to the rule is the recently described "mammalian meat allergy" mediated by IgE antibodies to galactose-alpha-1,3-galactose (alpha-gal), a carbohydrate commonly expressed on mammalian proteins. In this special case, delayed symptoms including anaphylaxis occur 3 to 6 hours after ingestion of beef, pork, or lamb.

Table 16-1 Classic Food Allergy Versus Food Intolerance

	Classic Food Allergy	Food Intolerance
Examples	Peanut anaphylaxis	Migraines, irritable bowel syndrome, acne
Cause	Misguided immune reaction to structure of specific food	Usually unknown Lactose intolerance due to low level of enzyme
Symptoms	Most have hives or swelling May have respiratory compromise, emesis, irregular HR, syncope	Variable Bowel irregularity, bloating, mood disturbance, headache, fatigue
Severity	Can be life threatening	Not life threatening, but can be absolutely miserable
Timeline	Usual onset within minutes, can take up to 2 hours to develop, peak of reaction ~30 minutes	Variable, usually delayed
Reproducible	Intake of food (in the same form) always triggers reaction, although severity may differ	Variable
Form of food	Some baked forms can be tolerated especially for milk and egg	Variable
Trace Amounts	Can trigger severe reactions	Generally tolerated
Avoidance	Asymptomatic	Improved
Validated Tests	Skin tests, IgE testing, observed food challenge	None
Treatment	Avoidance, antihistamines, epinephrine, steroids	Treat the primary problem. Often, trigger food exacerbates another process. Tolerance usually increases with improvement in primary condition.

- Anaphylaxis describes life-threatening reactions and usually includes cutaneous manifestations in addition to respiratory, gastrointestinal, or cardiovascular findings. In contrast, food intolerance reactions vary in presentation and reproducibility and are not life threatening.

DIFFERENTIAL DIAGNOSIS

Food intolerance, bloating, chronic urticaria, pollen food allergy syndrome (oral allergy syndrome), irritable bowel syndrome, food protein–induced enterocolitis, gastroenteritis, atopic dermatitis, secondary gain/behavioral issues, Crohn's disease, ulcerative colitis, celiac disease, bacterial overgrowth, gastroesophageal reflux disease (GERD)

PATHOPHYSIOLOGY

- Binding of IgE receptors to food antigen triggers an inflammatory cascade.
- Classic food allergy is governed by a Type I or immediate hypersensitivity reaction in which B cells secrete IgE that binds to mast cells and basophils. Exposure to the specific offending food protein then triggers these cells to degranulate and induce a TH-2-mediated inflammatory cascade. However, IgE alone is not sufficient to cause disease. In nonallergic individuals, the presence of detectable IgE represents "sensitization" as they lack manifestations of immediate hypersensitivity. IgG to food specific proteins is not typically pathogenic, although celiac disease is a notable exception.

DIAGNOSIS

Food challenge is diagnostic. Risk is based on history, skin test, and in vitro assays.

- Both "skin prick" tests and IgE assays of the specific allergen or its components have a high negative predictive value (> 90%) and, although dependent on the history, positive predictive values can be as low as 50%.
- Frequently, a food challenge is required to confirm or refute the presence of a food allergy. The gold standard for diagnosis is a double-blind placebo-controlled food challenge. However, these are resource intensive. Open food challenges offer a more practical approach. Food challenges should only be performed at facilities staffed and equipped to recognize and treat anaphylaxis.
- There are no screening tests for food intolerance, with lactose intolerance as an exception, and IgG testing should not be performed.

TREATMENT

Affected individuals should always carry antihistamines and an epinephrine autoinjector.

- Currently there is no treatment available for food allergies, other than supportive care.
- Strict avoidance and management of adverse reactions with antihistamines, epinephrine, and systemic steroids remain the standard of care.

- Improvements in labeling and preparation of foods have decreased accidental reactions from cross contamination.
- If symptoms are limited to the skin, an oral antihistamine may suffice. For anaphylaxis, one should immediately self-administer epinephrine and call 911. Treatment in the emergency department should include systemic steroids to prevent late-phase reactions.
- If a food allergy is suspected, two epinephrine autoinjectors should be prescribed, and patients should carry epinephrine and antihistamines at all times. For those weighing less than 30 kg, 0.15 mg epinephrine is the recommended dose, and for all others, 0.3 mg is the recommended dose.

REFERENCES

1. NIAID-Sponsored Expert Panel, Boyce JA, Assa'ad A, et al. Guidelines for the diagnosis and management of food allergy in the United States: report of the NIAID-sponsored expert panel. *J Allergy Clin Immunol*. 2010; 126(6 Suppl):S1–58.
2. Commins SP, Satinover SM, Hosen J, et al. Delayed anaphylaxis, angio-edema, or urticaria after consumption of red meat in patients with IgE antibodies specific for galactose-alpha-1,3-galactose. *J Allergy Clin Immunol*. 2009;123(2):426–33. Epub 2008 Dec 13.
3. Bock SA, Sampson HA, Atkins FM, et al. Double-blind, placebo-controlled food challenge (DBPCFC) as an office procedure: a manual. *J Allergy Clin Immunol*. 1988;82(6):986–97.

CHAPTER 17 ■ IRRITABLE BOWEL SYNDROME AND SMALL INTESTINAL BACTERIAL OVERGROWTH

Folasade P. May, MD, MPhil and Lynn S. Connolly, MD, MSCR

OVERVIEW

- Irritable bowel syndrome (IBS) is a symptom complex characterized by abdominal pain or discomfort that occurs in association with altered bowel habits for a period of greater than 3 months.
- IBS is the most prevalent gastrointestinal condition and is associated with significant impairment in health-related quality of life (HRQOL).
- Women are 1.5 times more likely than men to carry the diagnosis.
- There are three subtypes: IBS-constipation predominant (IBS-C), IBS-diarrhea predominant (IBS-D), and mixed IBS (IBS-M).

PRESENTATION

- Abdominal pain is typically crampy in nature, periodic, and can vary broadly in location and severity.
- Pain or discomfort is often exacerbated by PO (by mouth) intake, anxiety, and stress, and it is alleviated by bowel movement and flatus.
- Patients may present with infrequent stools, frequent stools, or both.
  - **IBS-C:** infrequent, hard, or pellet-like stools lasting for days to months. Stools are often associated with incomplete evacuation and defecation straining. Bristol stool scale types 1 and 2.
  - **IBS-D:** frequent loose stools, often after meals. Stools may contain mucus, be explosive in nature, and/or associated with abdominal cramping and urgency. Bristol stool scale types 6 and 7.
  - **Mixed IBS:** constipation that alternates with loose stools. Often, patients will describe several days of constipation followed by 1 to 2 days of loose stools.
- Up to 80% of IBS patients report food-related symptoms.
- Bloating and abdominal distention occur in over 50% of IBS patients.
- Other symptoms include gas, belching, and nausea.
- IBS is often associated with other comorbid pain conditions such as interstitial cystitis, fibromyalgia, dyspareunia, migraine headaches, and chronic pelvic pain. It is also linked to depression and anxiety.
- Weight loss, anorexia, nocturnal stools, bloody stools, and anemia are not typical of IBS and warrant evaluation for other clinical conditions.

- Postinfectious IBS is a condition characterized by the development of IBS symptoms after an acute infectious enteritis. Risk factors include female gender, under 60 years of age, chronic stress at time of initial illness, severe initial illness, and prolonged duration of initial episode.

DIFFERENTIAL DIAGNOSIS

- IBS-C: functional constipation, gastroparesis, colonic obstruction, and hypothyroidism
- IBS-D: celiac disease, dietary intolerance (lactose, sugar alcohols), small intestinal bacterial overgrowth, hyperthyroidism, ulcerative colitis, Crohn's disease, and microscopic colitis

SMALL INTESTINAL BACTERIAL OVERGROWTH

- Small intestinal bacterial overgrowth (SIBO) is a condition characterized by excessive colonic bacteria in the small intestine ($\geq 10^5$ bacteria per mL of proximal jejunal aspiration).
- Alterations in the natural composition of intestinal microflora can lead to bacterial imbalance, inflammatory changes, increased intestinal permeability, fermentation, and malabsorption.
- There has been significant debate about the relationship between IBS and SIBO and whether SIBO is more common in IBS patients compared to healthy individuals.
- Symptoms include nausea, abdominal bloating and discomfort, excessive flatus, weight loss, and loose stools.
- The gold standard for diagnosis of SIBO is jejunal aspirate; however, hydrogen and methane breath tests are more clinically assessable and more widely used.
- Lactulose hydrogen and glucose breath tests are used as surrogate markers for SIBO but are limited by a high false-positive rate. Positivity may reflect orocecal transit time rather than SIBO.
- If suspicion for SIBO is high, empiric treatment for 10–14 days may be favored over diagnostic testing.
- Treatment for SIBO may improve abdominal pain and altered stool form in some individuals with IBS.
- Antibiotic regimens to reduce intestinal bacterial load include:
  - Rifaximin: 550 mg BID or TID
  - Ciprofloxacin: 500 mg BID
  - Metronidazole: 250 or 500 mg TID
  - Norfloxacin: 400 mg BID
  - Neomycin: 500 mg QID
  - Amoxicillin-clavulanic acid: 500 mg TID

Chapter 17: Irritable Bowel Syndrome

- Recurrence is common and can be treated with another course of antibiotics.
- The evidence for use of probiotics in SIBO is limited, and probiotics are not recommended at the present time.

PATHOPHYSIOLOGY

- The pathophysiology of IBS is not completely understood; however, the condition is felt to involve both abnormal gastrointestinal motility and enhanced visceral sensitivity.
- Studies have also implicated a role for alterations in the composition of intestinal flora, small intestinal bacterial overgrowth, chronic low-grade inflammation, alterations in the immune system, and central dysregulation.

DIAGNOSIS

- Several diagnostic criteria for IBS exist; however, the accuracy of proposed diagnostic criteria may be limited.
- The Rome III criteria are recurrent abdominal pain/discomfort for at least 3 days per month in the past 3 months associated with two or more of the following: improvement with defecation, onset associated with a change in frequency of stool, and/or onset associated with a change in stool form.
- In all disease subtypes, physical examination is often normal.
- In the absence of alarm symptoms (fever, weight loss, rectal bleeding, anemia, or a family history of IBD [inflammatory bowel disease], celiac disease, or colon cancer), routine diagnostic testing (complete blood count, serum chemistries, thyroid tests, stool tests, and abdominal imaging) has low yield and is not recommended.
- Patients with IBS-D should also undergo screening for celiac disease.
- Patients who are either over age 50 or presenting with alarm symptoms should have further investigation with colonoscopy.

TREATMENT (SEE FIGURE 17-1)

- There is no cure for IBS. Therapies are aimed to relieve symptoms and improve quality of life.
- Treatment will vary by IBS subtype and severity of symptoms.
- Patient education, patient reassurance, and an open patient–provider relationship are essential to management. Providers should also establish reasonable expectations with patients when possible.

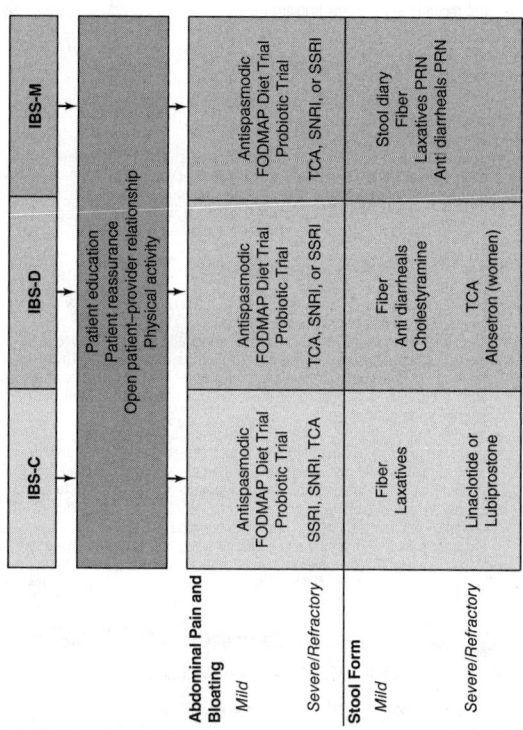

Figure 17-1 Treatment options for IBS

FODMAPs = fermentable, oligo-, di-, monosaccharides, and polyols; PRN = as needed; SNRI = serotonin-norepinephrine reuptake inhibitor; SSRI = selective serotonin reuptake inhibitor; TCA = tricyclic antidepressant

Chapter 17: Irritable Bowel Syndrome

- **Dietary modification:** evidence for dietary modification is limited, although empiric elimination of lactose, sugar alcohols like xylitol and sorbitol, gas-forming foods and fermentable, oligo-, di-, monosaccharides, and polyols (FODMAPs) from the diet may reduce symptoms. Elimination of gluten improves symptoms in some individuals, even in the absence of celiac disease. Food diary may reveal other trigger foods that can also be eliminated. Referral to a nutritionist or dietician should be considered.
- **Fiber:** an initial trial of 0.5 to 1 tablespoon of fiber per day can be considered, although side effects may include gas and bloating.
- **Probiotics:** clinical studies and meta-analyses suggest that some strains of probiotics can decrease global IBS symptoms. Probiotics with potentially beneficial effects include *Lactobacillus* species, VSL#3, and *Bifidobacterium* species.
- **Laxatives:** both osmotic laxatives (polyethylene glycol; PEG) and stimulant laxatives (Senokot and Dulcolax) may improve stool form in IBS-C.
- **Cholestyramine:** consider a trial of cholestyramine, one packet BID, in the setting of prior cholecystectomy and/or a potential component of bile acid diarrhea.
- **Antidiarrheals:** loperamide (2 mg QD to 4 mg QID) or diphenoxylate/atropine (Lomotil) (5 mg QD to QID) can reduce stool frequency and urgency in IBS-D. These medications may be most effective when doses are timed with meals. Dose should not exceed 16 mg daily and 20 mg daily, respectively.
- **Antispasmodic agents:** hyoscyamine 0.125 to 0.25 mg SL TID-QID, dicyclomine 20–40 mg QID, chlordiazepoxide and clidinium (Librax) 1–2 capsules TID–QID, and peppermint oil can provide short-term relief of abdominal pain and bloating.
- **Antidepressants:** low-dose tricyclic antidepressants (TCAs), selective serotonin reuptake inhibitors (SSRIs), and selective serotonin and norepinephrine reuptake inhibitors (SNRIs) have been used to treat IBS.
  - **TCAs:** desipramine, amitriptyline, and nortriptyline reduce pain in IBS patients in randomized trials. Consider starting at 10 mg QHS and titrate to 50 mg QHS. Side effects may include constipation and somnolence.
  - **SSRIs:** fluoxetine, paroxetine, and citalopram improved overall well-being although not pain or stool form in clinical studies. Dose should start at 20 mg QD and can be titrated to 60 mg QD.
  - **SNRIs:** of the SNRIs, duloxetine 15–60 mg QD has shown some clinical efficacy.
- **Alosetron** (0.5 mg QD to 1 mg BID): a 5-hydroxytryotamine-3 receptor antagonist that can reduce pain, urgency, and diarrhea in IBS-D. Use of the medication is only approved in women with severe IBS-D. Potential side effects include ischemic colitis and severe constipation.
- **Intestinal secretagogues:** both lubiprostone (8 mcg BID) and linaclotide (145 or 290 mcg daily) are approved for the treatment of

refractory IBS-C. These agents accelerate colonic transit and facilitate defecation by stimulating a net efflux of ions and water into the intestinal lumen. Side effects include diarrhea, headaches, and nausea. A negative pregnancy test is required before initiation of these medications.
- Use of a stool diary will direct the balance of laxatives and antidiarrheals in IBS-M.
- In addition to these therapies, cognitive behavioral therapy, physical activity, and acupuncture have improved symptoms in some individuals.

REFERENCES

1. Brandt LJ, Chey WD, Foxx-Orenstein AE, et al. An evidence-based position statement on the management of irritable bowel syndrome. *Am J Gastroenterol.* 2009;104(Suppl 1):S1–S35.
2. Ford AC, Spiegel BM, Talley NJ, Moayyedi P. Small intestinal bacterial overgrowth in irritable bowel syndrome: systematic review and meta-analysis. *Clin Gastroenterol Hepatol.* 2009;7:1279–1286.

CHAPTER 18 ■ GASTROINTESTINAL ISSUES IN THE IMMUNOCOMPROMISED HOST

Rini Abraham, MD and Michael A. Poles, MD, PhD

OVERVIEW

- Immunocompromise can be primary or acquired.
- Immunodeficiencies can also be categorized according to which components of the immune mechanism are affected—which will impact the clinical manifestations experienced.
- The gastrointestinal (GI) tract is disproportionately affected by immunocompromise, and the more comprehensive the immunologic defect, the more severe the clinical gastrointestinal consequences.

PRIMARY IMMUNODEFICIENCY

- Loss of one component of the humoral immune response: selective IgA deficiency
  - The most common primary immunodeficiency, seen in up to 1 in 500–700 patients.
  - Caused by a genetic defect in IgA B-cell maturation, resulting in loss of IgA production.
  - IgA is the dominant immunoglobulin produced by mucosal B cells, but because this defect only affects this immunoglobulin subtype, it is rare for patients to present with significant disease manifestations.
  - Given its role as a mucosal protectant, clinical manifestations usually involve mucosal surfaces, such as the GI, respiratory, and genitourinary tracts.
    - Diarrhea, especially from *Giardia* and small bowel bacterial overgrowth (SIBO).
    - Increased prevalence of celiac disease (10–30%).
    - Patients may develop severe infusion reactions, including anaphylaxis, when transfused with IgA-containing blood.
  - May be diagnosed by quantitative immunoglobulin measurement of the blood.
  - There is no treatment of the underlying disease so treatment of the mild comorbid conditions is necessary when they develop.
- Greater loss of the humoral immune response: common variable immunodeficiency (CVID)
  - Second most common primary immunodeficiency.

- Heterogeneous group of primary immunodeficiencies, each characterized by panhypoglobulinemia with decreased secretion of IgG, IgA, and/or IgM.
- The greater impairment in humoral immunity commonly leads to recurrent respiratory and GI infections by extracellular pathogens, such as bacteria and protozoa.
- Patients develop chronic and recurrent diarrhea, especially caused by *Giardia, Cryptosporidium, Campylobacter,* and *Salmonella.*
- Patients may develop SIBO and small bowel villous atrophy, resembling celiac disease.
- Increased risk of neoplastic consequences, including GI carcinoma or lymphoma.
- Diagnosis is usually made demonstrating low immunoglobulin levels in the blood.
- Treatment, when necessary, consists of treating the comorbid conditions and passive immunization with intravenous immunoglobulin (IVIG) or with subcutaneously administered immunoglobulin treatment.
- Loss of both humoral and cell-mediated immunity: severe combined immunodeficiency (SCID)
  - Rare, affecting approximately 1 in 50,000 live births.
  - Characterized by absence of functional T cells and a defective antibody response.
  - Because it affects both arms of the adaptive immune response, these patients are subject to severe infections by all pathogens, including bacterial, viral, fungal, and protozoal.
  - Typically fatal in infancy due to infection (including diarrhea, mucosal candidiasis) if not treated with hematopoietic stem cell transplantation.

ACQUIRED IMMUNODEFICIENCY

Acquired immunodeficiency can result in susceptibility to systemic or localized infections, of which the GI tract may be a dominant site. Depending on the immune component targeted and the degree of immunosuppression, infections may be bacterial, viral, fungal, or parasitic in origin. Patients may acquire immunodeficiency due to a variety of factors, including:

- Human immunodeficiency virus (HIV).
- Post-transplant, both of solid organs and stem cells (hematopoietic stem cell transplants; HSCT), usually due to the immunosuppressive medication use.
- Medication-induced immunosuppression, including immunosuppressive agents (steroids, immunomodulators [thiopurines, calcineurin inhibitors, and methotrexate]) and biological agents (including tumor necrosis factor-alpha inhibitors and chemotherapeutics). Medications can also cause immunosuppression through adverse effect such as neutropenia.
- Advanced age, due to immune senescence and malnutrition.

Chapter 18: Gastrointestinal Issues in the Immunocompromised 95

HIV is a prototypical acquired immunodeficiency and serves as an excellent exemplar for the effects of acquired immunodeficiency in the GI tract. HIV preferentially targets cells expressing the CD4 receptor and the CCR5 or CXCR4 co-receptors. The GI mucosa is the primary site of residence of these cells, which are readily infected in HIV and are efficiently destroyed. This causes a significant degree of mucosal immunosuppression and a greater susceptibility to opportunistic infection. Up to 90% of all patients with acquired immune deficiency syndrome (AIDS) have GI complaints at some point in their disease course, which may affect all GI sites.

ESOPHAGEAL INVOLVEMENT

The target of many infections in HIV, esophageal involvement typically results in odynophagia and dysphagia, which may cause food avoidance and exacerbate malnutrition.

- *Candida* (monilial) esophagitis
  - The most common infectious manifestation in HIV and in transplant patients.
  - Readily diagnosed by endoscopy, it is more cost-effective to give empiric antifungals to immunosuppressed patients with esophageal symptoms, reserving endoscopy for those who do not have a response.
- Cytomegalovirus (CMV) esophagitis
  - CMV esophagitis is the second most common cause of esophageal symptoms in severely immunosuppressed HIV patients (CD4 cell count is usually < 50 cells/µL). Also common in patients receiving solid organ transplants.
  - It should be considered in patients who have failed a course of empiric antifungal treatment.
  - Endoscopy is necessary for diagnosis.
    - The endoscopic appearance is typically that of a solitary linear ulcer in the mid-distal esophagus.
    - Occasionally esophageal ulcers may be multiple or diffuse.
    - Biopsy, looking for the typical owl's eye inclusions, is necessary to make the diagnosis.
    - Biopsies are best taken from the ulcer base. Immunohistochemical techniques will increase the sensitivity.
  - In HIV, the best treatment approach for CMV ulcers, as well as all opportunistic infections, is effective HIV therapy. Specific therapy with ganciclovir or foscarnet is also effective for CMV and should be used for immunosuppressed transplant patients.
- Herpes simplex virus (HSV) esophagitis
  - Common viral cause of esophagitis in HIV-infected and transplant patients.
  - Endoscopic biopsy is the primary means of diagnosis.
    - HSV ulcers tend to be smaller, round, and discrete from the distal esophagus.
  - Usually responds to intravenous or oral therapy with acyclovir.

Table 18-1 Esophageal diseases among the immunosuppressed

Fungal	Bacterial	Viral
Candida species	*M. tuberculosis*	CMV
Pneumocystis jirovecii	MAC	HSV 1 and 2
Histoplasma capsulatum	*Actinomyces*	EBV
		Papovavirus
Neoplastic	**Miscellaneous**	**Protozoal**
Lymphoma	GERD	*Cryptosporidia*
Kaposis sarcoma	Pill esophagitis	*Microsporidia*
	Aphthous ulcer	*Isospora belli*
		Cyclospora

- Idiopathic (aphthous) esophageal ulcers
  - Ulcers that are not clearly due to any obvious pathogen
  - Unknown pathogenesis, but may be a consequence of HIV itself
- Graft-versus-host disease (GVHD) after a hematopoietic stem cell transplantation may be associated with nonspecific esophageal motility disorders and esophageal webs and rings due to submucosal fibrosis and strictures.
- Additional causes of esophageal disease among the immunosuppressed, are shown in **Table 18-1**.

GASTRIC DISEASE

Subject to same disease processes as esophagus. There is also some overlap with duodenal pathologic entities.

SMALL AND LARGE INTESTINE INVOLVEMENT

- Diarrhea is the most common GI manifestation experienced by patients with HIV and after stem cell transplantation.
- The factor most predictive of diarrhea among HIV patients is the degree of immunosuppression.
  - The risk is greatest when the CD4 T-cell count falls below 50 cells/μL.
- Be suspicious of every conceivable disease because new pathogens have appeared in common places and common pathogens in new places.
- Patients may harbor multiple pathogens, so treating one may not result in diarrhea resolution.
- Parasitic and fungal infections are less frequent causes of diarrhea in patients who have received organ transplantation.
- CMV may cause diarrhea—not only in HIV and status post-transplant, but can also occur in patients with severe or refractory inflammatory bowel disease (IBD) who are using corticosteroids or other immunosuppressants.

Chapter 18: Gastrointestinal Issues in the Immunocompromised

- Some of the diagnostic considerations for infectious diarrhea are shown in **Table 18-2**.
- One diagnostic algorithm, shown in **Figure 18-1**, includes fat malabsorption and small intestinal bacterial infection, which may occur more commonly in HIV.
- It is important to remember that not all problems are HIV-related and HIV patients are subject to the same diseases as age- and gender-matched patients without HIV.
- When an organism is found, treatment should be initiated.
- In HIV, the response to treatment is often decreased, relapse is frequent, and maintenance therapy may be required unless the CD4 cell count can be normalized with effective antiretroviral therapy.

Table 18-2 Diagnostic considerations for infectious diarrhea

Small bowel	Large bowel	Miscellaneous
Crytposporidium	Cytomegalovirus	Drugs
Microsporidium	Herpes simplex virus	Idiopathic AIDS enteropathy
Isospora belli	Adenovirus	Graft versus Host Disease
Giardia	Rotavirus	(post HSCT)
MAC	Cryptosporidium	Lymphoproliferative
Salmonella	Campylobacter jejuni	disease (post SOT)
Campylobacter	Shigella; group D	Neoplasms ie Lymphoma,
Strongyloides stercoralis	Ecoli	Kaposi
Norovirus	Entamoeba histolytica	Pancreatitis
	Clostridium difficile	Lactose intolerance
	MAC	Neutropenic enterocolitis
	Chlamydia Trachomatis	IgA deficiency
	Pneumocystis carinii (rare)	SCID
	Histoplasma capsulatum	CVID
	Blastocystis hominis	

PANCREAS/BILIARY DISEASE

- Pancreatitis is common in HIV.
- Typically asymptomatic, but may present with abdominal pain, nausea/vomiting.
- Certain HIV drugs/immunomodulators/immunosuppressive drugs can cause pancreatitis.
- Opportunistic infections have been implicated as well, including CMV, HSV, *Cryptosporidium, Toxoplasma, Mycobacterium avium* complex (MAC), *Pneumocystis*.
- Patients receiving hematopoietic stem cell transplants are at increased risk of cholecystitis, gallstones, sludge, pancreatitis, pancreatic insufficiency.

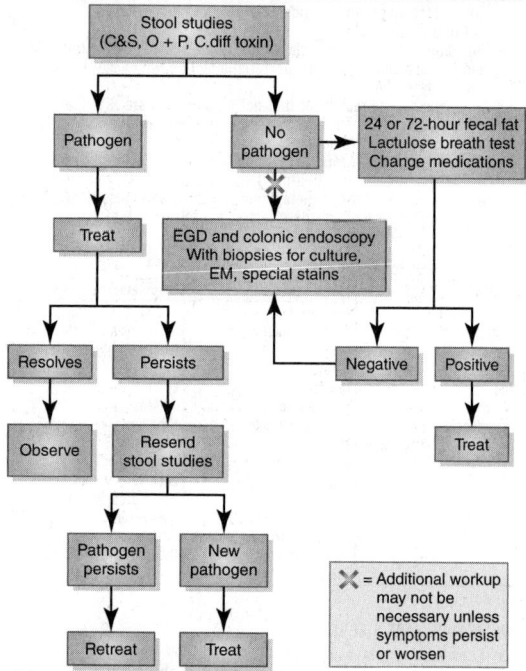

Figure 18-1 Diagnostic algorithm for possible infectious diarrhea.

LIVER DISEASE

- Given the shared epidemiologic risks, patients infected with HIV are very commonly co-infected with hepatitis B virus (HBV) and hepatitis C virus (HCV), which may be associated with worse outcomes in the immunosuppressed.
- Antiretroviral mediations used by HIV-seropositive patients are often hepatotoxic, contributing to hepatic damage.

- With increasing immunosuppression, HIV patients are at an increased risk of infection with opportunistic viral (including HSV and CMV), fungal (including *Histoplasma, Cryptococcus, Coccidioides*), bacterial (*Bartonella*), and protozoal (*Microsporidia, Cryptosporidia*) pathogens, and neoplastic manifestations.
- MAC infection is a common cause of cholestatic serologies.
- Hematopoietic stem cell recipients may experience hepatic GVHD, which presents as acute hepatocellular injury, as well as varicella zoster virus (VZV) or HSV hepatitis, fungal abscesses, nodular regenerative hyperplasia, and drug-induced liver injury.
- Additional hepatobiliary entities
  - Hepatomegaly
  - Lactic acidosis syndrome characterized by marked hepatomegaly, steatosis, lactic acidosis and liver failure, which may be caused by use of nucleoside reverse transcriptase inhibitor antiretrovirals
  - AIDS cholangiopathy

Liver diseases seen in hematopoietic stem cell patients

- Hepatic GVHD, which presents as acute hepatocellular injury
- VZV, HSV hepatitis
- Fungal abscess
- Nodular regenerative hyperplasia
- Biliary obstruction
- Drug-induced liver injury
- Hepatocellular carcinoma

RISK OF GI MALIGNANCY IN IMMUNOSUPPRESSED PATIENTS

HIV

- Kaposi's sarcoma (KS) is seen in 5–25%, especially among men who have sex with men (MSM)
- Non-Hodgkin's lymphoma (NHL)
  - Typically, B-cell derivation and may be seen throughout the GI tract.
  - Late event of HIV infection.
  - May present with B-symptoms and GI symptoms (weight loss, abdominal pain, fever, diarrhea or perianal pain, GI bleed).
  - Multifocal.
  - May appear as polypoid, bulky lesions or well defined.

POST-ORGAN TRANSPLANTATION (HSCT OR SOLID)

- May develop Kaposi's sarcoma and hepatobiliary carcinoma
- Post-transplant lymphoproliferative disorders (PTLD) includes lymphoproliferative entities ranging from reactive hyperplasia to malignant lymphoma

- Most cases are B-cell lymphoma.
- Half occur within 12 months with a second peak occurring 5–10 years after transplantation.
- Common symptoms include fever, pain, weight loss, bowel perforation.
- The liver is involved in 30–50%, and the luminal GI tract in up to 25%.
- Diagnostic evaluation includes Epstein-Barr virus (EBV) immunohistochemistry, esophagogastroduodenoscopy (EGD), colonoscopy, small bowel evaluation, abdominal ultrasound.

IBD

- Immunosuppressive agents such as azathioprine, 6-MP, cyclosporine, methotrexate, and infliximab increase the absolute risk to develop lymphoma, but the overall risk is low.
- Hepatosplenic T-cell lymphoma has been associated with anti-TNF (tumor necrosis factor), especially when administered with immunomodulators.

REFERENCES

1. Krones E, Hogenauer C. Diarrhea in the immunocompromised patient. *Gastroenterol Clin North Am.* 2012;41:677–701.
2. Thom K, Forrest G. Gastrointestinal infections in immunocompromised hosts. *Curr Opin Gastroenterol* 2006;22:18–23.
3. Kida A, McDonald GB. Gastrointestinal, hepatobiliary, pancreatic, and iron-related diseases in long-term survivors of allogeneic hematopoietic cell transplantation. *Semin Hematol.* 2012;49:43–58.
4. Agarwal S, Mayer L. Gastrointestinal manifestations in primary immune disorders. *Inflamm Bowel Dis.* 2010;16:703–711.
5. F Hoentjen, van Bodegraven AA. Safety of anti-tumor necrosis factor therapy in inflammatory bowel disease. *World J Gastroenterol.* 2009;15(17):2067–73.
6. Baroco AL, Oldfield EC. Gastrointestinal cytomegalovirus disease in the immunocompromised patients. *Curr Gastroenterol Rep.* 2008;10:409–16.

CHAPTER 19 ■ VASCULAR DISORDERS OF THE GASTROINTESTINAL TRACT

Nima Nassiri, BS and Peter F. Lawrence, MD

OVERVIEW

Adequate perfusion is central to the maintenance of the energy-demanding functions of the gastrointestinal (GI) tract, which include digestion, nutrient absorption, and maintenance of innate and adaptive branches of immunity.

BLOOD SUPPLY (SEE FIGURE 19-1)

- Arterial supply
  - Celiac artery supplies stomach, proximal duodenum, liver, spleen, and pancreas. Normal anatomic variations include gastrosplenic trunks and hepatosplenic trunks. The hepatic artery also exhibits normal variation and may arise from the left gastric artery or superior mesenteric artery (SMA).
  - SMA supplies distal duodenum, small intestine, cecum, ascending colon, and proximal transverse colon (*most important visceral vessel for gut perfusion*).
  - Inferior mesenteric artery (IMA) supplies the distal transverse colon to the proximal rectum.
  - The internal iliac and pudendal arteries supply the distal rectum.
  - The superior, middle, and inferior rectal arteries supply the anus.
- Venous drainage
  - Gastric and duodenal veins are tributaries to portal circulation.
  - Venous drainage of the colon and rectum follows the arterial supply.
  - Superior rectal vein drains the anus.

ISCHEMIC COLITIS

- The most common ischemic disorder of the GI tract, ischemic colitis affects the left side of the colon in 75% of cases. In patients who develop gangrene, mortality approaches 50–75% despite surgical intervention.
- Symptoms/findings vary from mild and transient abdominal pain, rectal bleeding, diarrhea, and fever to gangrene of the colon.
- Diagnosis: computed tomography (CT) scan with contrast is the primary imaging modality employed in diagnosis. Endoscopic evaluation via colonoscopy or flexible sigmoidoscopy is the diagnostic procedure

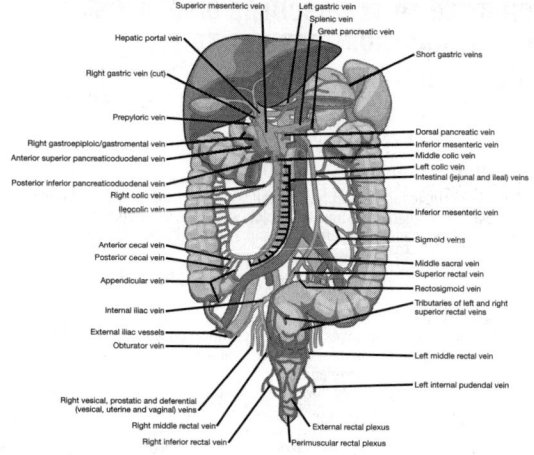

Figure 19-1 Anatomy

of choice when CT imaging is equivocal and in postop aortic aneurysm patients.
- Treatment: supportive care with intravenous (IV) fluids, bowel rest, and optimization of oxygenation. Nasogastric tube may be placed in the presence of ileus. In the presence of worsening signs, such as leukocytosis, fever, worsening abdominal pain, and increased bleeding, laparotomy with bowel resection is indicated.

ACUTE MESENTERIC ISCHEMIA (AMI)

- Symptoms/findings: sudden onset abdominal pain, nausea, vomiting, diarrhea, emptying, and abdominal distension.
- Late findings include hypoactive bowel sounds, abdominal guarding, and rebound tenderness. Classic description is *pain out of proportion to physical exam findings*.
- Rapidly progresses (hours to days), and if uncorrected, leads to acute intestinal infarction. Associated findings include fever, oliguria, dehydration,

Chapter 19: Vascular Disorders of the Gastrointestinal Tract

confusion, tachycardia and shock, leukocytosis, metabolic acidosis, elevated liver function tests (LFTs), and lactic acidemia.

- Occlusive AMI
  - Embolization to the SMA is the most common cause of AMI (40–50% of cases). Common sources of emboli include intracardiac mural thrombus, thrombus formed in proximal aortic aneurysms, and septic emboli from endocarditis. The SMA arises at a less acute angle from the aorta than the celiac and is thus more commonly affected. Emboli lodge distal to the middle colic artery, resulting in ischemic damage to the ascending colon with sparing of the colon distal to the splenic flexure.
  - Thrombosis constitutes the second most common cause of AMI. Atherosclerotic plaques can affect all visceral vessels and serve as a nidus for thrombosis. Thrombosis associated with higher mortality than embolic counterpart (77.4% and 54.1%, respectively).
- Non-occlusive mesenteric ischemia (NOMI)
  - Impaired intestinal perfusion in the absence of thromboembolic occlusion. Most commonly secondary to severe congestive heart failure (CHF) or atrial fibrillation with decreased left ventricular function and cardiac output.
  - Risk factors = hypovolemia, systemic vasoconstrictors, vasoactive drugs, aortic insufficiency, cardiopulmonary bypass, abdominal and cardiovascular surgery, and liver failure.
- Mesenteric venous thrombosis (MVT)
  - Symptoms/findings: fever, abdominal distension, and bloody stools are most common. Dehydration and profound fluid shifts can lead to hypovolemia.
  - Thrombosis is often limited to superior mesenteric vein, but may also involve inferior mesenteric vein and portal vein. Causes include hypercoagulopathy (most common), malignancy, trauma, abdominal surgery, hepatic failure, pancreatitis, and oral contraceptive (OCP) use. Edema and hemorrhage of the intestinal wall are frequently seen, and are followed by focal sloughing of the mucosa—with slow progression to ischemia. High rate of recurrence in the absence of long-term anticoagulation.
  - Treatment: anticoagulation with heparin remains first line, and surgical exploration is reserved for clinical deterioration (acute abdomen).

CHRONIC MESENTERIC ISCHEMIA (CMI)

- Most commonly caused by progressive atherosclerotic occlusive disease of the visceral arteries. More than two mesenteric vessels involved before symptoms develop.

- Symptoms/findings: insidious (months–years) development of postprandial abdominal pain (dull and crampy, mid-epigastric) and progressive weight loss. Cachexia and malnourishment (low albumin and pre-albumin) from sitophobia (fear of eating). Hyperactive bowel sounds without guarding or rebound tenderness. Frequently misdiagnosed as a GI disorder.
- Diagnosis
  - Duplex ultrasonography for noninvasive detection of chronic visceral ischemia. Positive findings include stenosis/occlusion of celiac and/or SMA with high velocities. Limited by obesity, excessive intraluminal bowel gas, and anatomical variation.
  - Computed tomography angiography (CTA) is an accurate modality for diagnosis of acute and chronic mesenteric ischemia and visualization of calcified plaques. Positive findings include asymmetric bowel wall thickening, ileus, ascites, and free peritoneal air.
  - Magnetic resonance angiography (MRA) used to diagnose mesenteric occlusive disease. Limited role in diagnosing AMI because relatively long duration of imaging.
  - Conventional angiography: "gold standard" for mesenteric arterial evaluation.

TREATMENT OF MESENTERIC ISCHEMIA

- Goal of therapy is restoration of blood flow to the visceral organs.
- Medical treatment
  - Preoperative restoration of adequate urine output with fluid resuscitation.
  - Prophylactic broad-spectrum IV antibiotics decrease mortality as bacterial translocation may occur with bowel ischemia.
  - Nasogastric decompression and bowel rest should also be instituted.
  - High-dose IV prostaglandin E1 (PGE1 0.01–0.02 µg/kg/min) for 5 days indicated when vasospasm of the mesenteric arteries is observed without evidence of obstruction or stenosis. Aggressive monitoring for hypotension is required.
  - Prompt initiation of systemic anticoagulation (heparin bolus followed by continuous infusion). Goal activated partial thromboplastin time (aPTT) is 50–70 seconds.
  - Thrombolytic therapy is associated with higher mortality compared to isolated systemic anticoagulation.
- Endovascular therapy
  - Appropriate for patients with both acute and chronic mesenteric ischemia. Balloon angioplasty and stenting are the most common interventions in this patient population. Retrograde mesenteric stenting during laparotomy for AMI is a newer approach with good technical success but uncertain long-term efficacy.

- Patients with NOMI benefit from direct infusion of intra-arterial vasodilators (papaverine, nitroglycerin), low-dose intra-arterial iloprost, and angioplasty with or without stenting.
- Surgical intervention
  - Laparotomy with open revascularization is the preferred therapy for AMI. Doppler evaluation of the mesenteric arteries is used to assess bowel perfusion. Most patients should undergo second-look laparotomy in 24 hours after the initial operation to evaluate for extent of bowel ischemia and resection of necrotic bowel. Special consideration: patients with embolic AMI should receive systemic heparinization prior to embolectomy.
  - Patients with CMI who undergo elective revascularization may need transaortic endarterectomy, antegrade mesenteric bypass, or retrograde mesenteric bypass.

CELIAC ARTERY PATHOLOGY

- Aneurysm:
  - Splenic artery is the second most common site of abdominal aneurysm, after the aortoiliac. Portal hypertension increases the aneurysmal propensity in the splenic artery. Though arteriosclerosis is the most common pathological finding, it is thought to occur as a post-aneurysmal phenomenon. Rupture occurs most commonly in pregnant women and is associated with high mortality (70–90%).
  - Symptoms/findings: usually asymptomatic, and < 30% present with abdominal pain.
  - Treatment: embolization is the favored approach. Open or laparoscopic surgery indicated when embolization is difficult or contraindicated by the proximity of the aneurysm to the spleen (risk of splenic infarction).
  - The celiac trunk is a rare site for aneurysm formation and is associated with a low rate of rupture. Surgical intervention requires reconstruction of the celiac trunk to the hepatic and splenic arteries using a saphenous vein graft.
- Compression
  - Median arcuate ligament syndrome occurs when there is compression of the celiac axis by the diaphragmatic median arcuate ligament.
  - Symptoms/findings: epigastric abdominal pain, persistent nausea, vomiting, and weight loss.
  - Diagnosis is made by conventional angiography or CTA, demonstrating a focal narrowing of the proximal celiac axis.
  - Treatment: decompression of the median arcuate ligament with or without visceral artery bypass. Endovascular treatment alone is ineffective because it does not relieve the extrinsic compression of the celiac artery.

SMA PATHOLOGY

- Thromboembolic occlusive disease (see earlier discussion of occlusive AMI).
- Isolated dissection with secondary visceral arterial occlusion occurs most commonly in the SMA. Associated risk factors involve atherosclerosis, medial degeneration, arterial trauma, fibromuscular disease, pregnancy, and arteriopathy.
  - Symptoms: majority of patients are asymptomatic, but some may present with abdominal pain that progresses to AMI. CTA is the diagnostic study of choice. Conservative management with serial CTA to assess for aneurysmal degeneration is adequate for asymptomatic or minimally symptomatic patients. SMA dissection can actually heal or resolve with time. Repair is required in the setting of mesenteric ischemia, aneurysmal degeneration, or rupture. Both open and endovascular approaches may be used.
- SMA syndrome defines the compression of the third portion of the duodenum by the abdominal aorta (AA) and overlying SMA.
- Nutcracker syndrome (NS) defines the entrapment of the left renal vein (LRV) between the AA and SMA. Most frequently occurs in females age 30–50 years.
  - Symptoms/findings: hematuria, left flank pain radiating to the buttock, varicocele (men), and rarely, myelitis and syringomyelia. Pain elicited by standing—the weight of the bowel exacerbates acuity of SMA–AA angle.
  - Diagnosis is made by duplex ultrasonography measuring the diameter and peak flow of the LRV at the site of stenosis, and the SMA–AA angle. CTA or MRA can delineate the relationship of the LRV with surrounding structures and reveal LRV compression with proximal dilation.
  - Treatment: re-implantation of LRV is surgical treatment of choice and should be considered in patients with severe symptoms. Stenting of the LRV has not been associated with restenosis and may be used. Renal autotransplantation and LRV bypass may be considered. Children should be treated conservatively as spontaneous remission may occur during growth.

IMA PATHOLOGY

Involves the general principles outlined earlier under *acute mesenteric ischemia* and *chronic mesenteric ischemia*. Isolated IMA pathology of non-thromboembolic etiology is rare.

VASCULITIDES: MEDIUM TO SMALL VESSELS

- Wegner's granulomatosis may affect the GI tract, particularly the mesenteric arteries, leading to ischemic injury. The disease classically affects middle-aged males. The necrotizing granulomatous vasculitis involves the nasopharynx, lungs, and kidneys.
- Patients present with sinusitis, nasopharyngeal ulceration, hemoptysis with bilateral nodular lung infiltrates, or hematuria from rapidly progressive glomerulonephritis. Degree of serum c-ANCA (anti-neutrophil cytoplasmic antibodies) positivity correlates with disease severity. Histology demonstrates large necrotizing granulomas with adjacent necrotizing vasculitis. Treatment involves corticosteroids and cyclophosphamide; however, relapses commonly occur.
- Approximately 50% of patients with polyarteritis nodosa (PAN) have celiac and mesenteric involvement. PAN is a necrotizing vasculitis of multiple organs, most commonly affecting young adults with a positive serum hepatitis B antigen (HBV). Patients present with hypertension, abdominal pain with melena, neurological disturbances, or skin lesions. Importantly, the lungs are spared. Histology reveals lesions of varying stages producing a "string of pearls" appearance characterized by alternating transmural inflammation with fibrinoid necrosis and fibrosis. Treatment involves corticosteroids and cyclophosphamide. The disease is fatal if left untreated.

VASCULAR MALFORMATIONS

- Colonic angiodysplasia is an acquired dilation of mucosal and submucosal capillary beds in the lower GI tract. Incidence increases with age, and the right colon and cecum are most vulnerable due to high wall tension in these segments. It is a common cause of lower GI bleeding in the elderly. Bleeding occurs secondary to vessel rupture and is chronic and recurrent. Classically, it presents as hematochezia, with massive hemorrhage occurring in a minority of patients. Treatment of ruptured vessels is accomplished through therapeutic endoscopy. Therapeutic angiography with super-selective embolization may also be used to control bleeding. Surgical resection is reserved for patients with uncontrollable bleeding.
- Osler-Weber-Rendu syndrome (hereditary hemorrhagic telangiectasia; HHT) is an autosomal dominant thinning of blood vessel walls, typically affecting the upper GI tract. Rupture presents as proximal GI bleeding. Patients may present with hematemesis, melena, heme-positive stools, and less commonly, hematochezia. Treatment involves estrogen therapy, endovascular embolization, electrocautery or laser surgery, and open surgery.

REFERENCES

1. Cronenwett JL, Johnston KW, Rutherford RB. Mesenteric vascular disease. In Cronenwett JL, Johnston KW, eds. *Rutherford's Vascular Surgery*, 7th ed. Philadelphia: Saunders-Elsevier; 2010.
2. West B, Mitchell KA. Vascular disorders of the GI tract. In Odze RD, Goldblum JR, Crawford JM, eds. *Surgical Pathology of the GI Tract, Liver, Biliary Tract, and Pancreas*. Philadelphia: Saunders-Elsevier; 2004.

CHAPTER 20 ■ UPPER GI BLEEDING

Alireza Sedarat, MD

OVERVIEW

- Upper gastrointestinal (GI) bleeding traditionally refers to hemorrhage from the GI tract proximal to the ligament of Treitz. It is perhaps more useful to categorize GI bleeding into foregut, midgut, and hindgut causes to reflect endoscopic approaches (esophagogastroduodenoscopy, [EGD], enteroscopy, or colonoscopy, respectively). For the purposes of this chapter, unless otherwise stated, upper GI bleeding (UGIB) refers to foregut bleeding.
- The initial management of all patients with bleeding depends on effective airway management, volume resuscitation, risk stratification, management of medical comorbidities, and careful selection of patients who would benefit from urgent endoscopy.
- Comorbidities that should be assessed include presence of portal hypertension, significant cardiopulmonary or renal disease, history of malignancy, and use of anticoagulation or antiplatelet therapy. Nonsteroidal anti-inflammatory drug (NSAID) use history should also be sought.
- Severe GI bleeding is defined as hematemesis, melena, hematochezia, or positive gastric lavage with associated hemodynamic compromise, drop in hemoglobin level of > 2 g/dL, or transfusion of > 2 units of packed red blood cells (PRBCs).

PRESENTATION

- UGIB can present as hematemesis, melena, and/or hematochezia. Although traditional teaching states that sources as far distally as the proximal colon can result in melenic stool, in practice this is highly uncommon in the ambulatory patient. About 80% of patients with melena will have a source identifiable with push enteroscopy (i.e., proximal jejunum or higher).
- Hematochezia often results from a midgut or hindgut source of bleeding, but foregut bleeding can cause hematochezia often enough (17%) that it should be considered in every patient, especially with a history of cirrhosis or peptic ulcer disease.
- Patients presenting with bleeding as the admitting diagnosis have a better prognosis than those who have been hospitalized for another illness and develop bleeding.

DIFFERENTIAL DIAGNOSIS

Peptic ulcer disease (PUD; 38%), gastric or esophageal varices (16%), esophagitis (13%), neoplasia, angioma, Mallory-Weiss tear, Dieulafoy's lesion, hemobilia, hemosuccus pancreaticus, vascular-enteric fistula

PRE-ENDOSCOPY MANAGEMENT

- Airway protection, adequate vascular access, volume resuscitation, reversal of coagulopathy as necessary, and management of comorbid conditions take priority.
- If cirrhosis or portal hypertension is present or suspected, pre-EGD treatment with IV octreotide (50 µg bolus and 50 µg/hr drip for 72 hours) and antibiotics (ceftriaxone, norfloxacin, ciprofloxacin).
- Post-EGD proton pump inhibitor (PPI) infusion improves rebleeding rates and outcomes of ulcers with high-risk features. Pre-EGD PPI may downgrade the endoscopic lesion, but no clear benefit of infusion prior to endoscopy has been shown for patient outcomes (although this is often done in practice).
- Risk stratification tools (such as the Rockall, Blatchford, or AIMS65 scores) can be used to prognosticate and may help select patients more likely to benefit from urgent EGD.
- Nasogastric (NG) tube lavage can provide diagnosis and prognosis of UGIB (especially in the absence of hematemesis), but routine use and effect on patient outcomes have been challenged.

ENDOSCOPY

- Urgent endoscopy (i.e., within 12–24 hours of presentation) is indicated for patients with severe bleeding and evidence of ongoing acute blood loss.
- Goal of endoscopy is definitive diagnosis of the bleeding lesion and application of the appropriate hemostasis to prevent ongoing bleeding or rebleeding.
- In a proportion of severe bleeding, clots can obscure the bleeding site and impair definitive diagnosis and hemostasis. Approaches include suction through a large channel endoscope, attaching suction directly to the instrument channel, dilution with hydrogen peroxide, use of an overtube, mechanical removal, patient repositioning (with airway protected), and pre-EGD IV promotility agents.
- Risk stratification
  - Ulcers (rebleeding rate without endoscopic therapy): arterial spurting (90%) > nonbleeding visible vessel (50%) > adherent clot (33%) > oozing (10%) > flat pigmented spot (7%) > clean based (3%)

Chapter 20: Upper GI Bleeding

- Varices: active bleeding > platelet plug > red marks (vein-on-vein, cherry spot, red wale, etc.)
- Hemostasis maneuvers for selected lesions
  - Ulcers: combination therapy with:
    - 1:10000 epinephrine injection in 1 cc aliquots.
    - Multipolar electrocautery: 10Fr bipolar probe, 12–16W, 8–10 sec pulses of coaptive coagulation until obliteration of vessel.
    - Hemoclips.
    - Adherent clots can be gently cold snared off down to the pedicle to reveal the underlying stigmata and apply hemostasis.
  - Esophageal or junctional varices
    - Endoscopic rubber band ligation (EBL) starting distally and applying at least two bands per column
    - Sclerotherapy: intra- and/or paravariceal injection of 1–2 cc aliquots of sclerosant (such as 2 cc ethanolamine + 1 cc ethanol)
  - Gastric varices
    - Intravariceal injection of cyanoacrylate or thrombin is effective, but not Food and Drug Administration (FDA)–approved in the United States outside of research protocol, and there is a risk of serious embolism.
    - Sclerosant injection may be effective for immediate hemostasis, but the rebleeding rate is high.
    - EBL alone for large gastric varices is not recommended because post-EBL bleeding can be massive and life-threatening.
    - Transjugular intrahepatic portosystemic shunt (TIPS) or balloon-occluded retrograde transvenous obliteration (BRTO) is often considered when endoscopic means are unavailable or ineffective.

POST-ENDOSCOPY MANAGEMENT

- For high-risk ulcers: IV PPI infusion should be continued for 72 hours and then oral PPI for 12 weeks.
- For esophageal varices: IV octreotide should be continued for 72 hours, antibiotics for 5–7 days, repeat EGD for EBL in 7–10 days, oral PPIs continued until variceal obliteration is confirmed. Consider beta blockers for those that will tolerate.
- Routine second-look endoscopy is not recommended but may be considered if effective hemostasis was not performed or if visualization was suboptimal due to obscuring blood/clots.
- *Helicobacter pylori* status should be determined for all PUD patients and treatment to eradication administered if positive.
- Repeat endoscopy for additional hemostasis is indicated for evidence of acute rebleeding. In cases where endoscopic therapy is ineffective, angiographic or surgical approaches are considered next.

REFERENCES

1. Barkun AN, Bardou M, Kuipers EJ, et al. International consensus recommendations on the management of patients with nonvariceal upper gastrointestinal bleeding. *Ann Intern Med.* 2010;152:101–13.
2. Savides TJ, Jensen DM. Gastrointestinal bleeding. In: Feldman M, Friedman LS, Brandt LJ, eds. *Sleisinger and Fordtran's Gastrointestinal and Liver Disease.* Vol. 1. 9th ed. Philadelphia: Elsevier; 2010: 293–4.

CHAPTER 21 ■ LOWER GI BLEEDING

Parambir S. Dulai, MBBS and Gareth S. Dulai, MD

OVERVIEW

- Lower gastrointestinal (GI) bleeding (LGIB) is defined as bleeding that emanates from the colon or rectum.
- LGIB can be broadly classified as overt (hematochezia or melena) versus occult, painful versus painless, and acute (≤ 3 days) versus chronic.
- Acute overt painless LGIB is common in adults and most cases will resolve spontaneously, thereby allowing for a nonurgent evaluation.
- Severe LGIB is defined by ongoing bleeding often associated with hemodynamic instability, anemia, and the need for packed red blood cell transfusion.
- Adult patients with severe acute overt painless LGIB require urgent evaluation as outlined in this chapter.

INITIAL ASSESSMENT

- Key features of the history include duration and frequency of bleeding, color of stools, and symptoms of hemodynamic compromise (e.g., fatigue, tachypnea, syncope). Use of antithrombotic medications, comorbidity, and prior history of bleeding, surgery, or radiation therapy should be noted.
- The physical exam may help to quantify the extent of blood loss, with tachycardia (> 100/min), hypotension (systolic < 115 mmHg), and postural changes being the most predictive. A careful digital rectal exam should be done to exclude anorectal pathology.
- Initial laboratory evaluation should contain a complete blood count, a coagulation profile, and a sample for blood type and cross match.
- Consider nasogastric tube (NGT) lavage to exclude upper GI source. If negative, consider leaving NGT in place to facilitate bowel purge.

INITIAL MANAGEMENT

- Two large-bore peripheral IV catheters or a central venous line are recommended.
- Volume resuscitation should be done using crystalloid solutions (i.e., normal saline or lactated Ringer's).
- Supplemental oxygen should be given via nasal cannula.

- Blood transfusion should be given based on patient's hemodynamics, age, bleeding rate, and comorbidity.
- Many clinicians use a cut-point value of Hgb < 9–10 g/dL for transfusion, aware of the limitations of initial Hgb values prior to intravenous (IV) fluid resuscitation and equilibration.
- Thrombocytopenia and coagulopathy should be corrected with platelets and fresh frozen plasma. A heuristic goal is platelet count > 50,000 and international normalized ratio (INR) < 1.5.
- Patients should be triaged to the appropriate level of care (monitored or intensive care unit [ICU] bed) based on the severity of bleeding, age, and comorbidity.

DIFFERENTIAL DIAGNOSIS

After initial resuscitation efforts and triage, a more detailed history can be obtained to help elucidate the underlying etiology (see **Table 21-1**).

Table 21-1 Common Causes of Severe Painless Lower Gastrointestinal Bleeding

Etiology	History
Diverticular disease	Incidence increases with age; stops spontaneously in most; right > left colon; high rate of recurrence.
Post-polypectomy	Acute (within 24 hours) or delayed (within 2 weeks of colonoscopy); use of anticoagulant or antiplatelet meds
Radiation proctitis/telangiectasia	History of abdominal-pelvic radiation therapy
Sporadic vascular ectasia	May have had prior normal endoscopy; may have ESRD, vWD, AS, or anticoagulant/antiplatelet use; characteristic red fern appearance; often multiple; often in right colon

ESRD = end-stage renal disease; vWD = von Willebrand disease; AS = aortic stenosis

DIAGNOSIS (SEE FIGURE 21-1)

- Early colonoscopy (within 12–24 hours) following a rapid bowel purge (4–8 liters polyethylene glycol over 3–4 hours orally or via nasogastric tube until rectal effluent is clear) is safe, improves diagnostic yield, and may improve outcomes through targeted therapy.
- Metoclopramide, 10 mg intravenously, may be given before the purge and repeated every 3–4 hours to facilitate gastric emptying and reduce nausea.
- Mesenteric angiography can be diagnostic and therapeutic for patients who are unable to undergo endoscopy due to hemodynamic instability or those who fail endoscopic therapy.

Chapter 21: Lower GI Bleeding

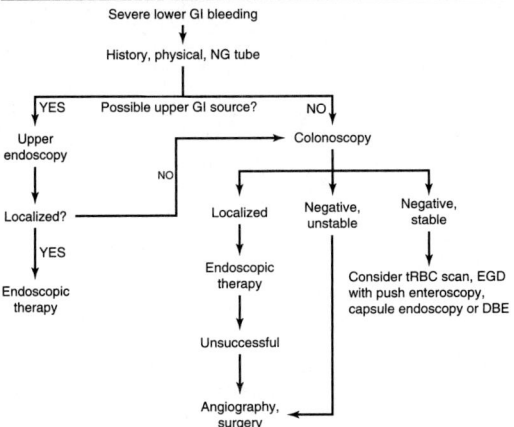

Figure 21-1 Diagnostic algorithm for adults with severe acute painless lower gastrointestinal bleeding

DBE = double balloon enteroscopy; EGD = esophagogastroduodenoscopy

- Nuclear scintigraphy (technetium-99m pertechnetate tagged red blood cell [RBC] scan) may be a useful diagnostic test in cases of recurrent bleeding when other methods have failed to localize a bleeding site.
- CT angiography may be a sensitive alternative to scintigraphy or angiography, particularly for angiodysplasia.

TREATMENT

Several common endoscopic treatment modalities can be used to achieve hemostasis when the source of the LGIB is identified (see **Table 21-2**).

DIVERTICULAR BLEED
- Left-sided lesions are more common, but right-sided diverticula are more likely to bleed.
- Treat endoscopically if stigmata identified (bleeding and nonbleeding visible vessels, adherent clots), but do not treat if presumed diverticular bleed.

Table 21-2 Common Endoscopic Treatments for Hemostasis

Treatment	Important points
Sub-mucosal epinephrine	- Temporary control - May improve visualization and facilitate definitive treatment
Coagulation techniques	- risk of colonic damage and perforation with both contact (e.g. BICAP) and non-contact (e.g. APC) modalities. Treatment of choice for vascular ectasia. Useful for diverticular and post polypectomy stigmata when unable to deploy clips.
Hemostatic clips	- Durable with no thermal risk

- Choice of intervention will depend on location and comorbid conditions, with coagulation techniques generally being avoided when the hemorrhage is located at the base of the diverticulum due to the risk of perforation.
- Once hemostasis has been achieved, a submucosal tattoo should be placed around the lesion to allow identification of the site in case repeat colonoscopy or surgery is required.

POST-POLYPECTOMY BLEED

- Treat endoscopically if stigmata of ulcer or hemorrhage are seen.
- Immediate bleeding after polypectomy can be stopped by regrasping the pedicle with a snare and holding pressure on the pedicle to stop blood flow.
- Massive immediate and delayed post-polypectomy bleeding can be also treated with loops or band ligation.

SPORADIC VASCULAR ECTASIA

Endoscopic treatment for active bleeding and consider treatment for non-bleeding ectasias when an alternative bleeding site cannot be identified.

REFERENCES

1. Ghassemi KA, Jensen DM. Lower GI bleeding: epidemiology and management. *Curr Gastroenterol Rep.* 2013;15(7):333–5.
2. Lhewa DY, Strate LL. Pros and cons of colonoscopy in management of acute lower gastrointestinal bleeding. *World J Gastroenterol.* 2012;18(11):1185–90.

CHAPTER 22 ■ ESOPHAGEAL CANCER

Svetlana Kotova, MD and Jay M. Lee, MD

OVERVIEW

- Esophageal cancer is relatively uncommon, accounting for ~18,000 diagnoses in 2013.
- Adenocarcinoma and squamous cell carcinoma comprise the majority of cases.
- Multidisciplinary care is often needed for successful management. Tumor staging is critical for a personalized approach to treatment.

PRESENTATION

- Most common histologic types of esophageal cancer are adenocarcinoma and squamous cell carcinoma—accounting for 90%. Lymphoma, carcinoid, melanoma, and leiomyosarcoma of the esophagus rarely occur.
- Slowly progressive dysphagia from tumor obstruction is the most common symptom (~75%) irrespective of type of cancer, and it is frequently accompanied by significant weight loss. Severity of malnutrition correlates with worse overall prognosis. Other symptoms such as odynophagia, early satiety, fullness, and cough are much less common but, if present, are likely due to locally advanced disease.
- Patient profile can be helpful in predicting the type:
  - Adenocarcinoma: history of reflux, Barrett's esophagus, prior history of radiation; usually located in distal esophagus and gastroesophageal junction.
  - Squamous cell carcinoma: history of smoking, alcohol use, head and neck cancers, achalasia, corrosive injury, prior radiation; mid-esophageal location.

PATHOPHYSIOLOGY

Lymphatics of the esophageal wall are located in submucosal layer (see **Figure 22-1**) and allow for early tumor metastasis to the lymph nodes (LN). LN involvement increases with depth of tumor—6% for T1a, 31% for T1b, 77% for T2, and 85% for T3—thus making LN assessment an important part of clinical staging.

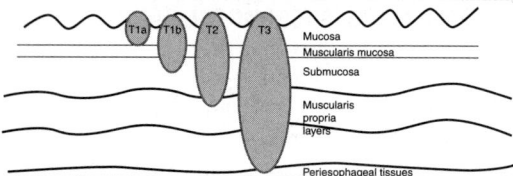

Figure 22-1 Tumor staging (T) of esophageal cancer

DIFFERENTIAL DIAGNOSIS IN PATIENTS WITH DYSPHAGIA

- Benign causes: leiomyoma, diverticulum, esophagitis, Schatzki ring, hiatal hernia, stricture (corrosive or peptic), esophageal motility disorders.
- Malignant causes: esophageal cancer and metastatic cancers of other origin must always be kept in mind based on patient's profile.

EVALUATION AND STAGING

- Esophagogram/upper GI series: will show a stricture or an irregularly shaped mass. It will help to rule out esophageal diverticulum, rings, or hiatal hernia. Leiomyoma will have a characteristic smooth appearance.
- Endoscopy (esophagogastroduodenoscopy; EGD): documents location of the mass (upper/mid/lower esophageal), presence of mucosal changes such as Barrett's esophagus, and biopsy to secure tissue diagnosis.
- Staging approach is summarized in **Figure 22-2**. Staging is based on TNM, which is obtained from the following studies:
  - Endoscopic ultrasound (EUS): determines extend of tumor (T) and local invasion of adjacent organs (pleura, aorta, vertebral bodies). It also documents involvement of local and regional LNs (N). Hypoechoic or enlarged LNs during EUS are considered abnormal.
  - Computed tomography (CT) of chest/abdomen (with IV and oral contrast): esophageal tumor is not visualized well, but CT allows one to evaluate regional lymph node involvement (N), organ invasion, and distant metastasis (M). Biopsy of suspicious lesions can be performed either with CT guidance or during EUS.
  - Positron emission tomography (PET): esophageal cancer is typically very fluorodeoxyglucose (FDG) avid. Similar to CT, PET evaluates distant disease (M) and areas of local disease (N), which are not in close proximity to the primary tumor. Its best application is as an

Chapter 22: Esophageal Cancer

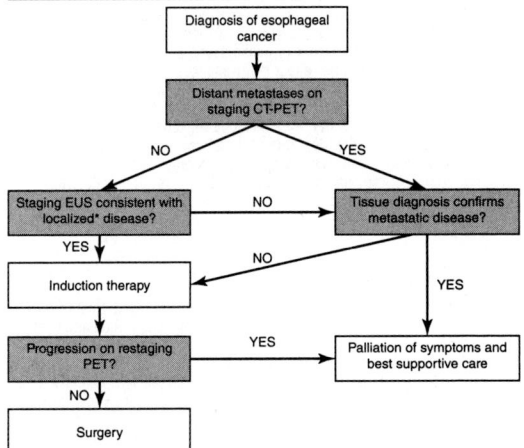

Figure 22-2 Esophageal cancer evaluation.

* Localized disease: T2N0/1, T3N0/1

initial staging tool and restaging after a course of induction therapy to monitor response and guide further therapy.
- Additional studies: bronchoscopy (evaluate airway invasion) and laparoscopy (suspected peritoneal spread of the primary tumor) can be done in select cases.

TREATMENT

Correct clinical staging is crucial because choice of treatment depends on clinical stage.

LOCALLY ADVANCED CANCER (T2N1, T3N0/1)

- Most patients with dysphagia will present with locally advanced disease, but as long as there is no evidence of metastases, they will be candidates for resection after induction/neoadjuvant therapy.

- The current approach is trimodality therapy—chemotherapy, concurrent radiation, and surgical resection—in patients with good performance status. Benefit of neoadjuvant therapy has been demonstrated in several studies and a meta-analysis.
- Cisplatin/fluorouracil is the most common regimen used. Alternative is carboplatin/paclitaxel. Radiation doses vary from 35 to 50 Grey. Survival up to 35–45% at 5 years can be expected.
- For patients who are not able to undergo surgery due to medical comorbidities, definitive chemo-radiotherapy can be considered. Induction course for patients with T2N0 is debated. However, because chances of having pathological LN involvement are over 70%, we believe these patients will benefit from induction systemic therapy.

METASTATIC CANCER
- About one-third of patients will have metastases at the time of initial diagnosis. In these patients, focus is on symptom palliation and control of tumor.
- Self-expandable metal stents (SEMS) have an important role in symptom palliation in patients with metastatic disease but should not be used routinely in patients who are anticipated to proceed with surgery. Five-year survival is under 5%.

EARLY CANCER
- Small number of patients will be diagnosed as a result of endoscopic surveillance for Barrett's esophagus at a very early stage (T1a/b on EUS). Endoscopic mucosal resection (EMR) should be performed because it can be curative when carcinoma is intramucosal and there is no LN involvement.
- If deep margin contains carcinoma after EMR, patients should proceed to surgical resection. Neoadjuvant therapy is usually omitted in early stage. Five-year survival is about 80%.

CONSULTATIONS

Successful treatment of esophageal cancer depends on multispecialty approach to coordinate prompt care and address all aspects of staging and treatment. The following specialties should be involved from the time of diagnosis to ensure best care: medical and radiation oncologist, gastroenterologist, thoracic surgeon, nutritionist/dietician, and palliative care specialist.

REFERENCES

1. Rice TW, Blackstone EH, Rusch VW. 7th edition of the AJCC Cancer Staging Manual: esophagus and esophagogastric junction. *Ann Surg Oncol*. 2010;17:1721–24.
2. van Hagen P, Hulschof MC, van Lanschot JJ, et al. Preoperative chemoradiotherapy for esophageal and junctional cancer. *N Engl J Med*. 2012;366(22):2074–84.
3. Sjoquist KM, Burmeister BH, Smithers BM, et al. Survival after neoadjuvant chemotherapy or chemoradiotherapy for resectable oesophageal carcinoma: an updated meta-analysis. *Lancet Oncol*. 2011;12:681–92.

CHAPTER 23 ■ GASTRIC CANCER

Mariela Macias, MD and Zev Wainberg, MD

OVERVIEW

- Gastric cancer is the fourth and fifth most common malignancy in males and females, respectively, and the second leading cause of cancer death worldwide. In the United States the incidence in 2013 was roughly 21,000 cases with approximately 11,000 cancer-related deaths. Globally, gastric cancer is more common in Asia, Eastern Europe, and South America than in Western Europe and the United States.
- These regional differences are seen anatomically as well. In the United States, the most common sites of gastric cancers are proximal in locations (gastroesophageal junction, gastric cardia), and in Asia most gastric cancers present in the body and distal parts of the stomach.
- More than 90% of gastric cancers are adenocarcinomas, with the remainder being lymphomas, sarcomas (e.g., gastrointestinal stromal tumor; GIST), or neuroendocrine tumors. Furthermore, pathological variants of adenocarcinomas can be divided by the Lauren classification into the following histological subtypes: *intestinal* type more commonly seen in endemic and high *Helicobacter pylori* areas, *diffuse* seen more commonly in the Western world and more common in hereditary syndromes.
- Globally, the incidence of gastric cancer has been declining by about 2% per year, which is likely partially due to the eradication of *H. pylori* bacterial infection. Other modifiable risk factors such as changes in dietary habits that improved after the wide use of refrigeration (e.g., decrease in salt consumption, pickled and/or smoked foods), and increased consumption of fresh fruits and vegetables have also contributed to this decline.
- Nonmodifiable risk factors for gastric cancer include male sex, atrophic gastritis, advanced age, blood type A, primary family history, and rare genetic syndromes (i.e., hereditary diffuse gastric cancer related to defects in E-cadherin).

PRESENTATION

- May present with unintentional weight loss, early satiety, and abdominal pain. Early stage disease is often asymptomatic. Red flags that should warrant further workup are: new onset dyspepsia in older adult (> 55 years), family history of gastric cancers, unintentional weight

loss, midepigastric pain persisting despite proton pump inhibitor, dysphagia, unexplained iron-deficiency anemia, and gastrointestinal bleeding.
- Palpable supraclavicular and periumbilical lymph nodes (Virchow's and Sister Mary Joseph nodules) are rarely seen and represent metastatic disease.

DIFFERENTIAL DIAGNOSIS

Includes peptic ulcer disease, gastric polyps, and other types of malignancies: lymphomas, sarcomas, carcinoid tumors, and metastatic carcinomas.

PATHOPHYSIOLOGY

While there is no consensus, may include the initiation of inflammatory pathways mediated by *H. pylori* infection, which leads to interaction of micro-environment and activation/disruption of regulatory transcription factors leading to tumorigenesis.

DIAGNOSIS

- There are currently no standard population screening programs in low endemic areas such as the United States, and the diagnosis is driven by the clinical presentation. Ultimately, diagnosis requires direct imaging of gastric mucosa with an esophagogastroduodenoscopy (EGD) and *multiple biopsies* of suspicious lesions with at least six to eight tissue samples.
- If biopsies from a suspicious lesion are negative, repeat endoscopy with more extensive biopsies and possibly endoscopic ultrasound (EUS) may be needed to avoid sampling error. Once gastric cancer is established, EUS and positron emission tomography (PET)/computed tomography (CT) imaging can be added to determine staging and surgical resectability.

TREATMENT (SEE TABLE 23-1)

- Can be grouped into three categories: immediately surgically resectable, midstage disease requiring multimodality treatment for resectability, and unresectable/metastatic gastric cancer for palliation. A multimodality treatment plan should include medical oncology, gastroenterology, radiation oncology, and surgical oncology. Early disease can be treated with potential endoscopic mucosal resection (EMR) if

Chapter 23: Gastric Cancer

Table 23-1 Treatment Strategies for Gastric Cancer

Gastric Cancer Stage	Type of Surgery Margins	LN Dissection (>15 LN)	Neo-adjuvant Chemotherapy	Adjuvant Chemotherapy (Cis/5FU+/− Epirubicin)	Adjuvant Chemoradiaton (5 FU Derivative)
Early (T1-T2, N0) Resectable	R0	Yes/ No	Sometimes (EGJ)	Yes	Only if LN +
	R1/R2	Yes/No	Sometimes	Yes	Yes, Preferred
Early Advanced Resectable (T3-T4 N1)	R0	Yes/ No	Yes	Yes	Yes, Preferred
	R1/R2	Yes/ No	Yes	Yes	Yes, Preferred
Advanced/ Mets	N/A	N/A	N/A	N/a	Chemotherapy +/− HER2 inhibitor (trastuzumab)

tumors are less than 1.5 cm, have low-grade histology, and are confined to the mucosa.
- Subtotal gastrectomies are comparable to total gastrectomies with less morbidity. The goal of surgery is to achieve an R0 resection with negative surgical margins of 3–4 cm. If R0 margins are achieved along with adequate lymph node (LN) dissection of at least 15 LN (D1 plus lymph node dissection of perigastric LN *plus* further dissection such as left gastric, or celiac LN, which are usually done in D2, a more extensive LN dissection), then adjuvant chemotherapy without radiation is recommended.
- Postoperative chemoradiation is usually done for microscopically or macroscopically involved margins and LN positivity and is usually done with fluoropyrimidine-based treatment.
- Perioperative chemotherapy (neo and adjuvant) can be done for high-risk disease and gastroesophageal junction tumors. In advanced or metastatic disease, the preferred regimens involve doublet therapy including platinum salts and fluoropyrimidines. The HER2 oncogene is considered positive in about 20% of gastric cancers, and if immunohistochemistry is 3+ or 2+, trastuzumab should be added to the regimen.

REFERENCES

1. Wadhwa R, Taketa T, Sudo K, Blum MA, Ajani JA. Modern oncological approaches to gastric adenocarcinoma. *Gastroenterol Clin N Am.* 2013;42(2):359–9.
2. Chung HW, Lim JB. Role of the tumor microenvironment in the pathogenesis of gastric carcinoma. *World J Gastroenterol.* 2014;20(7):1667–80.

CHAPTER 24 ■ PANCREATIC CANCER

Alexandra Drakaki, MD

OVERVIEW

- Pancreatic cancer remains the fourth leading cause of cancer-related deaths in the United States. The incidence of the disease approximates the mortality rate, which ultimately reflects the poor prognosis for this tumor.
- Most patients are over 65 years old at diagnosis, and African Americans have the worst prognosis.

PRESENTATION

- Patients typically present with a vague, nonspecific abdominal pain, and dyspepsia. Up to 70% will have biliary tract obstruction, and they may also have jaundice, pruritus, nausea, and vomiting.
- New onset diabetes often precedes the diagnosis of pancreatic cancer, and characteristic symptoms are those related to depression and thrombophlebitis (Trousseau's syndrome).
- As in most malignancies, patients will eventually present with fatigue, anorexia, and weight loss that often leads them to seek medical attention.

DIFFERENTIAL DIAGNOSIS

- Pancreatic malignancies are divided into two categories, the exocrine and the neuroendocrine cancers.
- The exocrine tumors are adenocarcinoma (up to 90%), acinar cancer (usually in younger patients), and cystic tumor—which is less aggressive.
- It is important to distinguish between exocrine and endocrine malignancies because the neuroendocrine tumors are more indolent.

RISK FACTORS

- Several risk factors have been linked to pancreatic cancer. Tobacco smoking or chewing history exists in up to 30% of the cases while the rest are chronic pancreatitis—either familial or acquired—(5%), increasing age (> 60 years), male gender, and family history (5–10%).

- There is a weaker association with factors such as high-fat diet, diabetes, post-cholecystectomy, and post-gastrectomy.
- The familial syndromes with the involved genetic abnormalities are Lynch syndrome (hMLH1, h MSH2), familial atypical mole melanoma syndrome (CDKN2A), familial pancreatitis syndrome (RPSS1), Peutz-Jaegers syndrome (STK11/LKB1), hereditary breast-ovarian syndrome (BRCA1, BRCA2, PALB2), cystic fibrosis (CFTR), familial polyposis syndrome (FAP), ataxia-telangiectasia (ATM), Li-Fraumeni syndrome (p53), and familial pancreatic cancer.

DIAGNOSIS

- *Computed tomography (CT) scan with pancreatic protocol* is the most commonly used diagnostic modality, given that patients with tumors located in the head of the pancreas may present with biliary obstruction.
- *Endoscopic retrograde cholangiopancreatography (ERCP)* is desired because it helps with diagnosis (brushings for cytology and/or tumor biopsy) and temporary symptom control (stent placement).
- *Endoscopic ultrasound* is used especially for tumors in the tail of the pancreas.
- *Magnetic resonance cholangiopancreatography (MRCP)* gives more detailed information of the surrounding tissues and helps determine the resectability of larger tumors.
- *Percutaneous biopsy* could be part of the diagnostic workup (especially for lesions that are deemed unresectable). Ultimately, tissue diagnosis is required prior to discussing the different treatment options.
- *CA 19-9* is a mucinous glycoprotein that is used as a tumor marker typically included in the initial diagnostic workup. Of note, not all patients have elevated levels (patients who are Lewis antigen negative cannot synthesize CA 19-9), and there are other nonmalignant causes that could elevate it (e.g., pancreatitis, cholangitis, biliary obstruction).

STAGING

TNM system is used for staging; however, in practice, a newly diagnosed pancreatic cancer falls into one of the following four groups: (1) localized resectable, (2) localized borderline resectable, (3) locally advanced unresectable, and (4) metastatic. This categorization is clinically important and dictates the management.

PROGNOSIS

Factors that are linked to poor prognosis are large tumor size, positive margins postoperatively, lymph node involvement (especially if multiple lymph nodes), poorly differentiated tumors, and CA19-9 that is significantly elevated preoperatively—and does not decrease or normalize postoperatively.

TREATMENT (SEE FIGURE 24-1)

- The appropriate approach for a newly diagnosed pancreatic cancer is primarily dependent on the resectability of the tumor. The input of the surgeon and the radiologist is critical in that decision making.
- What determines resectability is absence of extra-pancreatic disease and retroperitoneal lymph node involvement; patency of the superior mesenteric, splenic, and portal veins; and no evidence of encasement of the celiac or superior mesenteric artery.

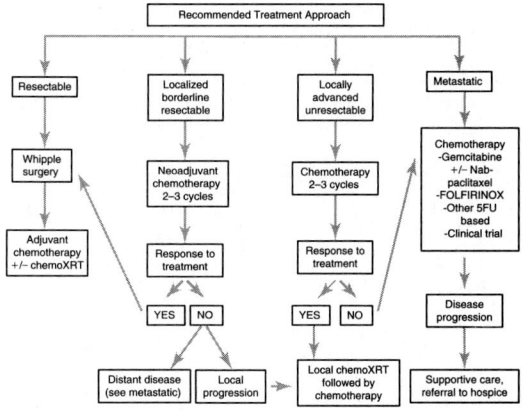

Figure 24-1 Recommended treatment approach for patients with pancreatic cancer.

- Patients with early stage localized disease who do not have other comorbidities, and with good performance status, typically undergo Whipple surgery followed by adjuvant single-agent gemcitabine chemotherapy (with or without adjuvant 5-FU based chemoradiation).
- For borderline resectable tumors, a common approach is to start with neoadjuvant chemotherapy such as gemcitabine or FOLFIRINOX depending on patient characteristics. If after two to three cycles there is response to treatment based on radiographic and clinical findings, then the patient should have the option of surgery (if complete resection will be feasible) followed by adjuvant chemotherapy combined with chemoradiotherapy targeting the surgical bed.
- Patients with locally advanced, but unresectable disease, typically receive a few cycles of chemotherapy. If the restaging imaging does not reveal any signs of metastatic disease, then based on an expert's opinion, patients may benefit from concomitant radiation continued by more chemotherapy—which will be chosen based on patient's characteristics and response to the initial chemotherapy regimen.
- The cornerstone of care for metastatic disease is gemcitabine, which primarily improves quality of life. Recent data support the use of gemcitabine in combination with nab-paclitaxel. FOLFIRINOX should be used in patients with good performance status, because while it improves survival it is more toxic.
- Other regimens, including 5-FU based or irinotecan, can be considered. Eventually, patients with disease progression should be evaluated either for a clinical trial or for enrollment to hospice.

REFERENCES

1. Conroy T, Desseigne F, Ychou M, et al. *N Engl J Med.* 2011 May 12;364(19):1817–25.
2. National Comprehensive Cancer Network (NCCN). *Clinical Practice Guidelines in Oncology. Version 1: Pancreatic Adenocarcinoma.* Fort Washington, PA: NCCN; 2013.

CHAPTER 25 ■ PANCREATIC CYSTS

Rabindra R. Watson, MD

OVERVIEW

- Pancreatic cysts are a heterogeneous group of lesions that encompass a spectrum of benign, premalignant, and malignant diagnoses (see **Table 25-1**).

Table 25-1 Cyst Types and Characteristics

	IPMN	MCN	SPN	SCN	CPEN	PC
Age	60–70	40–60	20–40	60–70	Any	Any
Sex	M = F	F > M	F > M	F > M	M = F	M = F
Location	Head > body/tail	Body/tail > head	Any	Body/tail > head	Any	Any
Treatment	MD – surgery SB – variable	Surgery	Surgery	PRN	Surgery	PRN

IPMN = intraductal papillary mucinous neoplasms, MD = main duct, PRN = as needed, SB = side branch, MCN = mucinous cystic neoplasm, SPN = solid pseudopapillary neoplasm, SCN = serous cystadenoma, CPEN = cystic pancreatic endocrine neoplasms, PC = pseudocysts

- Pancreatic cystic neoplasms (PCNs) are increasingly recognized due to advances in imaging techniques and increasing awareness, with an estimated prevalence of 10–20% in cross-sectional imaging studies.
- The prevalence of PCNs increases with age, with up to 20–40% of patients harboring pancreatic cysts in the 7th to 8th decades of life.
- The aim of diagnostic work up is to differentiate between premalignant and benign cyst types, and identify malignant lesions.
- When cross-sectional imaging is equivocal, endoscopic ultrasound with fine-needle aspiration (EUS-FNA) is useful for cyst fluid analysis (**Table 25-2**).

Table 25-2 EUS-FNA Cyst Fluid Analysis

	IPMN	MCN	SPN	SCN	CPEN	PC
CEA	↑	↑	↓	↓	↓	↓
Amylase	↑	↓	↓	↓	↓	↑
Appearance	Clear, viscous	Clear, viscous	Clear, bloody	Thin, bloody	Clear, bloody	Yellow, brown, thick

CEA = carcinoembryonic antigen, IPMN = intraductal papillary mucinous neoplasms, MCN = mucinous cystic neoplasm, SPN = solid pseudopapillary neoplasm, SCN = serous cystadenoma, CPEN = cystic pancreatic endocrine neoplasms, PC = pseudocysts

DIFFERENTIAL DIAGNOSIS AND TREATMENT OF DIFFERENT PCNs

INTRADUCTAL PAPILLARY MUCINOUS NEOPLASMS (IPMNs)

- IPMNs are classified as main duct type (MD-IPMN), side branch duct type (BD-IPMN), or mixed type (involving both side branch and main ducts).
- IPMNs are typically diagnosed in the 6th to 7th decades of life; there is no gender predilection.
- MD-IPMNs arise in the proximal duct in two-thirds of patients, commonly presenting with abdominal pain (55%), weight loss (45%), jaundice (17%), and pancreatitis (15%).
- MD-IPMNs are characterized by dilation of the main pancreatic duct (> 6 mm), with a pathognomonic "fish-mouth" appearance of the ampulla filled with mucin (present in < 15% of cases).
- MD-IPMNs harbor malignancy in up to 40% of cases at diagnosis, with a poor 5-year survival (31–54%).
- Surgical resection is the treatment of choice, either by Whipple resection or distal pancreatectomy based on lesion location.
- In contrast, BD-IPMNs are typically asymptomatic, may be multifocal in 21–41%, and may appear as a single cyst or multicystic lesions.
- Unifocal BD-IPMN is the most common incidentally diagnosed PCN.
- Treatment of BD-IPMN is governed by the Fukuoka guidelines published in 2012.
- Immediate surgical resection is indicated by the presence of "high-risk stigmata" of malignant disease including: obstructive jaundice, enhancing solid component in the cyst, main duct size > 10 mm, rapidly growing cyst size, and high-grade cellular atypia.
- In the absence of high-risk stigmata, "worrisome features" are sought that include: pancreatitis, cyst size > 3 cm, thickened or enhancing cyst wall, nonenhancing mural nodule, main pancreatic duct diameter 5–9 mm, abrupt change in main duct caliber with distal pancreatic atrophy and lymphadenopathy.

- The presence of worrisome features is an indication for EUS-FNA for confirmation of these findings and cyst fluid analysis.
- In the absence of high-risk stigmata or worrisome features, surveillance with serial imaging and/or EUS is required, with intervals determined by cyst size.
- Multifocal SB-IPMN theoretically carries a higher risk of malignancy, though the lesion at highest oncologic risk per SB-IPMN protocol dictates treatment.
- Mixed types demonstrate pathologic involvement of both the main duct and side branches and are treated as main duct IPMNs.

MUCINOUS CYSTIC NEOPLASMS (MCNs)

- MCNs comprise 25% of all PCN and arise commonly in women (> 95%) in the 5th decade, in the pancreatic body and tail (> 95%), and carry malignant potential.
- They are typically asymptomatic though may present with pain or pancreatitis.
- MCNs appear as a solitary cyst, although they may be septated and have peripheral calcifications.
- The treatment for all MCNs is surgical resection in light of the malignant risk.

SOLID PSEUDOPAPILLARY NEOPLASMS (SPNs)

- SPNs are indolent tumors with malignant potential but an excellent long-term prognosis (5-year postoperative survival of > 95%) appearing as a heterogeneous mass with solid and cystic components.
- They are diagnosed incidentally or may present with mass effect and jaundice.
- SPNs are typically diagnosed in women in the 2nd to 4th decades.
- Surgical resection is indicated in all cases.
- Lifelong postoperative imaging surveillance is indicated due to the risk of recurrence.

SEROUS CYSTADENOMAS (SCAs)

- SCAs are most often incidentally diagnosed in women (75%) in the 6th to 7th decades and comprise 16% of resected PCNs.
- They have a characteristic microcystic appearance, and, when present, a central stellate scar is pathognomonic (30–40%).
- SCAs are benign, thus surgical resection is reserved for symptomatic lesions only.

CYSTIC PANCREATIC ENDOCRINE NEOPLASMS (CPENs)

- CPENs are most commonly diagnosed as part of MEN I, though may arise de novo.

- They comprise 10–17% of resected pancreatic endocrine neoplasms.
- They are often associated with a solid hypervascular mass lesion on CT.
- Surgical resection is indicated for all CPENs.

PSEUDOCYSTS (PCs)

- Pseudocysts arise as sequelae of acute pancreatitis and are not true cysts in that they lack a true epithelial lining.
- They may present with symptoms due to mass effect such as jaundice, early satiety, nausea, and pain.
- In the absence of symptoms, follow-up imaging is sufficient regardless of cyst size, though larger cysts (< 5 cm) are less likely to resolve spontaneously.
- If symptomatic, drainage can be achieved by endoscopic cystogastrostomy or percutaneous drainage. The presence of necrosis requires debridement, either endoscopically or surgically.

REFERENCES

1. Tanaka M, Fernandez-del Castillo C, Adsay V, et al. International consensus guidelines 2012 for the management of IPMN and MCN of the pancreas. *Pancreatol.* 2012;12:183–97.
2. Talukdar R, Reddy DN. Treatment of pancreatic cystic neoplasms: surgery or conservative? *Clin Gastro Hepatol.* 2014;12:145–51.

CHAPTER 26 ■ PANCREATITIS

Andrew H. Nguyen, MD and Timothy R. Donahue, MD

OVERVIEW

- Acute pancreatitis is a disease characterized by localized inflammation of the pancreas.
- Alcohol use and gallstones are the most common causes, although many other etiologies such as metabolic disturbances, obstruction, or medications may less frequently cause pancreatitis.
- The classic presentation is acute onset of mild to severe epigastric pain radiating to the back with associated nausea.
- While most patients follow a mild course of disease, 15–20% of patients may progress to severe acute pancreatitis characterized by organ dysfunction. The initial phase of severe acute pancreatitis is due to a systemic inflammatory response with the later phase due to local pancreatic destruction. The overall mortality rate of acute pancreatitis is about 2–3% and is highest in the subset of patients with severe disease.
- Supportive therapy with intravenous hydration and pain control remains the mainstay of treatment.
- Recurrent pancreatitis can lead to chronic pancreatitis, characterized by irreversible parenchymal fibrosis and damage to the pancreatic duct.

PRESENTATION

- Up to 70% of patients with acute pancreatitis have the classic pattern of symptoms: epigastric pain radiating to the back with associated nausea and vomiting.
- In mild acute pancreatitis, epigastric tenderness on deep palpation may be elicited.
- Severe acute pancreatitis may be present with abdominal rigidity, hypotension, and signs of organ dysfunction. Signs of retroperitoneal hemorrhage may include bruising around the umbilicus (Cullen's sign), along the flanks (Grey Turner's sign), or along the inguinal ligaments (Fox's sign).

DIFFERENTIAL DIAGNOSIS

Cholecystitis, cholangitis, gastritis, duodenal ulcer, small bowel obstruction, viral hepatitis, myocardial infarction, pneumonia, ruptured or dissecting aortic aneurysm

PATHOPHYSIOLOGY

- The inflammatory process of acute pancreatitis is thought to begin in the pancreatic acinar cells with colocalization of pancreatic zymogens and lysozymes in the cytoplasm, resulting in inappropriate activation and "autodigestion."
- This process leads to acinar cell damage, followed by a robust infiltrate of leukocytes, further propagating this inflammatory process.

DIAGNOSIS

- Diagnosis relies on the patient's presentation of epigastric pain accompanied by nausea, followed by clinical suspicion for pursuing a diagnosis of pancreatitis.
- Amylase is a commonly used biochemical marker to diagnose acute pancreatitis. A level of three times the upper limit of normal may be used as the cutoff for diagnosis.
- Serum lipase is a better diagnostic study compared to amylase as it is more sensitive and specific. Lipase tends to remain elevated for as long as a week after onset of disease.
- Abdominal ultrasound may identify an enlarged, hypoechoic pancreas, although about a third of studies are limited by bowel gas, obscuring visualization of the pancreas and peripancreatic areas.
- Computed tomography (CT) is the most valuable imaging modality in diagnosis, and the assessment of severity of acute pancreatitis. All patients scanned for pancreatitis should receive oral and intravenous contrast and follow a pancreatic protocol. Severity may be determined by CT imaging findings of pancreatic edema, fluid collections, and necrosis.

TREATMENT

- Early management of acute pancreatitis should include fluid resuscitation, control of symptoms, and a rapid assessment of severity.
- Prognostication of severity typically relies on evaluation of Ranson's criteria (see **Table 26-1**) within the first 48 hours of admission or APACHE II score for more critically ill patients. A Ranson's criteria score of > 3 has previously been used as a marker of severe disease. Evaluation of

Chapter 26: Pancreatitis

Table 26-1 Ranson's Criteria

At admission	At 48 hours
Age: > 55 years old	Calcium: < 8 mg/dL
WBC: > 16,000 /μL	BUN change: > 1.8 mmol/L (5 mg/dL)
Glucose: > 200 mg/dL	HCT fall: > 10%
LDH: > 350 U/L	Base deficit: > 4 mEq/L
Aspartate aminotransferase (AST or SGOT): > 250 U/L	PaO$_2$: < 60 mmHg
	Fluid seq: > 6 L s

disease severity with CT imaging may be a valuable adjunct to other clinical parameters. It should be noted that neither amylase nor lipase are predictive of disease severity.
- Intravenous fluid resuscitation should be performed to maintain organ perfusion. Close monitoring of vital signs and urine output may assist appropriate resuscitation.
- Parenteral analgesia with morphine, hydromorphone, or other narcotics is most commonly used in acute pancreatitis for controlling pain, especially in patients with poor oral tolerance. Occasionally patient-controlled analgesia and even epidural analgesia may be required in severe cases.
- Antiemetics, such as ondansetron, may alleviate nausea symptoms. With persistent emesis, nasogastric decompression may be necessary.
- Mild hypoxia occurs frequently in severe disease and a chest X-ray should be performed. Nasal cannula oxygen delivery may be appropriate in mild lung dysfunction. In severe disease, endotracheal intubation may be required.
- With prolonged disease where patients are unable to tolerate oral intake for over 7 days, nutritional support with total parenteral nutrition or enteral feeding, preferably via a nasojejunal tube, may be considered.
- Severe acute pancreatitis may result in pancreatic necrosis, which may be identified by contrast-enhanced computerized tomography (CT) scan. Pancreatic necrosis is frequently sterile but can become infected via translocation of intestinal bacteria. If an infection is suspected, it should be documented with a fine needle aspiration and antibiotics (imipenem) started. Infected fluid or necrosis often requires drainage with a percutaneously placed drain or surgical debridement.
- Patients with mild-to-moderate gallstone pancreatitis should undergo cholecystectomy within the index hospitalization; endoscopic sphincterotomy is reserved as an alternative for patients who are unfit to undergo an operation. In patients with severe acute gallstone pancreatitis, endoscopic retrograde cholangiopancreatography (ERCP), and sphincterotomy should be performed within 48 hours of presentation; cholecystectomy should be delayed until symptoms resolve.

- Long-term complications include pancreatic pseudocyst and chronic pancreatitis. Pancreatic pseudocysts by definition do not occur until 4–6 weeks after the onset of symptoms and occasionally spontaneously resolve. Persistent, symptomatic pseudocysts may be drained by imaging-guided, endoscopic, or surgical approaches. Chronic pancreatitis may cause persistent pain, occasionally requiring surgical therapy for definitive alleviation of symptoms. Patients with chronic pancreatitis occasionally benefit from pancreatic enzyme supplementation due to exocrine insufficiency.

REFERENCE

1. Forsmark CE, Baillie J. AGA Institute technical review on acute pancreatitis. *Gastroenterol.* 2007;132(5):2022–44.

CHAPTER 27 ■ GALLBLADDER DISEASE

James X. Wu, MD and F. Charles Brunicardi, MD

OVERVIEW

- The gallbladder lies on the inferior surface of the liver between segments I and IV. The blood supply is the cystic artery, a branch of the right hepatic artery. Bile flows from the right and left hepatic ducts, which join into the common hepatic duct. Bile enters the gallbladder via the cystic duct. The common hepatic duct and cystic duct form the common bile duct, which drains into the duodenum.
- Gallbladder fills by contraction of sphincter of Oddi at ampulla of Vater.
  - Sphincter is stimulated by morphine, relaxed by glucagon.
  - Cholecystokinin (CCK), secretin, vagal tone increase bile excretion.
  - Vasoactive intestinal peptide (VIP), somatostatin, sympathetic tone decrease bile excretion.
- Normal gallbladder wall thickness is 3–4 mm.
- Normal common bile duct diameter is 4 mm + 1 mm per decade over age 40.

WORKUP OF GALLBLADDER DISEASE

Workup of gallbladder disease should include basic serum electrolytes and complete blood count (CBC), liver function tests (LFTs), amylase/lipase, and abdominal ultrasound. May require further workup with magnetic resonance cholangiopancreatography (MRCP), endoscopic retrograde cholangiopancreatography (ERCP), hepatobiliary iminodiacetic acid (HIDA) scan, or abdominal computed tomography (CT). See **Table 27-1**.

- Magnetic resonance cholangiopancreatography (MRCP): noninvasive imaging of biliary and pancreatic ducts using magnetic resonance imaging (MRI) technology.
- Endoscopic retrograde cholangiopancreatography (ERCP): an endoscope is used to access ampulla and inject contrast into bile ducts, visualized with fluoroscopy. Advantages include ability to perform interventions.
- Hepatobiliary iminodiacetic acid (HIDA) scan: a nuclear medicine study where the tracer is excreted into the biliary tract and normally stored by the gallbladder. Obstruction of cystic duct or inadequate excretion will show inadequate filling of the gallbladder.

Table 27-1 Common Clinical Features of Different Types of Gallbladder Disease

Disease Process	Symptoms	WBC	AST/ALT	T. Bili	Ultrasound Findings	Additional Tests	Management
Asymptomatic Cholelithiasis	None	NL	NL	NL	Gallstones	None	None
Symptomatic Cholelithiasis	Intermittent RUQ pain; precipitated by fatty foods; nausea/vomiting	NL	NL	NL	Gallstones	None	Elective cholecystectomy
Acute Cholecystitis	Constant RUQ pain; + Murphy's sign; nausea/vomiting	↑↑	↑↑/NL	NL	Gallstones; gallbladder wall Thickening; +/− pericholecystic fluid	None	Urgent cholecystectomy
Choledocholithiasis	RUQ/epigastric pain; +/− jaundice; nausea/vomiting	NL	↑↑/NL	↑↑	Gallstones; dilated common bile Duct; CBD stone often not seen	ERCP if total bilirubin. remains elevated	+/− ERCP, cholecystectomy +/− intraoperative cholangiogram
Gallstone Pancreatitis	Epigastric pain; nausea/vomiting	↑↑/NL	NL	NL	Gallstones	Elevated amylase, lipase	Resuscitation, pain control, cholecystectomy prior to discharge
Ascending Cholangitis	Fever, jaundice, RUQ pain (Charcot's triad); hypotension, altered mental status (Reynaud's pentad)	↑↑	↑↑/NL	↑↑	Gallstones; +/− fluid around bile ducts	None	Decompression with ERCP or cholecystostomy tube, cholecystectomy when stable
Gallstone Ileus	Small bowel obstruction; nausea/vomiting	↑↑/NL	NL	NL	Gallstones	AXR/abdominal CT	Enterostomy with stone removal, cholecystectomy
Mirizzi Syndrome	Jaundice; RUQ pain	NL	↑↑/NL	↑↑	Gallstones	MRCP/ERCP	Cholecystectomy +/− biliary reconstruction

CBD = common bile duct; ERCP = endoscopic retrograde cholangiopancreatography; MRCP = magnetic resonance cholangiopancreatography; NL = normal

GALLSTONE DISEASE

- Gallstones are crystalline precipitations of cholesterol, bile salts, bilirubin, and calcium salts formed within the gallbladder.
- Asymptomatic cholelithiasis: most patients with gallstones are asymptomatic.
- Symptomatic cholelithiasis: gallstones that intermittently obstruct the neck of the gallbladder, causing distension of the gallbladder and subsequent abdominal pain, nausea, and vomiting.
- Acute cholecystitis: obstruction of gallbladder leading to inflammation, gallbladder wall edema, areas of hemorrhage and necrosis, and ultimately suppuration depending on duration and degree of obstruction.
- Choledocholithiasis: gallstone that lodges in and obstructs the common bile duct.
- Gallstone pancreatitis: transient reflux into pancreatic duct caused by gallstone obstruction leading to pathologic activation of pancreatic enzymes in the pancreas causing inflammation.
- Ascending cholangitis: bacterial infection of bile ducts, typically caused by obstructive gallstone.
- Gallstone ileus: typically associated with formation of gallbladder-duodenal fistula, excretion of gallstone that leads to small bowel obstruction, most commonly at the terminal ileum.
- Mirizzi syndrome: obstructive jaundice caused by two major subtypes:
  - A large stone in gallbladder neck that compresses the common bile duct
  - Fistulous connection of cystic to common bile duct

NON-GALLSTONE GALLBLADDER DISEASE

- Acalculous cholecystitis: cholecystitis without cholelithiasis, caused by thick gallbladder secretions. Usually seen in critically ill patients due to dehydration or biliary stasis.
  - HIDA scan will reveal inadequate gallbladder filling.
- Biliary dyskinesia: impaired sphincter of Oddi tone leading to poor excretion
  - HIDA with less than 40% gallbladder volume excreted after 1 hour with CCK administration is diagnostic; treat with cholecystectomy.
- Choledochal cysts: congenital bile duct malformations that increase risk of cholangitis and malignancy; treat with resection and hepaticojejunostomy if necessary.
- Gallbladder polyps: concern for increased cancer risk if > 1 cm in size; treat with cholecystectomy.
- Common iatrogenic injuries include common bile duct injury, common bile duct transection leading to cholangitis, bile leaks, and biliary strictures following instrumentation.

GALLBLADDER MALIGNANCY

- Gallbladder adenocarcinoma: rare form of gastrointestinal (GI) malignancy, can present with jaundice, weight loss, fatigue, abdominal pain in right upper quadrant.
  - Porcelain gallbladder is a radiographic finding of calcification of the gallbladder wall, and palpation of a distended, non-tender gallbladder. It is associated with gallbladder carcinoma, but only a small minority of porcelain gallbladders contain malignancy.
- Cholangiocarcinoma: rare adenocarcinoma of bile ducts. Can present with jaundice, weight loss, fatigue. Can have elevated CEA or CA 19-9 levels. Increased risk in patients with primary sclerosing cholangitis or choledochal cysts.

REFERENCE

1. Kimura Y, Takada T, Strasberg SM, et al. TG13 current terminology, etiology, and epidemiology of acute cholangitis and cholecystitis. *J Hepatobiliary Pancreat Sci.* 2013;20(1):8–23.

CHAPTER 28 ■ COLORECTAL CANCER SCREENING

Christine Yu, MD and Bennett E. Roth, MD

OVERVIEW

- Colorectal cancer (CRC) is the third most common cancer diagnosed and the second leading cause of cancer-related deaths in both men and women in the United States (third when considered separately).
- Five-year survival rates for localized, regional, and distant disease are 90.3%, 70.4%, and 12.5%, respectively. Hence, early detection is crucial.
- Traditional concepts of CRC progression: small → large adenomas → cancer over about 10 years.
- Serrated adenoma sequence: development of high-grade dysplasia → cancer may be more rapid.
- Since 1985, mortality from CRC has declined in large part related to enhanced screening and advances in treatment options.

SCREENING STRATEGIES

- Modalities for CRC screening include guaiac-based fecal occult blood test (gFOBT), fecal immunochemical test (FIT), computed tomography (CT) colonography (CTC), flexible sigmoidoscopy (FSIG), and colonoscopy (CSPY).
- Modalities that demonstrated reduction in CRC incidence and mortality:

    gFOBT: 17–20% incidence, 11–33% mortality

    FSIG: 32% incidence, 50% mortality

    CSPY: 76–90% incidence, 53% mortality

    CTC: not yet approved for routine screening

- Relative sensitivity and specificity is as follows:

    Sensitivity: gFOBT < FIT < FSIG < CSPY

    Specificity: gFOBT < FIT < FSI = CSPY

STOOL-BASED STUDIES: GFOBT, FIT, STOOL DNA

- gFOBT sensitivity of single testing 30%; repeat testing 64–79%. However, after the first year, adherence to testing declines by nearly half. Specificity is poor.
- Advantages: widely available, inexpensive with no special resources required (may be best used in patients with limited access to care), can be performed at home.
- Disadvantages: may provide false reassurance given low sensitivity for polyps and even advanced adenomas. Polyps, and even cancers, do not consistently bleed, resulting in false-negative tests. High rate of false positivity; limited in diagnostic capabilities, because positive screens require further workup with colonoscopy.
- gFOBT with sigmoidoscopy is preferred over gFOBT alone; yet combined modality failed to detect advanced colonic neoplasia in 24% of patients. > 40% of polyps are above reach of sigmoidoscope and may not bleed.
- FIT is specific to human hemoglobin and does not detect upper gastrointestinal (GI) bleeds as the globin is digested in transit. Requires fewer stool samples, but is more expensive than gFOBT. Sensitivity decreases with delay in processing. Optimal screening interval is unknown.
- Stool DNA: investigational, expensive, requires collection of an entire bowel movement, and repeat intervals are unknown. Detects specific mutations. May miss approximately 50% of advanced polyps and CRC detected by colonoscopy.

CT COLONOGRAPHY

- Sensitivity for detection of polyps ≥ 6 mm (threshold for colonoscopy referral) is 78–90%, specificity 86–88%.
- Advantages: less invasive than colonoscopy, examines entire length of colon, no sedation required.
- Disadvantages: requires aggressive bowel prep, cumulative radiation exposure, flat/sessile polyps more likely to be missed, significant findings require second procedure (colonoscopy), unclear management of patients with polyps < 6 mm, appropriate screening intervals are unknown, and increased costs for workup of incidental extra-colonic findings. Risk of perforation is estimated to be 0–6/10,000 studies. Least cost-effective modality.

FLEXIBLE SIGMOIDOSCOPY

- Sensitivity: 58–86%.
- Advantages: direct visualization, identification and possible biopsy of distal lesions in an office-based setting with minimal preparation, no sedation. Rate of perforation is about half that of colonoscopy. Accessibility and compliance may be increased.

- Disadvantages: invasive with associated discomfort, requires a limited bowel preparation, examines only distal 60 cm of bowel. Serious complications occur in approximately 3.4/10,000 procedures. Large percentage of polyps (especially serrated adenomas) are in the right colon, do not bleed, and are beyond the reach of sigmoidoscopy.

COLONOSCOPY

- Sensitivity: 77–100%, varies depending on technique and experience of the endoscopist.
- The National Polyp Study showed that colonoscopic polypectomy decreased the CRC incidence by 76–90% and mortality by 53% as compared to the expected rate.
- Quality of colonoscopy may vary and can be measured by adenoma detection rate, cecal intubation rate, documentation of careful examination during withdrawal, and appropriate follow-up recommendations based on findings and quality of preparation.
- Advantages: diagnosis and therapy in one exam, examines entire length of colon.
- Disadvantages: high initial cost, invasive, and requires bowel preparation, sedation, special resources, and expertise. Risk of perforation is an estimated 3.8/10,000 procedures. Serious complication requiring hospitalization (perforation, major bleeding) or death attributable to colonoscopy occurs in approximately 25/10,000 procedures. With advancing age, benefit risk ratios suggest that routine screening can cease beyond 75 to 80 years of age in most patients. Compliance issues remain, with only ~55% of eligible people completing an examination.

GUIDELINES FOR CRC SCREENING (SEE FIGURE 28-1)

- Recommendations are made by various expert groups including the U.S. Preventive Service Task Force (USPSTF), American College of Gastroenterology (ACG), American Society for Gastrointestinal Endoscopy (ASGE) based on factors including effectiveness, sensitivity, false-positive rate, safety, cost, cost-effectiveness, and patient preference.
- Screening and surveillance guidelines are dependent upon determination of risk based upon personal or family history. For those without increased risk, initiation of screening is recommended at age 50.
- Screening is recommended until 75 years of age with individual consideration for 75-to-85-year olds.
- Increased risk:
  - Single first-degree relative with CRC above age 60: begin screening at age 40.

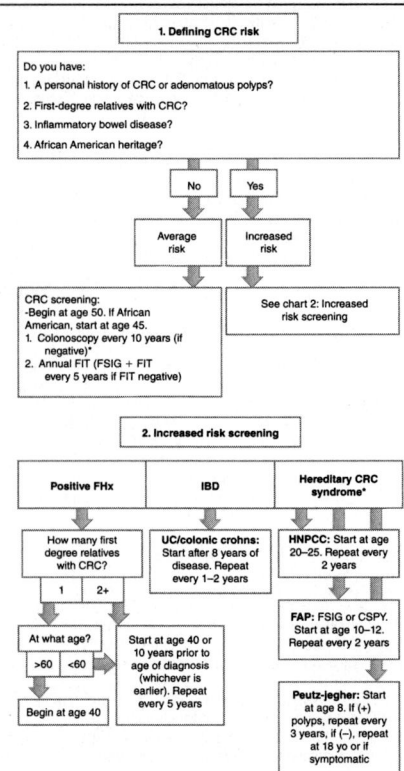

Figure 28-1 Algorithm for screening and surveillance.

*Recommendations for surveillance vary pending findings on initial screening colonoscopy

Note: For high-risk individuals, colonoscopy is the recommended screening modality.

*Genetic testing for index case and family members is preferable when availble

3. Colorectal cancer surveillance	
Findings	**Recommended follow-up interval**
History of 1–2 tubular adenomas <1 cm in size	every 5 years
3 or more tubular adenomas	every 3 years
Adenoma 1 cm or more in size	
Adenoma with advanced histology (villous features or serrated adenoma)	
History of CRC	1 and 3 year f/u after initial diagnosis, then every 5 years thereafter if negative exam

Figure 28-1 Algorithm for screening and surveillance (*continued*).

- Two or more first-degree relatives with CRC or one with onset before age 60: begin screening at age 40 or 10 years prior to age of onset of index cancer.
- African American heritage: begin routine screening at age 45.
- High-risk criteria
  - Familial adenomatous polyposis (FAP)
  - Hereditary noncolorectal cancer polyposis syndrome (HNPCC)
- Colonoscopy is currently the preferred CRC screening modality.

REFERENCES

1. Lieberman DA. Clinical practice. Screening for colorectal cancer. *N Engl J Med*. 2009;361(12):1179–87.
2. Rex DK, Johnson DA, Anderson JC, et al. American College of Gastroenterology guidelines for colorectal cancer screening 2009 [corrected]. *Am J Gastroenterol*. 2009;104(3):739–50.
3. Lieberman DA, Rex DK, Winawer SJ, et al. Guidelines for colonoscopy surveillance after screening and polypectomy: a consensus update by the US Multi-Society Task Force on Colorectal Cancer. *Gastroenterol*. 2012;143(3):844–57.
4. Zauber AG, Winawer SJ, O'Brien MJ, et al. Colonoscopic polypectomy and long-term prevention of colorectal-cancer deaths. *N Engl J Med*. 2012;366(8):687–96.

CHAPTER 29 ■ BOWEL OBSTRUCTION

Nelya Melnitchouk, MD and James Yoo, MD

OVERVIEW

- Bowel obstruction is a common problem that is defined as a partial or complete interference with passage of stool in small or large intestines.
- Bowel obstruction can be divided into small and large bowel obstruction, partial or complete, strangulated or not.
- Pseudo-obstruction, or Ogilvie syndrome, is a paralytic ileus of the large intestine that usually presents in debilitated, immobile patients. If untreated, colonic ischemia and perforation can occur.
- Bowel obstruction is common after previous abdominal surgery, and can be differentiated into an early and late postoperative obstruction.
- Small bowel obstruction (SBO) accounts for 20% of all acute surgical admissions.
- Large bowel obstruction (LBO) is an emergency condition that requires early identification and intervention, and the prevalence increases with age.

PRESENTATION

- Depending on the exact location and severity, bowel obstruction can present with a wide spectrum of symptoms.
- The most common symptoms are abdominal distention, nausea, vomiting, obstipation, and abdominal pain.
- A bowel obstruction can have associated signs of hypovolemia, renal failure, and associated electrolyte disturbances.
- Peritonitis is a late sign, suggesting perforation or ischemia.

DIFFERENTIAL DIAGNOSIS

- The differential diagnosis includes ileus, pancreatitis, pseudo-obstruction, appendicitis, diverticulitis, perforated peptic ulcer, ischemic colitis, mesenteric ischemia, malrotation, radiation enteritis, gastroenteritis, inflammatory bowel disease (IBD), pelvic inflammatory disease (PID), urinary tract infection (UTI), kidney stone, biliary disease, endometriosis.
- A multitude of abdominal pathologies can present with similar symptoms.

PATHOPHYSIOLOGY

- A bowel obstruction can be due to adhesions, tumor (both intrinsic and extrinsic), strictures, volvulus, hernias, a foreign body, gallstones, intussusception, diverticulitis, inflammatory bowel disease, and fecal impaction.
- The most common cause of small bowel obstruction is adhesions, followed by tumors, hernias, and IBD. Some studies report Crohn's disease as the third most common cause.
- Surgeries most closely associated with SBO are colorectal surgery, appendectomies, gynecologic, and upper gastrointestinal (GI) surgery.
- The most common cause of large bowel obstruction is tumor, followed by diverticular disease, volvulus, and IBD.
- Obstructions by tumor are gradual in onset.
- The pathophysiology of Ogilvie syndrome is not clear but it is thought to result from an autonomic imbalance, which results from decreased parasympathetic tone or excessive sympathetic output.

DIAGNOSIS

- The diagnosis starts with a careful history and physical exam.
- The history should be focused on possible etiologies of the obstruction, the duration of symptoms, prior episodes, history of malignancy, prior operations, and prior radiation therapy.
- The physical exam should include a complete abdominal exam, noting the degree of distention, tenderness, signs of peritonitis, presence of scars and hernias (ventral, umbilical, inguinal, femoral), and a rectal exam.
- The aim of the initial evaluation should be to assess the degree of metabolic derangement and volume depletion and to determine the possible need and timing of surgery.
- Plain films (upright and supine) can show pneumoperitoneum, an increase in bowel diameter, dilated bowel loops, air-fluid levels, a distended stomach. They can also show the typical appearance of sigmoid ("bent inner tube" or "coffee bean sign") or cecal (kidney-shaped mass or "comma-shaped") volvulus.
- A computed tomography (CT) scan can provide important information about the cause, degree, and site of obstruction, and the presence of a closed-loop obstruction, ischemia, or perforation.
- When large bowel obstruction is present, a diatrizoic acid (Gastrografin) enema study may be helpful to differentiate pseudo-obstruction from mechanical obstruction. Barium should be avoided in this situation.
- In patients with Crohn's disease, enterography may be helpful to look for the presence of strictures.

Chapter 29: Bowel Obstruction

TREATMENT

- Treatment is based on the presumed cause of the obstruction.
- Initial management should consist of fluid resuscitation, correcting electrolyte abnormalities, bowel rest, and GI decompression with a nasogastric tube (NGT).
- The decision to operate is dependent on a multitude of factors including the probable etiology, stability of the patient, abdominal exam, history of prior surgery, first occurrence versus recurrence, partial versus complete obstruction, and presence of a closed loop.
- Conservative management can be attempted if the patient is stable, the abdominal exam is not concerning for ischemia or perforation, and no closed-loop obstruction is suspected.
- Surgery should be strongly considered for patients who are clinically stable but do not respond to initial conservative measures and for patients with no prior surgical history, because adhesions are much less likely and an incarcerated hernia or tumor should be considered.
- Surgical management can consist of lysis of adhesions, reduction and repair of a hernia, bowel resection, bowel bypass, or ostomy.
- Laparoscopy has been shown to be safe and effective in selected cases of bowel obstruction.
- The management of Ogilvie syndrome includes correction of electrolyte abnormalities, mobilizing the patient, monitoring with daily plain films to measure the diameter of the bowel, neostigmine, and endoscopic decompression.
- Endoscopic decompression and reduction should be attempted for sigmoid volvulus if no ischemia is present.
- Endoscopic stent placement can be considered for distal large bowel obstruction—caused by tumor or stricture.

REFERENCES

1. Arnaoutakis GJ, Eckhauser FE. Small bowel obstruction. In: Cameron JL, Cameron AM, eds. *Current Surgical Therapy*. 10th ed. Philadelphia: Elsevier Saunders; 2011.
2. Webb A. L.B, Fink AS. Large bowel obstruction. In: Cameron JL, Cameron AM, eds. *Current Surgical Therapy*. 10th ed. Philadelphia: Elsevier Saunders; 2011.

CHAPTER 30 ■ DIVERTICULITIS

Jeffrey R. Lewis, MD

OVERVIEW

- By age 80, at least 50% of the population has diverticulosis. However, only a minority of patients with diverticulosis (< 5–10%) develop diverticulitis.
- Acute diverticulitis results from microperforation within a diverticular sac—producing local inflammation.
- Acute diverticulitis can be simple or complicated. Complicated diverticulitis arises when there is an associated abscess, fistula, perforation, or obstruction.
- Treatment includes antibiotic therapy (either oral or intravenous), nil per os (NPO; nothing by mouth) status or liquid diet, and abscess drainage and/or surgery if there is a local complication.

PRESENTATION

- Most patients with acute diverticulitis present with abdominal pain. The pain is usually in the left lower quadrant. However, pain can also be suprapubic as the sigmoid colon lies in close relationship to the bladder in the pelvis.
- Patients may have smoldering symptoms for days before coming to medical attention.
- If there is an associated fistula with the bladder, pneumaturia or fecaluria may be present.

DIFFERENTIAL DIAGNOSIS

- Ischemic colitis: patients typically present with hematochezia and have risk factors for vascular disease including diabetes, smoking, hypercholesterolemia, and other end-organ vascular disease (coronary artery disease, peripheral vascular disease).
- Inflammatory bowel disease (ulcerative colitis or Crohn's disease): patients typically present with a history of hematochezia, chronic diarrhea, and possibly perianal disease.
- Colon cancer: patients can present with left lower quadrant pain and, if extensive, can present with colonic obstruction or perforation.

- Other gastrointestinal conditions that can mimic diverticulitis include appendicitis and infectious colitis. Nongastrointestinal etiologies of left lower quadrant pain that can mimic diverticulitis include tubo-ovarian abscess, ovarian cyst, ectopic pregnancy, nephrolithiasis, and pyelonephritis.

PATHOPHYSIOLOGY

- Patients by definition have preceding diverticulosis—sac-like protrusions of mucosa and submucosa in the colon wall where penetrating vasa recta enter the circular muscle layer of the colon.
- Pathologically, diverticulitis represents a contained microperforation that arises when the colon wall becomes eroded due to elevated intraluminal pressure, food, or fecal matter. Most commonly the subsequent inflammatory response results in a walled-off, or contained, microperforation. However, in complicated diverticulitis, this microperforation can lead to abscess formation or macroperforation, resulting in free intraperitoneal air and even fecal peritonitis.

DIAGNOSIS

- Physical examination most commonly reveals left lower quadrant tenderness or suprapubic tenderness. Care needs to be taken to evaluate for peritoneal signs that signify perforation. Diverticular disease may be limited to the right colon in some patients.
- Computed tomography (CT) of the abdomen and pelvis with intravenous (IV) and oral (PO) contrast is the most commonly employed study to diagnose acute diverticulitis. This imaging modality also allows the provider to exclude other causes of abdominal pain. Diverticulitis presents as a segment of bowel wall thickening with associated diverticulosis and pericolonic fat stranding.
- Colonoscopy is relatively contraindicated in the setting of acute diverticulitis as there is a theoretical concern that air insufflation could precipitate colonic wall perforation. Colonoscopy is recommended at least 6 weeks after an episode of acute diverticulitis to exclude an underlying malignancy, a large colon polyp, or other such triggers as the etiology of symptoms and abnormal CT scan findings.

TREATMENT

- Antibiotics are the mainstay of treatment for diverticulitis. Patients with uncomplicated diverticulitis who are able to tolerate liquids can be discharged from the emergency room with oral antibiotics. Those with systemic signs of inflammation, complicated diverticulitis, and those

unable to consume food or liquid by mouth require hospitalization and intravenous antibiotics.
- Common outpatient antibiotic regimens include ciprofloxacin (500 mg PO twice daily) with metronidazole (500 mg PO three times per day), amoxicillin-clavulanate (875/125 mg PO twice daily), and trimethoprim-sulfamethoxazole (1 double-strength tab twice daily) *with* metronidazole (500 mg PO three times per day) for 10 to 14 days.
- Common inpatient antibiotics include piperacillin-tazobactam, ampicillin-sulbactam, and ciprofloxacin *with* metronidazole.
- Abscesses require drainage, either surgically or through CT-guided aspiration.
- Peritonitis, bowel obstruction, and fistula formation in complicated diverticulitis most commonly require operative management.

REFERENCE

1. Stollman NH, Raskin JB. Diagnosis and management of diverticular disease of the colon in adults. *Am J Gastroenterol.* 1999;94(11):3110–21.

CHAPTER 31 ■ GASTROENTERITIS

Nikhil Agarwal, MD and Mark Ovsiowitz, MD

OVERVIEW

- *Gastroenteritis* is a general term to describe an acute irritation and inflammation of the stomach and intestines.
- This condition is commonly referred to as "stomach flu," but can be due to bacterial, viral, and protozoal infections.
- Symptoms usually begin abruptly within 12–72 hours after contacting the infectious agent and are self-limited and resolve within a week.
- People at risk for gastroenteritis include travelers, immunosuppressed patients, and those who live in common quarters (students in dormitories, nursing home residents, military personnel, etc.).
- For acute nausea, vomiting, and diarrhea that is self-limited, think of acute gastroenteritis!

PRESENTATION

- Typically, gastroenteritis presents with the abrupt onset of nausea, vomiting, crampy abdominal pain, and diarrhea.
- Additional symptoms may include headache, fever, muscle aches, and fatigue.
- Bloody diarrhea, fever, severe abdominal pain, or signs of dehydration or hypovolemia may indicate a more severe illness and warrant further diagnostic evaluation.

DIFFERENTIAL DIAGNOSIS

Crohn's disease, ulcerative colitis, celiac disease, irritable bowel syndrome

ETIOLOGY

- The most common etiology of acute gastroenteritis is viral; however, up to 50% of the time no specific etiology is found.
- Norovirus is the most common infectious agent and is transmitted by consuming contaminated food or by contacting contaminated objects. This virus is the common etiology for "cruise ship gastroenteritis."

- Rotavirus is a common cause of severe diarrhea in infants and young children.
- Adenovirus, parvovirus, and astrovirus are other common etiologies of viral gastroenteritis.
- *Campylobacter jejuni* is the primary cause of bacterial gastroenteritis and is usually traced to poultry, meat, or dairy products.
- If a short incubation period of less than 6 hours is noted, think of ingestion of a preformed toxin of *Staphylococcus aureus* or *Bacillus cereus*.
- If recent antibiotic use or recent hospitalization, think *Clostridium difficile*.
- Bloody diarrhea can be seen with *Escherichia coli* O157: H7 and *Shigella* and *Salmonella* species.
- Traveler's diarrhea is commonly from enterotoxigenic *E. coli* (ETEC).
- Parasites and protozoal infections are less likely but can be considered in patients with prolonged diarrhea or risk factors: drinking or swimming in freshwater lakes or pools.
- *Giardia* is the most common cause of waterborne diarrhea.
- *Cryptosporidium* should be considered in immunocompromised individuals.

DIAGNOSIS (SEE FIGURE 31-1)

- Most cases of gastroenteritis should be diagnosed from taking a careful history. Timing of symptom onset, exposure to other family members or friends, or recent travel may help provide clues to a specific etiology.
- Stool studies for culture, leukocytes, ova and parasites, and *C. difficile* should be considered in individuals who are over age 65, immunocompromised, have taken recent antibiotics, have a prolonged illness lasting more than 1 week, or have other signs of severe illness.

TREATMENT

- Most cases of acute gastroenteritis are self-limited and do not require specific antibiotic therapy.
- The most critical element of therapy is hydration and repletion of electrolytes. Patients should be instructed to drink plenty of fluids and to intake solute-rich foods or supplements.
- Inability to tolerate liquids or to be able to keep up with hydration may warrant hospitalization for intravenous repletion.
- Symptomatic therapy with loperamide, bismuth, or diphenoxylate can be considered if fluid intake is adequate.
- Empiric antibiotics can be considered in those with signs of severe diarrhea or in hospitalized patients while stool studies are pending.
- Antibiotics should be avoided in patients in whom enterohemorrhagic *E. coli* (EHEC) is suspected.

Chapter 31: Gastroenteritis

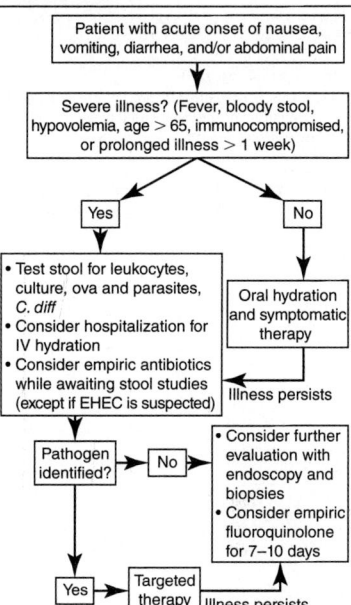

Figure 31-1 Management algorithm for acute gastroenteritis.

C. diff = *Clostridium difficile*, IV = intravenous, EHEC = enterohemorrhagic *E. coli*

- Empiric antibiotic therapy for *C. difficile* infections is generally not recommended and therapy should be delayed until a diagnosis can be confirmed.
- Specific antibiotic therapy is warranted when a treatable pathogen is identified in stool samples.

REFERENCES

1. Musher DM, Musher BL. Contagious acute gastrointestinal infections. *N Engl J Med*. 2004;351:2417–27.
2. Dupont HL. Guidelines on acute infectious diarrhea in adults. The Practice Parameters Committee of the American College of Gastroenterology. *Am J Gastroenterol*. 1997;92(11):1962–75.

CHAPTER 32 ■ COLON POLYPS

Andrew Ho, MD and Daniel D. Cho, MD

OVERVIEW

- Colon polyps typically represent indolent lesions of the colonic mucosa that have the potential of undergoing malignant transformation.
- The histologic feature, shape, and size of a colonic polyp determine their clinical relevance.
- Adenomatous polyps represent the most common neoplasm encountered during colorectal cancer screening. Adenomas are low-grade dysplastic lesions associated with a higher risk of progression to colorectal cancer.
- Advanced adenomas include adenomas that are greater than 10 mm in size, feature a villous component, or contain high-grade dysplasia.
- Advanced adenomas carry a higher risk of colon cancer, but they are less prevalent than other adenoma subtypes.
- Surveillance guidelines are provided in **Table 32-1**.

Table 32-1 AGA Surveillance Guidelines for Average-Risk Individuals

Baseline Colonoscopy	Recommended Surveillance Interval (years)
No polyps	10
Small (< 10 mm) hyperplastic polyps	10
1–2 small (< 10 mm) tubular adenomas	5–10
3–10 tubular adenomas	3
> 10 adenomas	< 3
One or more tubular adenomas > 10 mm	3
One or more villous adenomas	3
Serrated lesions	
Sessile serrated polyp(s) < 10 mm with no dysplasia	5
Sessile serrated polyp(s) > 10 mm OR Sessile serrated polyp with dysplasia OR Traditional serrated adenoma	3

PRESENTATION

- Colon polyps rarely cause symptoms. Often patients will be unaware they have polyps until they are detected on colonoscopy or other imaging studies.
- One of the main goals of a screening colonoscopy is to detect and remove polyps to obviate the risk of colorectal cancer.
- Larger polyps are more likely to cause symptoms including rectal bleeding, changes in bowel habits, abdominal discomfort, or intestinal obstruction.

DIFFERENTIAL DIAGNOSIS

Hyperplastic polyps, tubular adenomas, tubulovillous adenomas, villous adenomas, serrated polyps, adenocarcinoma, lipomas, fibromas, carcinoids, hamartomas, inflammatory pseudopolyps

PATHOPHYSIOLOGY

- Colonic polyps can be divided into three main categories: hyperplastic polyps, serrated lesions, and adenomas.
- Hyperplastic polyps most commonly occur in the rectosigmoid region, are small (< 5 mm), and are not dysplastic.
- Serrated lesions can be subdivided into sessile serrated polyps and traditional serrated adenomas. Sessile serrated polyps typically lack dysplasia while traditional serrated adenomas have cytologic dysplasia.
- Adenomas can be divided into three types by histology: tubular, tubulovillous, and villous.

DIAGNOSIS

- Colonoscopy and flexible sigmoidoscopy are modalities most often utilized to detect colorectal polyps and colorectal cancer. If polyps are found during colonoscopy, these polyps can be removed by various modalities and then sent for histologic examination.
- Histology examination differentiates between hyperplastic, serrated lesions, and adenomatous polyps.
- For screening colonoscopy, an adenoma detection rate (ADR) of 25% and 15% are recommended benchmarks in men and women, respectively. The ADR reflects the proportion of screening colonoscopies performed by a physician that detect one or more adenomas.

TREATMENT

- Removal with a forceps biopsy device: appropriate for many polyps.
- Snare polypectomy: pedunculated polyps (and larger sessile polyps) are removed by snaring them with a wire loop that cuts the polyp and cauterizes it to prevent bleeding.
- Endoscopic mucosal resection (EMR): larger or flat polyps that are more challenging to remove can be resected with various commercially available devices.
- Surgery: for polyps that are too large to resect endoscopically, or in cases of inherited syndromes such as familial adenomatous polyposis (FAP), surgery may be warranted.

REFERENCES

1. Lieberman DA, Rex DK, Winawer SJ, et al. Guidelines for colonoscopy surveillance after screening and polypectomy: a consensus update by the US Multi-Society Task Force on Colorectal Cancer. *Gastroenterol.* 2012;143:844–57.
2. Levin B, Lieberman DA, McFarland B, et al. Screening and surveillance for early detection of colorectal cancer and adenomatous polyps, 2008: a joint guideline from the American Cancer Society, the US Multi-Society Task Force on Colorectal Cancer and the American College of Radiology. *Gastroenterol.* 2008;134(5):1570–95.

CHAPTER 33 ■ ULCERATIVE COLITIS

Jennifer M. Choi, MD

OVERVIEW

- Ulcerative colitis (UC) is a chronic inflammatory disease limited to the colon and characterized by diffuse mucosal inflammation. 95% of cases involve the rectum.
- First described in 1875 by Wilks and Moxon, this is a form of inflammatory bowel disease (IBD). Crohn's disease (CD) is another type of IBD that is distinct from UC and can involve the entire gastrointestinal (GI) tract.
- Inflammation involving the colonic mucosa extends proximally in a continuous, symmetric, and circumferential pattern.
- Classifications are based on the extent of disease: proctitis (limited to the rectum), proctosigmoiditis (involving the rectum and sigmoid colon), left-sided colitis (involving the rectum to descending colon up to the splenic flexure), and pancolitis (involving the entire colon).

PRESENTATION

- The classic clinical symptom is bloody diarrhea, commonly associated with rectal urgency, frequency, and tenesmus. Patients may also report mucus in stools, abdominal pain, fever, malaise, and weight loss.
- The clinical course is often punctuated with periodic exacerbations or flares of disease between periods of remission.
- Extraintestinal manifestations may include dermatologic (e.g., erythema nodosum), rheumatologic (arthralgias), ophthalmologic, hepatobiliary (e.g., primary sclerosing cholangitis), and hematologic involvement.
- Complications may include severe bleeding, bowel perforation, toxic megacolon, and epithelial dysplasia, or malignancy.
- UC patients have a higher risk for colorectal cancer than the general population. The degree of increased risk is related to the duration, extent, and severity of disease. More frequent surveillance colonoscopy is recommended, generally every 1–2 years beginning 8 years after onset of disease.

DIFFERENTIAL DIAGNOSIS

Crohn's disease, chronic infections like *Clostridium difficile*, cytomegalovirus, tuberculosis, celiac disease, irritable bowel syndrome, ischemic colitis, microscopic colitis, drug- or radiation-induced colitis, diverticulitis, solitary rectal ulcer syndrome

PATHOPHYSIOLOGY

- There is no clear consensus opinion. Genetic factors, environmental factors (e.g., smoking, appendectomy), medications, infectious etiologies (e.g., alterations in the gut microbiota), mucosal immunity, and autoimmune factors have all been proposed.
- IBD is associated with smoking, high-fat and sugar-diets, medication use, stress, high socioeconomic status, and appendectomy. Of these, only cigarette smoking and appendectomy are reproducibly linked to ulcerative colitis. (Interestingly, the risk of developing ulcerative colitis is decreased in current smokers compared to people who have never smoked. Also, children who underwent appendectomy are less likely to develop ulcerative colitis later in life.)

DIAGNOSIS

- The diagnosis is suspected on clinical grounds based on medical history (including family history), physical examination, and tests. Initial diagnostic workup may include laboratory tests (complete blood count may reveal leukocytosis, anemia, and thrombocytosis; complete metabolic panel including electrolytes, renal and liver function tests; erythrocyte sedimentation rate, and C-reactive protein, which may be elevated in inflammatory conditions) and stool studies to rule out infectious causes. Perinuclear antineutrophil cytoplasmic antibodies (pANCA) are considered highly specific for ulcerative colitis. (Though a positive pANCA is not diagnostic, it may help to differentiate ulcerative colitis from Crohn's disease.)
- Diagnosis relies on endoscopic evaluation with colonoscopy or flexible sigmoidoscopy to assess the extent and severity of disease and biopsies to determine specific histopathologic characteristics.
- Endoscopy shows uniformly inflamed mucosa from the anorectal verge, extending proximally with transition to normal-appearing mucosa. Affected areas may demonstrate granularity, erythema, friability, and loss of vascular pattern, with erosions, ulcerations, spontaneous bleeding, and pseudopolyps.
- Histologic features may include crypt architectural distortion, inflammatory infiltrates (consisting of lymphocytes, plasma cells, and

granulocytes) in the lamina propria, cryptitis, crypt abscesses, diminished crypt density, goblet cell depletion, and ulcerations.
- Radiologic and ultrasonographic examinations may be useful, but are not critical.

TREATMENT

- There is no standard regimen. Treatment must be tailored to the individual, based on disease severity, disease location, medication side effects, prior response to medications, and medical comorbidities.
- Medical treatments aim to achieve clinical remission (defined as the absence of symptoms) through initial induction regimens, and then to maintain remission to prevent recurrence of symptoms and flares. Other goals of medical therapy include minimization of medication side effects (e.g., those from long-term corticosteroid use), hospitalizations, and surgery, and endoscopic/histopathologic improvement or mucosal healing (i.e., deep remission).
- Medications routinely used include aminosalicylates (e.g., sulfasalazine, mesalamine), corticosteroids (e.g., prednisone, budesonide), immunomodulators (e.g., 6-mercaptopurine, azathioprine), cyclosporine (a calcineurin inhibitor that selectively inhibits T-cell immunity), and biologics (e.g., infliximab, adalimumab, and golimumab, which are monoclonal antibodies that target tumor necrosis factor alpha).
- Unlike Crohn's disease, ulcerative colitis is cured by surgical colectomy. Standard surgical options include the ileal pouch-anal anastomosis (IPAA) procedure or total proctocolectomy with permanent ileostomy.

REFERENCES

1. Danese S, Fiocchi C. Ulcerative colitis. *N Engl J Med.* 2011;365(18): 1713–25.
2. Kornbluth A, Sachar DB. Ulcerative colitis practice guidelines in adults: American College of Gastroenterology, Practice Parameters Committee. *Am J Gastroenterol.* 1997;92(2):204–11.

CHAPTER 34 ■ CROHN'S DISEASE

Christina Ha, MD

OVERVIEW

- Crohn's disease (CD) is a chronic inflammatory disease of the gastrointestinal system characterized by periods of increased disease activity (flares) and remission.
- CD can involve any part of the luminal gastrointestinal (GI) tract with small bowel and colonic involvement being most common.
- The inflammatory process in CD can be transmural, involving all the layers of the intestine, and patchy, with areas of normal-appearing mucosa interspersed among sections of inflamed mucosa. These features are sometimes referred to as "skip lesions."
- Intestinal strictures, which can cause symptomatic narrowing of the small bowel or colon, and fistulas, which are abnormal connections between the intestine to another structure such as other parts of the intestine, genitourinary structures, and the skin, indicate more aggressive disease.
- Up to 30% of CD patients may also have perianal disease which can include fistulas, abscesses, fissures, anal strictures, or larger "elephant ear" perianal skin tags.

PRESENTATION

- Symptoms of CD may be dependent on disease phenotype.
  - Inflammatory disease presents with abdominal pain or tenderness, diarrhea (not always bloody), low-grade fever, and weight loss. Growth delay is often seen among pediatric-onset patients.
  - Stricturing disease presents with more obstructive symptoms with postprandial cramping, abdominal distention, borborygmi, nausea, vomiting, and weight loss.
  - Fistulizing disease symptoms depend on the location of the fistulae and can include abdominal pain with a fullness at a site of potential abscess or contained perforation; recurrent urinary tract infections; psoas abscess signs with hip, back, or thigh pain; fevers; or symptoms mimicking appendicitis or diverticulitis.

- Perianal disease symptoms include painful defecation, rectal bleeding, tenderness with sitting, urgency, or obstipation from anorectal strictures and drainage.
- Disease severity is determined by the change in number of bowel movements from baseline (when patients are feeling well), degree of abdominal pain, presence of a fullness of mass suggestive of abscess or obstruction, systemic signs of inflammation including fever, weight loss/malnutrition, anemia, and extraintestinal manifestations of disease.

- Extraintestinal manifestations of CD may occur and include oral aphthous ulcers or stomatitis, inflammatory arthropathies, pyoderma gangrenosum, erythema nodosum, uveitis, episcleritis, gallstones, oxalate kidney stones, and primary sclerosing cholangitis. CD patients are also at greater risk for venous thromboembolic events as well as osteopenia and osteoporosis, particularly with prolonged steroid exposure.
- The majority of patients with CD will undergo at least one surgery for aggressive or refractory disease during their lifetime. Postsurgical anatomy, depending on the type of surgery performed and the length of resection, can place patients at risk for bile-acid diarrhea, fat malabsorption, vitamin B_{12} deficiency, and small intestinal bacterial overgrowth.

DIFFERENTIAL DIAGNOSIS

Diverticulitis, appendicitis, endometriosis, pelvic inflammatory disease, intra-abdominal or tubo-ovarian abscess, medications (nonsteroidal anti-inflammatory drugs [NSAIDs], mycophenolate), vasculitis, infections (e.g., tuberculosis, *Yersinia*, *Mycobacterium avian-intracellulare*, cytomegalovirus), radiation enteritis, malignancy (e.g., small bowel or colorectal adenocarcinoma, lymphoma, carcinoid, metastatic disease, melanoma)

PATHOPHYSIOLOGY

- The etiology is not fully understood. However, it appears to occur as a result of the complex interplay of genetic predisposition and environmental influences leading to immune system dysregulation. As a result, immune-mediated changes occur within the epithelial barrier of the luminal gastrointestinal tract that lead to an aberrant inflammatory response and subsequent clinical manifestations of disease.
- Potential predictors of progressive and aggressive disease include young age at onset, early development of fistulizing disease, steroids requirement early during the disease course, and deep ulcerations identified during endoscopic or imaging studies.
- Disease duration, endoscopic, and histologic activity increase risk for colorectal cancer among patients with Crohn's colitis involving more

than one-third of the colon. Additional risk factors for colorectal cancer among patient with colonic CD include family history of colorectal cancer, primary sclerosing cholangitis, and a personal history of colon adenomas or cancer.

DIAGNOSIS

- There is no single test that establishes the diagnosis of CD.
- Relevant laboratory testing includes a complete blood count to look for anemia, inflammation, or infections; inflammatory markers (erythrocyte sedimentation rate, C-reactive protein); and stool studies to exclude infection such as *Clostridium difficile*. Stool biomarkers such as fecal calprotectin have been shown to correlate well with both endoscopic disease activity and differentiate inflammatory bowel disease from diarrhea-predominant irritable bowel syndrome.
- The CD diagnostic testing panel consists of a variety of serologic markers used to detect the titers of antibodies to certain microbial antigens that may help in the differentiation of indeterminate colitis and for prognostication. The presence of high titers of some or multiple antibodies may suggest complicated disease behavior or post-surgical complications such as pouchitis. However, it is not meant to be a standalone *diagnostic* test to determine the presence or absence of CD without additional supporting data.
- Small bowel imaging aids are used in establishing the diagnosis of CD, assessing disease activity, identifying disease-related complications such as strictures, fistulae, or abscesses, and assessing response to therapy over time.
  - Imaging modalities used include magnetic resonance enterography, computed tomography enterography, barium or gastrografn-based small bowel follow through, or capsule endoscopy.
  - CD patients tend to have higher imaging requirements due to the multiple behaviors of disease activity that may change over time, and increased radiation exposures due to frequent testing for symptoms have been reported. Choosing imaging modalities that decrease overall radiation exposure in the appropriate clinical setting is important to balance diagnostic accuracy and exposure for these patients.
- Ileocolonoscopy allows for endoscopic disease assessment as well as histologic assessment.
  - Disease activity is graded based on the presence of the erosions and ulcers, mucosal appearance, and presence of strictures or fistulas.
  - Endoscopic stricture dilation of short-segment (< 5 cm) strictures can be safely performed and offers the CD patients an option to avoid surgery.

TREATMENT (SEE FIGURE 34-1)

- The goals of therapy for CD are to induce and then maintain a steroid-free remission with resolution of clinical symptoms and, ideally, mucosal healing. Treatment options include medical (oral, topical, or injectable/infusion based) and/or surgical management.
- Medication selection is dependent on disease behavior, location, symptom severity, and endoscopic activity.
- Steroids have only short-term efficacy for CD with no role as a maintenance medication. The toxicity profile of corticosteroids makes them unacceptable for long-term use as they are associated with increased risks of death, infection, and disease-associated complications.
  - Calcium and vitamin D supplementation is essential while on corticosteroid therapy. Bone densitometry to look for early signs of osteopenia or osteoporosis is recommended for IBD patients who have received prolonged or repeated courses of steroids.
- The immunomodulators, 6-mercaptopurine (6MP), azathioprine, and methotrexate can be used to maintain a steroid-induced remission. They are also used in combination with the biologics (e.g., the anti-tumor necrosis factor-alpha [anti-TNF, agents]) to reduce immunogenicity, the development of antibodies to the biologic agents.

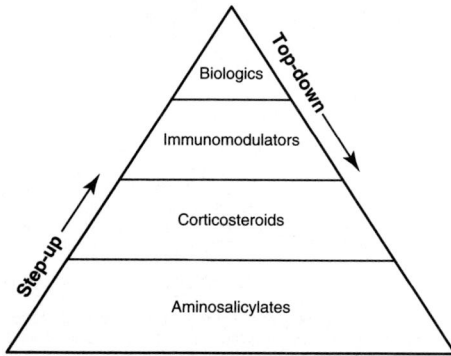

Figure 34-1 Crohn's disease treatment options.

Reproduced from Pharmacologic Therapies for the Management of Crohn's Disease: Comparative Effectiveness. Comparative Effectiveness Review No. 131. AHRQ Agency for Healthcare Research and Quality; February 2014.

- Before starting immunomodulators, it is recommended that thiopurine methyltransferase (TPMT) activity be tested to determine if thiopurines may be safely administered to the patient. 10% of the population has either low or intermediate TPMT activity, which may increase the risk of thiopurine-related myelotoxicity.
- Routine monitoring of complete blood counts and liver enzymes is recommended while on thiopurine or methotrexate therapy to monitor for medication-associated cytopenias and hepatotoxicity.
- Longer term use of thiopurines may also be associated with an increased risk of lymphoproliferative disorders and nonmelanoma skin cancers. Therefore, appropriate counseling and monitoring for these potential malignancies is important, particularly among older CD patients.
- Indications for biologics (e.g., anti-TNFs) include steroid-dependent or refractory CD, patients with persistent disease activity while on thiopurines, or patients presenting with moderate to severe or fulminant disease. Approved biologic agents for CD to date include infliximab, adalimumab, certolizumab pegol, and natalizumab.
  - Before starting anti-TNFs, it is recommended to check tuberculosis testing either with a purified protein derivative (PPD) skin test or QuantiFERON gold tuberculosis serum testing. Also, prior exposure to hepatitis B should be assessed pretreatment.
- Indications for surgery in CD include bowel perforation, hemorrhage, dysplasia/cancer, recurrent bowel obstruction, medically refractory disease, complex fistulizing disease, and complicated perianal disease.
  - Types of surgeries typically performed for CD patients include bowel resections, strictureplasties, incision and drainage of abscesses, fistulotomies, seton placement for perianal disease, and diverting ostomies.
- Healthcare maintenance is important for CD patients, particularly while on immunosuppression. Maintaining up-to-date vaccinations, routine dermatologic and ophthalmologic exams, and cancer surveillance is important for prevention of infection and disease or medication-related complications.

REFERENCES

1. Lichtenstein GR, Abreu MT, Cohen R, Tremaine W. American Gastroenterological Association Institute technical review on corticosteroids, immunomodulators, and infliximab in inflammatory bowel disease. *Gastroenterol.* 2006;130(3):940–87.
2. Lichtenstein GR, Hanauer SB, Sandborn WJ. Management of Crohn's disease in adults. *Am J Gastroenterol.* 2009;104(2):465–83.

CHAPTER 35 ■ POUCHITIS

Michelle Vu, MD and Puja Khanna, MD

OVERVIEW

- Proctocolectomy with ileal pouch-anal anastomosis (IPAA), the surgery of choice for ulcerative colitis (UC) patients with refractory symptoms or dysplasia, is a sphincter-sparing surgery that maintains intestinal continuity and optimizes continence via anastomosis of an ileal pouch to the anus.
- Pouchitis, or inflammation of the ileal reservoir, is the most frequent complication after IPAA and is characterized by a spectrum of manifestations ranging from an acute antibiotic-responsive attack to a chronic, treatment-refractory process.
- The risk of developing at least one episode of pouchitis post-IPAA for UC is approximately 50%, with as many as 40% of patients developing pouchitis within the first year after ileostomy takedown. Inconsistencies in reported prevalence (7%–46%) and incidence (up to 40%) rates are likely due to variation of diagnostic criteria.

PRESENTATION

Patients present with a wide range of symptoms such as increased stool frequency, tenesmus, altered stool consistency, fever, abdominal pain, and hematochezia.

DIFFERENTIAL DIAGNOSIS

Outlet obstruction, infection (bacterial, parasitic, viral), undiagnosed Crohn's disease, anal stenosis, abscess, cuffitis (especially with stapled anastomotic sites), functional bowel syndromes (i.e., irritable pouch syndrome)

PATHOPHYSIOLOGY

- The exact pathogenesis of pouchitis is unknown.
- Characteristic changes, including exposure of the ileal reservoir to an increased fecal load and subsequent adaptive colonic metaplasia, have been described.

- Colonic metaplasia in the pouch predisposes toward dysbiosis and inflammation.
- Analysis of pouch microbiota during acute pouchitis and in pouch-free phases showed decreased concentration of anaerobes and *Lactobacillus* species and a rise in pathogenic organisms such as *Clostridium perfringens* in an acute attack.
- Although certain types of pouchitis are responsive to antibiotics, this association has not been consistently attributed to any single pathogen.

DIAGNOSIS

- Diagnosis is confounded by the fluctuating disease course, where symptomatic patients may not immediately develop endoscopic evidence of pouchitis.
- Disease severity is evaluated via the pouchitis disease activity index (PDAI) and the pouchitis activity score (PAS), which use clinical symptoms, endoscopic changes, and histologic findings of inflammation.
- Pouchoscopy reveals a spectrum of findings: from normal-appearing mucosa to severe mucosal inflammation with erythema, edema, friability, hemorrhage, or ulcerations. Changes associated with chronic inflammation might include the presence of inflammatory polyps, decreased distensibility with insufflation, or loss of normal configuration of the pouch inlet and J portion.
- Biopsies can look for histologic changes that can confirm a diagnosis of pouchitis, characterize acuity/severity of inflammation, and evaluate for other pathologic findings such as granulomas, viral inclusions, dysplasia, ischemia, crypt apoptosis, or chronic inflammation.
- Abdominal/pelvic imaging can also evaluate ileal pouch disorders, especially if there are suspected structural abnormalities. A pouchogram can define anatomy and reveal local stricture, sinus, or fistula. Computed tomography or magnetic resonance imaging enterography can reveal proximal inflammation, strictures, fistulas, or abscesses. Anorectal ultrasound can detect anal sphincter injury in addition to identifying sinuses, strictures, or fistulas.

TREATMENT (SEE FIGURE 35-1)

- Prophylaxis
  - Probiotics, such as VSL #3 and *Lactobacillus rhamnosus* GG, have been evaluated in smaller trials as prophylactic agents against pouchitis after ileostomy closure, and shown to have some benefit. Larger studies with long-term data are not available.
- Acute pouchitis
  - New-onset pouchitis is typically responsive to antibiotic therapy.

Chapter 35: Pouchitis

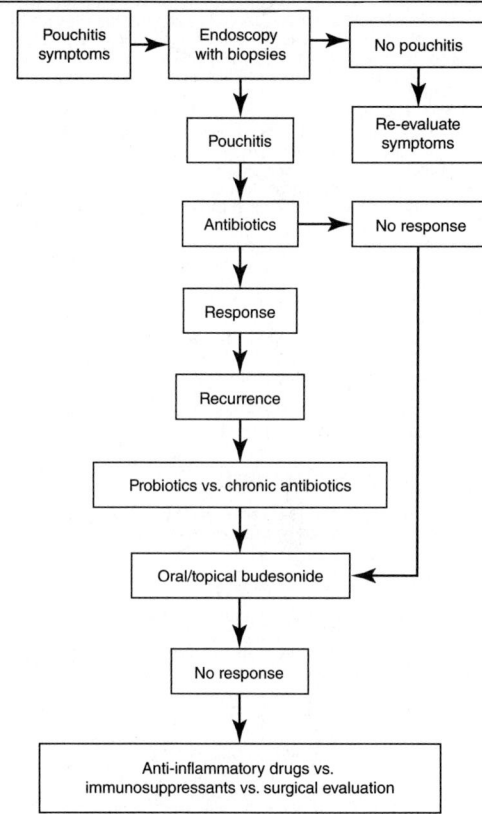

Figure 35-1 Treatment algorithm for pouchitis.

Source: Data from Pardi et al. *IBD* 2009;15:1424–31.

- Metronidazole taken in doses of 1–2 g daily for a week and ciprofloxacin at 1 g daily for a week are effective in treating acute pouchitis.
- For those who do not respond to ciprofloxacin or metronidazole, budesonide administered orally or rectally for 4 weeks may be effective.
- Recurrent pouchitis
  - As many as 19% of patients with acute pouchitis will develop antibiotic-refractory or recurrent disease. Studies of rifaximin as a maintenance agent show good short-term results in those with antibiotic-refractory pouchitis. Oral or topical mesalamine has shown some benefit in smaller studies. Larger studies with long-term data are not available.
- Chronic antibiotic-responsive pouchitis
  - For those who do not respond to traditional antibiotic therapy, a longer course of combination antibiotics may be needed. Common regimens include ciprofloxacin 1 g/day plus rifaximin 2 g/day for 15 days, ciprofloxacin 1 g/day plus metronidazole 1 g/day for 4 weeks, or ciprofloxacin 1 g/day plus tinidazole 15 mg/kg/day for 4 weeks.
  - A subset of patients will develop dependence on medications for pouchitis. Other therapeutic options include budesonide, immunomodulators, and anti-tumor necrosis factor-alpha (anti-TNF) agents. Use of these agents is generally limited to those with Crohn's disease-like complications such as pouch fistulae or structuring.

CANCER SURVEILLANCE

There have been very few cases of cancer within the pouch in post-IPAA UC patients, and as such there are no clear guidelines for cancer surveillance.

REFERENCES

1. Shen B. Pouchitis: what every gastroenterologist needs to know. *Clin Gastroenterol Hepatol*. 2013;11(12):1538–49.
2. Navaneethan U, Shen B. Diagnosis and management of pouchitis and ileoanal pouch dysfunction. *Curr Gastroenterol Rep*. 2010;12(6):485–94.

CHAPTER 36 ■ MICROSCOPIC COLITIS

Eric Esrailian, MD, MPH

OVERVIEW

- Microscopic colitis is the general term used to describe two specific conditions: lymphocytic and collagenous colitis. They have similar clinical presentations and treatment approaches.
- Similarities between lymphocytic colitis and collagenous colitis have been discussed for decades, and they could be two subtypes of the same disease. There is an increasing incidence in population-based studies, and it is no longer considered rare.
- Lymphocytic colitis and collagenous colitis are much more frequent in women—particularly in collagenous colitis. Most patients are older than 50 years of age, but younger patients are more common in collagenous colitis. Lymphocytic colitis is often associated with celiac disease.
- If a patient has chronic diarrhea, think about microscopic colitis!

PRESENTATION

- Typically, microscopic colitis presents as chronic, watery diarrhea. Bowel movements are nonbloody and have increased frequency and urgency. Patients have crampy pain and usually do not have fever, chills, nausea, or vomiting.
- These conditions may involve extraintestinal manifestations if comorbidities, such as celiac disease, are present.
- Nocturnal bowel movements are common.

DIFFERENTIAL DIAGNOSIS

Crohn's disease, ulcerative colitis, celiac disease, chronic infections like giardiasis or *Clostridium difficle*, irritable bowel syndrome

PATHOPHYSIOLOGY

- There is no clear consensus opinion. Autoimmune factors, environmental factors, medications, and infectious etiologies have all been proposed.

- Common medications such as nonsteroidal anti-inflammatory drugs (NSAIDs) and proton pump inhibitors (PPIs) are possible triggers.

DIAGNOSIS

- The diagnosis is definitively made by endoscopy with biopsies. In all cases of microscopic colitis, there is chronic inflammation in the lamina propria. In lymphocytic colitis, there are increased intraepithelial lymphocytes (IEL), and typically > 20 IEL per 100 epithelial cells. In lymphocytic colitis, there is also possible crypt distortion but no abscesses or granulomas.
- In collagenous colitis, there is a distinct thickening of the subepithelial collagen layer, and this band is diagnostic on histopathology.
- Although sigmoidoscopy may yield a diagnosis, the disease can be patchy. When in doubt, right-sided colonic biopsies should be considered with a full colonoscopy. Specimens must be properly described because the right colon can look inflamed in healthy patients and can be mistaken for "pseudo-inflammation" if thought to be from the distal colon.

TREATMENT (SEE FIGURE 36-1)

- Reassurance should be provided to the patient once a diagnosis is made, because microscopic colitis has a good long-term prognosis.
- Possible offending agents should be discontinued if identified (NSAIDs). In patients with celiac disease, adherence to a gluten-free diet should be confirmed.
- Microscopic colitis has a waxing and waning course so the focus should be on quality-of-life impact and symptom control.
- Antidiarrheal therapy should be the mainstay of treatment in mild-to-moderate disease, and relapse is common. Loperamide or diphenoxylate/atropine are first-line therapies, and either one can be titrated to control diarrhea and avoid constipation.
- Bismuth subsalicylate, 2 or 3 tablets (262 mg each) 3–4 times per day for 6–8 weeks, is another option for moderate disease.
- For more active disease, budesonide is the best studied drug in randomized-controlled trials and meta-analyses. A recommended dose for budesonide is 9 mg/day for 6 weeks with a planned taper off of therapy. It has been shown to be better than placebo and with fewer side effects than prednisone. The approach should be similar to its use in inflammatory bowel disease—avoid steroids and consider other agents if possible.

Chapter 36: Microscopic Colitis

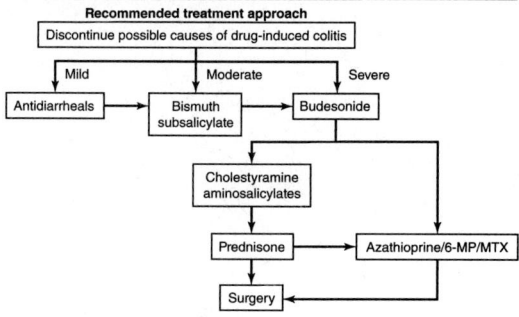

Figure 36-1 Treatment algorithm for microscopic colitis.

Source: Reprinted with permission from Elsevier: Pardi DS, Kelly CP. Microscopic colitis. *Gastroenterol.* 2011;140(4):1155–65.

- Some patients may require long-term therapy at lower doses (3 mg for example).
- There are less data for 5-aminosalicylate drugs, cholestyramine, and immunomodulators like 6-mercaptopurine.

REFERENCES

1. Pardi DS, Kelly CP. Microscopic colitis. *Gastroenterol.* 2011;140(4):1155–65.
2. Pardi DS. Miscellaneous colitides. *Curr Opin Gastroenterol.* 2012;28(1):76–81.

CHAPTER 37 ■ *CLOSTRIDIUM DIFFICILE* INFECTION AND TREATMENT

Ishan Patel, MD and Ciaran P. Kelly, MD

OVERVIEW

- *Clostridium difficile* is an obligate anaerobic, spore-producing, Gram-positive rod.
- *C. difficile* is the causative pathogen in most cases of antibiotic-associated colitis.
- According to the Centers for Disease Control and Prevention (CDC), *C. difficile* infection is linked to 14,000 deaths every year in the United States.

PRESENTATION

Symptoms of *C. difficile* infection (CDI) may include watery diarrhea (3 or more unformed stools within 24 hours), fever, nausea, anorexia, and abdominal pain. Patients with severe disease may develop small bowel and/or colonic ileus or toxic megacolon and present with abdominal pain and distension but minimal or no diarrhea. Peripheral leukocytosis is common but found in fewer than half of patients. Based on severity of illness, patients with CDI can be stratified into the following.

MILD-TO-MODERATE CDI

- Diarrhea (3 or more but < 6 unformed stools within 24 hours)
- Fever < 101°F (38.3°C)
- White blood count (WBC) < 15,000 cells/µL
- Serum creatinine < 1.5 times premorbid level
- Serum albumin > 2.5 mg/dL or unchanged from baseline
- Not a known case of inflammatory bowel disease (IBD)
- Not significantly immunocompromised

SEVERE CDI

- Diarrhea (> 6 unformed stools within 24 hours)
- Fever ≥ 101°F (38.3°C)
- WBC ≥ 15,000 cells/µL but < 20,000 cells/µL
- Serum creatinine ≥ 1.5 times premorbid level
- Serum albumin ≤ 2.5 mg/dL

- Known case of IBD
- Immunocompromised

SEVERE-COMPLICATED CDI

- Admission to ICU for CDI
- Ileus
- Megacolon
- Hemodynamic instability
- Pressor requirement
- Sepsis
- WBC ≥ 20,000 cells/μL
- Serum lactate (> 5 mmol/L)
- Confluent pseudomembranous colitis seen on colonoscopy
- Colonic perforation

DIFFERENTIAL DIAGNOSIS

- Simple antibiotic-associated diarrhea
- Other infectious causes like *Clostridium perfringens* type A, *Staphylococcus aureus*, and *Salmonella enterica*
- Noninfectious causes like postinfectious irritable bowel syndrome that occurs following a successfully treated initial CDI episode, osmotic diarrhea, etc.

PATHOPHYSIOLOGY

- Primary mode of *C. difficile* transmission is person-to-person spread through the fecal–oral route.
- Risk factors for CDI include:
    i. Antibiotic exposure
    ii. Hospitalization
    iii. Increasing age
    iv. Enteral feeding
    v. Gastrointestinal surgery
    vi. Cancer chemotherapy
    vii. Possibly, gastric acid suppressing medication like proton pump inhibitors (PPIs)
- The main risk factor for CDI is antibiotic exposure, which disrupts the colonic microflora and provides an opportunity for *C. difficile* to colonize in the large intestine and release two potent exotoxins: toxin A and toxin B responsible for causing CDI.

DIAGNOSIS

Testing for *C. difficile* or its toxins should be performed only on diarrheal (unformed) stool. A number of stool tests are available, including:

- Polymerase chain reaction (PCR)
  - Rapid and sensitive. Will also be positive in those with symptomless carriage
- Enzyme immunoassay (EIA) for *C. difficile* toxin A and B
  - Sensitivity (63–94%) and specificity (75–100%)
- Enzyme immunoassay (EIA) for *C. difficile* glutamate dehydrogenase (GDH)
  - Sensitivity (85–95%) with negative predictive value of 95–100% but low positive predictive value of 50%
- Cell culture cytotoxicity assay
  - High sensitivity (67–100%) but takes 24 to 48 hours and requires tissue culture facility
- Selective anaerobic culture
  - Highly sensitive and useful for epidemiologic studies but requires 48 to 72 hours for culture followed by confirmation of toxigenicity using a toxin assay

TREATMENT (SEE FIGURE 37-1)

MILD-TO-MODERATE CDI

- Oral metronidazole 500 mg every 8 hours for 10–14 days
- Oral vancomycin 125 mg every 6 hours for 10–14 days if there is a failure to respond to metronidazole within 5–7 days or metronidazole intolerance or metronidazole allergy or pregnancy or breastfeeding

SEVERE CDI

- Oral vancomycin 125 mg every 6 hours for 10–14 days.
- If vomiting or other risk of poor delivery of enteral vancomycin, consider IV metronidazole 500 mg every 8 hours for initial therapy.
- Intravenous tigecycline was shown to successfully treat a small number of patients with severe CDI refractory to standard treatment.
- Intravenous immunoglobulin (IVIG) (150–400 mg/kg) may be helpful in patients with hypogammaglobulinemia and in those not responding to other therapies in some cases.

SEVERE-COMPLICATED CDI

- Vancomycin 500 mg every 6 hours orally or by nasogastric tube plus metronidazole 500 mg every 8 hours intravenously

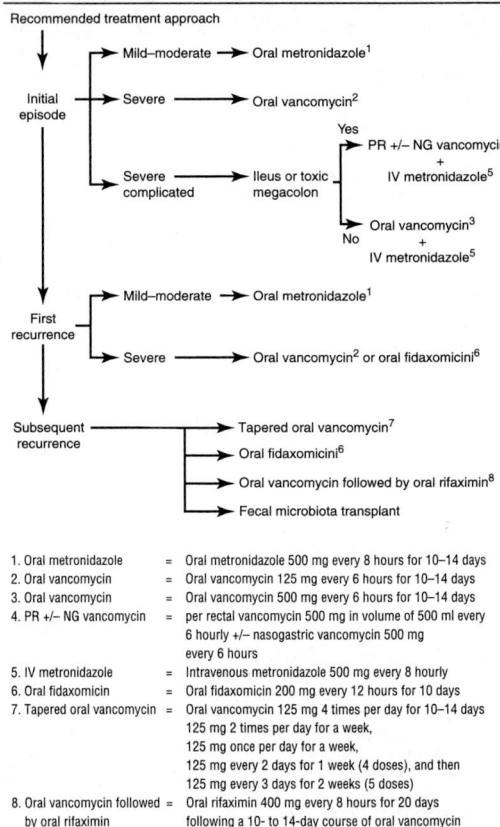

Figure 37-1 Recommended treatment approach for *Clostridium difficile* infection.

- In setting of ileus, consider rectal (500 mg in volume of 500 mL every 6 hours) and/or nasogastric (500 mg every 6 hours) instillation of vancomycin.
- Consult surgery for consideration of subtotal colectomy or diverting loop ileostomy with colonic lavage and intracolonic vancomycin instillation.

RECURRENT DISEASE

Occurs in ~25% of patients treated with metronidazole or with oral vancomycin.

- Initial recurrence:
  - Mild-to-moderate disease
    - Oral metronidazole 500 mg three times daily for 10–14 days
  - Severe or unresponsive to or intolerance of metronidazole
    - Oral vancomycin 125 mg four times daily for 10–14 days
- Subsequent recurrence
  - Tapered and pulsed regimen of oral vancomycin
    - 125 mg four times per day for 10–14 days then
    - 125 mg two times per day for a week then
    - 125 mg once per day for a week then
    - 125 mg every 2 days for 1 week (four doses) then
    - 125 mg every 3 days for 2 weeks (five doses)
  - Fecal microbiota transplantation (FMT) should be considered if there is a third recurrence after a pulsed vancomycin regimen and/or fidaxomicin therapy.
  - Oral rifaximin 400 mg three times per day for 20 days following a 10–14 day course of oral vancomycin.
  - There are limited and conflicting data on the efficacy of adjuvant probiotics in preventing recurrent CDI.
- Fidaxomicin became available in 2011 for treatment of CDI but its place in management has yet to be determined in major national guidelines.
  - Lower recurrence rate is seen with fidaxomicin therapy (200 mg orally twice daily for 10 days) when compared to vancomycin.
    - In an initial episode of CDI (15.4% vs 25.3%)
    - In non-NAP-1 infected subjects (7.8% vs 25.5%)
    - In subjects with a first recurrence of CDI (19.7% vs 35.5%)

REFERENCES

1. Kelly CP, LaMont JT. Antibiotic-associated diarrhea, pseudomembranous enterocolitis and *Clostridium difficile* associated diarrhea and colitis. In: Feldman M, Friedman LS, and Brandt LJ, eds. *Sleisenger & Fordtran's Gastrointestinal and Liver Disease*, 9th ed. Philadelphia: WB Saunders Co., 2010: 1889–1904.
2. Cohen SH, Gerding DN, Johnson S, et al. Clinical practice guidelines for *Clostridium difficile* infection in adults: 2010 update by the Society

for Healthcare Epidemiology of America (SHEA) and the Infectious Diseases Society of America (IDSA). *Infect Control Hosp Epidemiol.* 2010;31(5):431–55.
3. Surawicz CM, Brandt LJ, Binion DG, et al. Guidelines for diagnosis, treatment, and prevention of *Clostridium difficile* infections. *Am J Gastroenterol.* 2013;108(4):478–98.
4. Beth Israel Deaconess Medical Center. *Interdisciplinary Practice Guidelines for the Diagnosis and Treatment of* Clostridium difficile *Infection* (CDI). Boston: Author. March 16, 2011. Revised April 2012.
5. Cloud J, Noddin L, Pressman A, Hu M, Kelly C. *Clostridium difficile* strain NAP-1 is not associated with severe disease in a nonepidemic setting. *Clin Gastroenterol Hepatol.* 2009;7(8):868–73.
6. Herpers BL, Vlaminckx B, Burkhardt O, et al. Intravenous tigecycline as adjunctive or alternative therapy for severe refractory *Clostridium difficile* infection. *Clin Infect Dis.* 2009;48(12):1732–5.
7. Garey KW, Ghantoji SS, Shah DN, et al. A randomized, double-blind, placebo-controlled pilot study to assess the ability of rifaximin to prevent recurrent diarrhoea in patients with *Clostridium difficile* infection. *J Antimicrob Chemother.* 2011;66(12):2850–5.
8. Louie TJ, Miller MA, Mullane KM, et al. Fidaxomicin versus vancomycin for *Clostridium difficile* infection. *N Engl J Med.* 2011;364(5):422–31.
9. Cornely OA, Miller MA, Louie TJ, Crook DW, Gorbach SL. Treatment of first recurrence of *Clostridium difficile infection*: fidaxomicin versus vancomycin. *Clin Infect Dis.* 2012;55(Suppl 2):S154–61.

PART III HEPATOLOGY

CHAPTER 38 ■ APPROACH TO ABNORMAL LIVER TESTS

Nirupama Bonthala, MD and Saro Khemichian, MD

OVERVIEW

Abnormal liver tests are a common cause of referrals to subspecialists. A preliminary workup is often performed by primary care physicians or other healthcare providers. This chapter aims to provide a general understanding and guidance to begin an appropriate workup (see **Figure 38-1**). Please refer to the specific liver chapters for further information.

LIVER PANEL TESTS

LIVER ENZYMES
- Alanine aminotransferase (ALT, formerly serum glutamic pyruvic transaminase [SGPT]): more specific to liver.
- Aspartate aminotransferase (AST, formerly serum glutamic oxaloacetic transaminase [SGOT]): can also be found in skeletal muscle, heart, brain, kidney.
- Alkaline phosphatase; derived from liver, bones, and to a small extent small bowel; may also be increased in third trimester of pregnancy due to placental production.
- Gamma-glutamyl transpeptidase: found in hepatocytes and biliary epithelial cells, as well as in the kidney, seminal vesicles, pancreas, spleen, heart, and brain.
- 5' nucleotidase: found in the liver, intestine, brain, heart, blood vessels, and endocrine pancreas.

MAJOR TESTS OF HEPATIC SYNTHETIC FUNCTION
- Albumin
- Prothrombin time
- Bilirubin—See **Table 38-3** for causes of unconjugated and conjugated hyperbilirubinemia

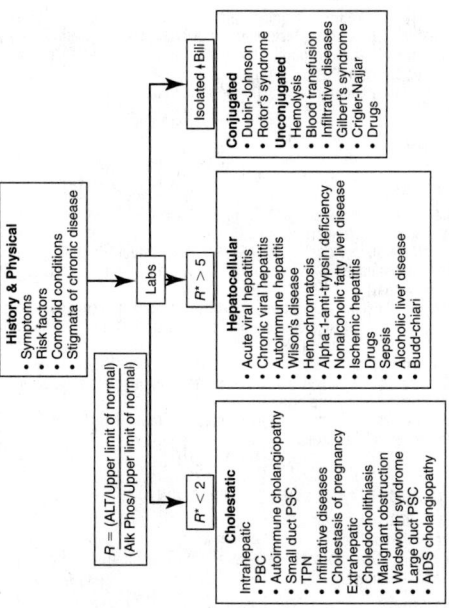

Figure 38-1 Summary of general approach in a patient with abnormal liver tests.

Chapter 38: Approach to Abnormal Liver Tests

PATTERNS OF INJURY

Liver panel abnormalities may fit certain patterns that help in differentiating different causes of liver disease or injury. An easier way to distinguish these patterns is to use them in an equation:

R value = (ALT/Upper limit of normal [ULN]) ÷ (Alk Phos/Upper limit of normal)

$R > 5$ = hepatocellular

$R < 2$ = cholestatic

$R > 2$ but < 5 = mixed hepatocellular/cholestatic

INITIAL APPROACH

An initial approach is to obtain a thorough history and physical examination.

HISTORY
- Evaluate for risk factors.
  - Exposure to hepatotoxins (alcohol, medications, herbs, over-the-counter medications, chemical exposures).
  - Drugs are typically a major cause of liver injury. There is a constantly evolving list of potential hepatotoxic medications that can be found at http://livertox.nih.gov.
  - Risk factors for viral hepatitis including blood transfusions, injection drug use, high-risk sexual behaviors, family history, travel to endemic areas.
  - Medical conditions such as obesity, diabetes mellitus, inflammatory bowel disease, celiac disease, thyroid disease, and neuromuscular diseases.
- Evaluate for symptoms: fatigue, jaundice, easy bruising, gastrointestinal bleeding, confusion.

PHYSICAL EXAM

If asymptomatic, may be normal. Findings to suggest chronic liver disease include spider nevi, palmar erythema, gynecomastia, distended abdominal veins and caput medusa, temporal and proximal muscle wasting, ascites, encephalopathy, jaundice, scleral icterus.

CAUSES OF INJURY (SEE TABLES 38-1 AND 38-2)

HEPATOCELLULAR INJURY
- ALT > AST with both > 10 × ULN (marked elevation): acute viral hepatitis, acute drug injury, ischemic injury, acute Wilson's, autoimmune hepatitis

Table 38-1 Causes of Hepatocellular Injury

Major Causes of Hepatocellular Injury	Indicated Initial Tests
Acute viral hepatitis	HAV IgM, HBsAg, HBcIgM, HCV Ab, HCV RNA
Chronic viral hepatitis	HCV Ab, HCV RNA, HBsAg, HBctotal
Autoimmune hepatitis	ASMA, ANA, immunoglobulin G
Wilson's Disease	Ceruloplasmin
Hemochromatosis	Ferritin
Alpha-1-anti-trypsin deficiency	Alpha-1-anti-trypsin phenotype
Nonalcoholic fatty liver disease, ischemic hepatitis, drugs, sepsis, alcoholic liver disease, Budd-Chiari syndrome, portal vein thrombosis, HELLP (hemolysis, elevated liver enzymes, low platelets in pregnancy), muscle disorders (polymyositis), malignant infiltration, celiac, Thyroid disease, congestive heart failure	Appropriate history, physical exam, laboratory, and imaging

Table 38-2 Causes of Cholestatic Injury

Intrahepatic Cholestasis	Extrahepatic Cholestasis
Primary biliary cirrhosis	Choledocholithiasis
Autoimmune cholangiopathy	Malignant obstruction
Primary sclerosing cholangitis (small duct)	Large duct primary sclerosing cholangitis
Cholestasis of pregnancy	AIDS cholangiopathy
Total parenteral nutrition	Wadsworth syndrome (biliary stenosis from chronic pancreatitis)
Paraneoplastic phenomenon	
Infiltrative diseases of the liver (fungal infection, tuberculosis, sarcoidosis, amyloidosis, malignancies)	

- AST > ALT 2:1 with both < 10 × ULN: potential alcohol abuse.
- AST >>> ALT: muscle disorders, strenuous exercise. Check creatinine kinase (CK).

CHOLESTATIC INJURY

Indicated initial tests:

- Extrahepatic cholestasis will typically show biliary abnormalities. Ultrasound is a good initial imaging modality to start. Further imaging can be done with MRCP, CT, or EUS.

Chapter 38: Approach to Abnormal Liver Tests

Table 38-3 Causes of Unconjugated and Conjugated Hyperbilirubinemia

Unconjugated Hyperbilirubinemia
• Increased bilirubin production (e.g., hemolysis, ineffective erythropoiesis, blood transfusion, resorption of hematomas)
• Decreased hepatocellular uptake (e.g., drugs such as rifampin)
• Decreased conjugation (e.g., Gilbert's syndrome, Crigler-Najjar syndrome, physiologic jaundice of the newborn, drugs)
Conjugated or Mixed Hyperbilirubinemia
• Dubin-Johnson syndrome
• Rotor's syndrome

- Intrahepatic cholestasis may not demonstrate any radiographic abnormalities. Further evaluation is indicated based on the clinical setting. Liver biopsy may also be helpful.

ABBREVIATIONS

ALT: alanine aminotransferase

SGPT: serum glutamic pyruvic transaminase

AST: aspartate aminotransferase

SGOT: serum glutamic oxaloacetic transaminase

ULN: upper limit of normal

CK: creatinine kinase

HAV IgM: hepatitis A virus immunoglobulin M

HbSAG: hepatitis B surface antigen

HBcIgM: hepatitis B core immunoglobulin M

HCV Ab: hepatitis C virus antibody

HCV RNA: hepatitis C virus ribonucleic acid

HBctotal: hepatitis B core total

ASMA: anti-smooth muscle antibody

ANA: anti-nuclear antibody

HELLP: hemolysis elevated liver enzymes low platelets

AIDS: acquired immunodeficiency syndrome

MRCP: magnetic resonance cholangiopancreatography

CT: computed tomography

EUS: endoscopic ultrasound

NAFLD: nonalcoholic fatty liver disease
Hep B: hepatitis B
Hep C: hepatitis C
US: ultrasound

REFERENCE

1. Pratt DS, Kaplan MM. Evaluation of abnormal liver-enzyme results in asymptomatic patients. *N Engl J Med*. 2000;342:1266.

CHAPTER 39 ■ HEPATITIS B VIRUS

Kali Zhou, MD, Dave Garg, and Steven-Huy B. Han, MD, AGAF, FAASLD

OVERVIEW

- There are approximately 350 million hepatitis B carriers worldwide and 1.25 million in the United States; 1 million die annually from hepatitis B virus (HBV)-related liver disease including cirrhosis, end-stage liver failure, and hepatocellular carcinoma (HCC).
- It is a member of the Hepadnaviridae family, enveloped, circular, partially double-stranded deoxyribonucleic acid (dsDNA).
- HBV virions characteristically undergo replication of the DNA genome by reverse transcriptase of an RNA intermediate that is generated within the nucleus of the cell and then transported to the cytoplasm.
- High-prevalence areas (Asian): vertical transmission, usually establishes lifelong infection in 90% of affected.
- Low-prevalence areas (Western): favors horizontal transmission during adolescence and early adulthood via sexual activity, injection-drug use, and occupational exposure.

PATHOPHYSIOLOGY

- HBV replication cycle is not directly hepatotoxic.
- Host immune response to HBV antigens on infected hepatocytes is primary means of cell injury by strong T-cell response in acute infection and decreased cytotoxic T-cell activity in chronic carriers with resultant secondary inflammation.

PRESENTATION

ACUTE INFECTION

- Common manifestations include jaundice, nausea, vomiting, body ache, fever, dark urine; symptoms present 60–150 days after exposure to HBV and can persist up to 6 months.
- HBsAg, HBeAg, and HBV DNA are detectable within 6 weeks of inoculation.

- Most primary infections in adults are self-limiting, with clearance from blood/liver with development of lasting immunity.
- Likelihood of progression to chronic infection is highest in infants/children acquiring infection perinatally, and decreases with the age of the patient at time of inoculation.
- Rarely develops into fulminant hepatitis. Fatality rate in acute cases is 0.5–1% according to the Centers for Disease Control and Prevention (CDC).

CHRONIC INFECTION (DOCUMENTED HBSAG POSITIVITY > 6 MONTHS)

- Phases of chronic HBV infection (see **Table 39-1**):
  - <u>Immune tolerant phase</u>: typically early on in patients infected at birth with high levels of HBV DNA (> 20,000 IU/mL), normal serum aminotransferase (ALT) levels, and no-to-minimal histological disease.
  - <u>Immune active (clearance) phase (HBeAg-positive chronic hepatitis B)</u>: virus is recognized as foreign with elevated ALT, high HBV DNA (> 20,000 IU/mL), and active histological disease.
    - 0.5–1% will clear HBsAg.
    - Most enter the "inactive carrier phase."
  - <u>Inactive carrier state</u>: characterized by persistently normal ALT, undetectable or low (< 2,000 IU/mL) HBV DNA, and inactive histological disease.
  - <u>Reactivation phase (HBeAg-negative chronic hepatitis B)</u>: due to development of precore or basal core promoter mutation causing spontaneous seroconversion from HBeAg-positive to HBeAg-negative/anti-HBe-positive infection; characterized by elevated, fluctuating ALT levels, moderate and fluctuating (> 2,000 IU/mL) HBV DNA, and active histological disease with variable amounts of fibrosis.
    - 10–40% experience reversions back to HBeAg seropositivity, associated with flares of hepatitis.

Table 39-1 Clinical Profiles of Chronic HBV Infection

	Immune Tolerant	HBeAg (+) CHB	Inactive HbsAg Carrier	HBeAg (−) CHB (Precore Mutant)
HBsAg	+	+	+	+
HBeAg	+	+	−	−
Anti-HBe	−	−	+	+
ALT	Normal	↑	Normal	↑
HBV DNA	> 20,000 IU/mL	> 20,000 IU/mL	< 200 IU/mL	> 2,000 IU/mL
Histology	Normal/Mild	Active	Normal	Active

Source: Data from Hoofnagle JH et al. *Hepatol*, 2007;45:1056–75.

Chapter 39: Hepatitis B Virus

- 20% of patients with chronic HBV infection will develop cirrhosis, characterized by marked fibrosis with regenerative nodules on liver biopsy, with development of hepatic insufficiency and portal hypertension.
- Of these patients, 6–15% will develop HCC and 20–23% will experience hepatic decompensation requiring consideration for liver transplantation.

DIAGNOSIS (SEE TABLE 39-2)

- Consider screening for HBV in immigrants, travelers from endemic regions, pregnant women, infants born to infected mothers or parents who were born in highly endemic areas, household/sexual contacts of HBsAg-positive persons, men who have sex with men, history of intravenous drugs, hemodialysis patients, healthcare workers, human immunodeficiency virus (HIV)/hepatitis C virus (HCV)–infected patients, immunosuppressed patients.
- HBV surface antigen (HBsAg): an envelope protein—marker of infection that becomes detectable in blood after incubation period of 4 to 10 weeks.
- HBV surface antibody (anti-HBs): marker of recovery from infection, vaccination, immunoglobulins. May be "falsely negative" during window period when HBsAg is gone but anti-HBs is not yet present.
- HBV core antigen (HBcAg): a structural nucleocapsid core protein—not detectable by commercial assays.
- HBV core antibody (anti-HBc): marker of exposure (anti-HBc IgM for acute infection and anti-HBc IgG in chronic infection).

Table 39-2 Diagnostic Interpretation of HBV Serologic Markers

Serologic Marker				
HBsAg	Total anti-HBc	IgM anti-HBc	Anti-HBs	Interpretation
−	−	−	−	Never infected and no evidence of immunization
+	+	−	−	Chronic infection
+	+	+	−	Acute infection
−	+	−	+	Recovered from past infection and immune
−	−	−	+	Immune after immunization
−	+	−	−	Past exposure with undetectable anti-HBs titers, previous chronic infection with loss of HbsAg or a false positive test

Source: Modified from Weinbaum CM et al. *MMWR*, 2008;57(RR08):1–20.

- HBV "e" antigen (HBeAg): a soluble nucleocapsid protein—marker of active viral replication.
- HBV "e" antibody (anti-HBe): marker of reduced viral replication, indicating lower level of infectivity. May be present in patients with HBeAg-negative chronic hepatitis B.

EVALUATION

- History: assess patient's current symptomology and ask about alcohol and drug use, sexual practices, family origin, family history of liver disease and/or HCC, risk factors for HCV, HIV testing, immunizations.
- Physical: examine eye and base of tongue for signs of jaundice, palpate liver edge, evaluate for signs of portal hypertension and end-stage liver disease.
- Labs/tests: complete blood count (CBC) with platelets, prothrombin time, hepatic panel to assess liver function; serology for HBV: HBsAg, anti-HBsAg, anti-HBcAg, HBeAg, anti-HBeAg, HBV DNA; anti-HCV, anti-HDV (hepatitis D virus), HIV testing to rule out co-infection with other viruses; baseline alpha fetoprotein (AFP).
- Imaging: ultrasonography assists in evaluation for cirrhosis along with screening for HCC.
- Liver biopsy: for grading of inflammation and staging of fibrosis.

TREATMENT (SEE TABLE 39-3)

- Goals of antiviral treatment are to suppress HBV DNA to low or undetectable levels to improve survival and prevent cirrhosis and HCC. Antiviral treatment is determined by the patient's HBeAg status, HBV DNA level, ALT level, and stage of liver disease. Treatment should be managed with specialist, given rapid changes in available therapies/guidelines.
- In patients without cirrhosis, antiviral therapy is indicated for patients with persistently elevated ALT levels *and* elevated HBV DNA levels according to specific criteria—which vary among specific guidelines (Table 39-3).
- In patients with cirrhosis, antiviral therapy is indicated if the patient has detectable HBV DNA by polymerase chain reaction (PCR).
- Antiviral therapy is *not* currently indicated for patients in the "immuno-tolerant phase" or "inactive carrier state."
- Several antiviral drugs are approved for treatment of chronic hepatitis B: interferon alfa-2b, pegylated interferon alfa-2a, and the oral nucleoside/nucleotide analogues adefovir, lamivudine, entecavir, telbivudine, and tenofovir.

Table 39-3 Treatment Criteria for Chronic Hepatitis B

Guideline	HBeAg+		HBeAg−	
	HBV DNA IU/mL	ALT U/L	HBV DNA IU/mL	ALT U/L
EASL 2009[1]	> 2,000	> ULN	> 2,000	> ULN
US Algorithm 2008[2]	≥ 20,000	> ULN or (+) biopsy	≥ 20,000	> ULN or (+) biopsy
APASL 2008[3]	≥ 20,000	> 2× ULN	≥ 2,000	> 2× ULN
AASLD 2009[4]	> 20,000	> 2× ULN or (+) biopsy	2,000–20,000	> 2× ULN or (+) biopsy

1. European Association for the Study of the Liver. *J Hepatol.* 2009;50:227–42.
2. Keeffe EB et al. *Clin Gastroenterol Hepatol.* 2008;6:1315–41.
3. Liaw Y-F et al. *Hepatol Int.* 2008;2:263–83.
4. Lok ABF, McMahon BJ. *Hepatology.* 2009;50:1–36.

- Long-acting pegylated interferon alfa-2a, injected once weekly for 1 year, is associated with comparable rates of HBeAg seroconversion to oral agents. However, oral agents typically require administration for > 1 year to achieve similar rates of HBeAg seroconversion. Advantages of pegylated interferon include a fixed 48-week period of therapy, no drug resistance, and high likelihood of durable response. However, interferon has many adverse side effects including flulike symptoms, marrow suppression, depression and anxiety, and autoimmune disorders. Interferon therapy is contraindicated in decompensated cirrhosis.
- Oral agents are effective in patients who previously did not respond to interferon therapy or have high/recent hepatitis B viremia. They are the only option for treating decompensated chronic HBV infection. Advantages of oral therapy include ease of administration and negligible side effect profile.
  - Entecavir and tenofovir are considered preferred first-line therapy given their high potency and lower rates of viral resistance. Lamivudine, telbivudine, and adefovir are not preferred as first-line therapy due to their high resistance profiles. Pegylated interferon is also considered preferred therapy.
- Duration of oral antiviral therapy:
  - In HBeAg-positive patients, treatment is continued 6 to 12 months after HBeAg seroconversion, then can be stopped, which results in a durable response in approximately 92% of patients. Because treatment is not always durable, continued monitoring is important to identify relapse.
  - In HBeAg-negative patients, oral antiviral therapy is indefinite, or until HBsAg loss, due to high relapse rates after stopping treatment.

- In patients with cirrhosis, oral antiviral therapy is indefinite, or until HBsAg loss, to maintain undetectable HBV DNA. Patients with decompensated cirrhosis should also be referred for liver transplantation.
- Screening for hepatocellular carcinoma should include ultrasound and serum AFP every 6 months in high-risk patients including: Asian men > FFEntecavir age 40 and women > FFEntecavir age 50, patients with cirrhosis, African Americans > FFEntecavir age 20, family history of hepatocellular carcinoma.

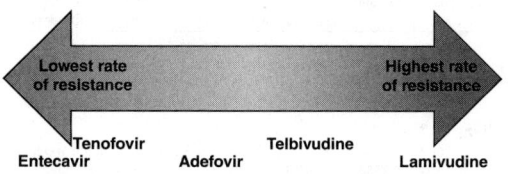

(First-line therapies) (Second-line therapies) (Third-line therapies)

Resistance does not appear to emerge during treatment with IFN α-2b or PEG-IFN α-2a

Figure 39-1 U.S. Treatment algorithm—resistance profile: first-line treatment options have the lowest resistance rates.

Source: Data from Keeffe EB, Dieterich DT, Han SH, et al. A treatment algorithm for the management of chronic hepatitis B virus infection in the United States: 2008 update. *Clin Gastroenterol Hepatol.* 2008;6(12):1315–41.

REFERENCES

1. Dienstag JL. Hepatitis B virus infection. *N Engl J Med.* 2008;359:1486–500.
2. Ganem D, Prince AM. Hepatitis B virus infection—natural history and clinical consequences. *N Engl J Med.* 2004;350:1118–29.
3. Lok AS, McMahon BJ. Chronic hepatitis B practice guidelines. *AASLD Practice Guidelines.* Alexandria, VA: American Association for the Study of Liver Diseases (AASLD); 2009.
4. McMahon BJ. Natural history of chronic hepatitis B. *Clin Liver Dis.* 2010;14:381–96.
5. Keeffe EB, Dieterich DT, Han S-H, et al. A treatment algorithm for the management of chronic hepatitis B virus infection in the United States: 2008 update. *Clin Gastroenterol Hepatol.* 2008;6:1315–41.

CHAPTER 40 ■ HEPATITIS C INFECTION

Alan J. Sheinbaum, MD

OVERVIEW

- An estimated 170 to 200 million people worldwide and 3 to 4 million people in the United States are infected with hepatitis C virus (HCV). These numbers may underestimate true prevalence when considering marginalized populations such as prisoners and the homeless.
- Since the 1990s, we have made slow but steady progress in the treatment of this infection.
- Drug development for HCV is dynamic, and recently approved drugs will alter our thinking and approach to this infection.

VIROLOGY AND EPIDEMIOLOGY

- HCV is a virus of the *Flaviviridae* family of viruses.
- Primitive virus consisting of an envelope and a positive single strand of ribonucleic acid (RNA).
- Primitive nature gives it many of its characteristics:
  - Remains in the cytoplasm of the liver cell and does not enter the nucleus. Infection is curable if the virus can be completely eradicated.
  - No extrahepatic reservoir of the virus.
  - Numerous viral mutations: may prove resistance to treatment.
- Six basic genotypes of this virus (numbered 1–6). These genotypes have subtypes called *quasispecies*.
- Transmission is from human to human via blood to blood.
- No apparent intermediate vectors known.
- Survival at room temperature outside the body for 16–96 hours.

TRANSMISSION AND SUSCEPTIBILITY

Sharing needles and drug-injecting equipment, recipients of human clotting factors prior to 1987 or blood transfusions or human allografts prior to 1992, tattoos or body piercings with unsterile equipment, patients with human immunodeficiency virus (HIV), dialysis patients, healthcare workers who have had needle-stick injuries, sexual contact and maternal–infant route (less than 5%)

NATURAL HISTORY

- Typically, HCV infection is silent and chronic.
- 70–85% of patients exposed develop lifelong infection.
- Acute infection is usually symptomless: minority may develop nonspecific, mild flu-like symptoms.
- 75% of the chronically ill in the United States do not know they have the disease.
- Inflammation and scarring slowly progressive over decades.
- Approximately 40–60% of patients will develop cirrhosis in 2 to 3 decades.
- Fibrosis maybe accelerated concomitant HIV or HBV or in those who regularly abuse alcohol.
- Cirrhosis increases risk of liver cancer and/or liver failure: mortality risk of about 4% per year.

EXTRAHEPATIC DISORDERS ASSOCIATED WITH HCV

Autoimmune disorders (auto-antibodies, Sjögren's syndrome, thyroiditis, autoimmune hepatitis, idiopathic thrombocytopenic purpura), dermatologic disorders (lichen planus, porphyria cutanea tarda, leukocytoclastic vasculitis), diabetes mellitus, glomerular renal diseases, hematologic disorders (B-cell lymph proliferative disorders, monoclonal gammopathies, essential mixed cryoglobulinemia)

COMMON DEFINITIONS TO KNOW WHEN TREATING HCV

- Null: null response has been historically defined as *inability* to achieve a 2 $\log_{10}$ decline in viral RNA by treatment week 12 (TW12).
- Partial: partial response has been historically defined as *ability* to achieve a 2 $\log_{10}$ decline in viral RNA by treatment TW12 but *inability* to clear virus completely by treatment week 24 (TW24).
- RVR: rapid viral response (no detectable virus after 4 weeks of therapy; previously used as a guide to response-guided therapy; may now be useful in detecting nonadherence to treatment regimen since current RVRs approach 100%).
- EOT: end-of-treatment response (typically reflects absence of virus on last day of treatment and is used to calculate relapse rates when virus is subsequently detected in serum).
- Relapse: EOT followed by reappearance of virus at some defined time after treatment is stopped.
- SVR_x: sustained viral response (no detectable virus × weeks after completing therapy). Current "gold standard" is SVR_{12}, which correlates well with prior standard of SVR_{24}.

Chapter 40: Hepatitis C Infection

CURRENT TREATMENTS AND CAVEATS

- Current and past therapies for hepatitis C have included pegylated interferon (PEG) and ribavirin (RBV) for 24–48 weeks depending upon the genotype of virus being treated. Interferon-free therapies have now been approved for certain types of infection and it is likely that interferon and ribavirin-based regimens will be phased out as newer all-oral direct acting antiviral (DAA) regimens are U.S. Food and Drug Administration (FDA)–approved in the coming years.
- In 2011 the first DAAs were approved and used in combination with pegylated interferon and ribavirin for patients with genotype 1 virus. The SVR rate for these medications ranged between 68% and 79%. These have been all but rendered obsolete with the advent of newer DAAs, which have a better safety profile and fewer side effects, are easier to use, and are more effective (see below).
- With the use of interferon/ribavirin, there were many obstacles to treatment to take into consideration prior to starting therapy.
- Only genotype and glomerular filtration rate (GFR) will likely become important as our treatment improves in the future. As some currently approved regimens still involve use of interferon, these pretreatment considerations will still be necessary. (Please refer to http://www.accessdata.fda.gov/drugsatfda_docs/label/2002/pegihof101602lb.htm for details regarding use of interferon and http://www.accessdata.fda.gov/drugsatfda_docs/label/2011/021511s023lbl.pdf for details regarding use of ribavirin.)

COMMON SIDE EFFECTS OF PEG/RBV THERAPY

Fatigue, headache, pyrexia, myalgia, rigors, insomnia, nausea, alopecia, irritability, arthralgia, anorexia, dermatitis, and depression

THERAPIES WITH PROTEASE INHIBITORS—BOCEPREVIR AND TELAPREVIR FOR GENOTYPE 1

While these drugs enhanced the viral response to interferon/ribavirin therapy for patients with genotype 1 HCV, they also added new side effects, difficult-to-follow treatment algorithms, drug–drug interactions, and an increased pill burden. Nevertheless, their improved effectiveness was indisputable and they became popular for several years until recently—when newer DAAs have replaced them.

RECENTLY APPROVED THERAPIES FOR HCV

▇ *Sofosbuvir (SOF) + ribavirin for genotype 2 and genotype 3 virus*

See http://www.gilead.com/~/media/Files/pdfs/medicines/liver-disease/sovaldi/sovaldi_pi.pdf for prescribing details.

- SOF is a DAA targeting the very important stage in viral replication where viral RNA is reproduced for the next generation of virus.

It does not target the virus enzyme responsible for RNA production (polymerase) but targets the newly forming RNA itself. Therefore, it is generally impervious to mutational resistance and is *effective for all genotypes*.
- Single pill per day and has very minimal side effects, the most prominent (> 10%) of which are fatigue, headache, nausea, and insomnia when used with ribavirin.
- SOF is not approved for patients with significant renal insufficiency (GFR < 30%) and because use with ribavirin is currently mandatory, it is not approved in women and partners of women who are pregnant or of childbearing potential and will not/cannot use two forms of contraception.
- SOF is approved in combination with weight-based ribavirin for 12 weeks of treatment in patients with genotype 2 disease who have never before been treated (treatment naïve, or TN) or who have been treated but have failed prior therapy because of ineffective viral response or intolerance to interferon (treatment experienced, or TE).
- SOF is approved in combination with weight-based ribavirin for 24 weeks of treatment in patients with genotype 3 disease who have never before been treated (TN) or who have been treated but have failed prior therapy because of ineffective viral response or intolerance to interferon (TE).

■ *Sofosbuvir + pegylated interferon + ribavirin for genotype 1 and genotype 4 virus*

- SOF is approved in combination with pegylated interferon and weight-based ribavirin for 12 weeks of treatment in patients with genotype 1 or genotype 4 infection who have never before been treated (TN) or who have been treated but have failed prior therapy because of ineffective viral response or intolerance to interferon (TE).
- SOF is approved in combination with weight-based ribavirin alone for 24 weeks of treatment in patients with genotype 1 or genotype 4 infection who have never before been treated (TN) or who have been treated but have failed prior therapy because of ineffective viral response or intolerance to interferon (TE) in patients who are interferon intolerant or for whom interferon is contraindicated.
- Efficacy in TN patients with genotype 1 infection treated for 12 weeks with SOF/PEG/RBV is 89% and in patients with genotype 4 infection is 96% and 80% (cirrhosis genotype 1 and 4 combined) SVR12.
- Efficacy in TN patients with genotype 1 infection treated for 24 weeks is 68–86% for patients in whom interferon is not tolerated or indicated due to comorbidities (SOF/RBV).

■ *Simeprevir (SMV) + pegylated interferon and ribavirin for genotypes 1a and 1b virus*

See http://www.olysio.com/shared/product/olysio/prescribing-information.pdf for prescribing details.

- SMV is a DAA targeting the stage in viral replication where the viral polyprotein is cleaved to produce the nonstructural proteins for the next generation of virus.
- It *does* target the virus protease enzyme responsible for polyprotein cleavage (NS3, 4a protease) and therefore it is generally susceptible to mutational resistance.
- Effective only for genotype 1 virus.
- Single pill per day and has side effects, the most prominent (> 10%) of which are rash (photosensitivity), pruritus, nausea, myalgia, and dyspnea when used with interferon and ribavirin.
- As a protease inhibitor, there are a number of drug–drug interactions that require careful consideration (see prescribing information at website above).
- Approved in combination with PEG and weight-based RBV as a once/day dose for 12 weeks followed by 12 weeks of PEG and weight-based RBV in patients who are treatment naïve or have previously relapsed on PEG and RBV. It is approved for 12 weeks followed by 36 weeks of PEG and RBV in patients who have had previous null response or partial response or who are cirrhotic.
- In addition, patients must meet certain on-treatment criteria (absence of quantifiable virus at treatment weeks 4, 12, and 24), which would otherwise require treatment discontinuation.

FUTURE OF HCV THERAPY

- Treatments for HCV are rapidly evolving and changing the approach to therapy and the very way we think about whom to treat and whom not to treat.
- Current and future therapies are extremely costly, and if current drug costs are not reduced, they will likely exceed $100,000.00 for even a 12-week course of treatment.
- In the coming years, we will likely see newer, more effective treatments approved by the FDA that may be taken alone or in combinations, which may raise the expectation of SVR closer to 100%.

REFERENCES

1. Ghany MG, Nelson DR, Strader DB, Thomas DL, Seeff LB. An update on treatment of genotype 1 chronic hepatitis C virus infection: 2011 practice guideline by the American Association for the Study of Liver Disease. *Hepatol.* 2011;54(4):1433–44.
2. Lawitz E, Mangia A, Wyles D, et al. Sofosbuvir for previously untreated chronic hepatitis C infection. *N Engl J Med.* 2013;368(20):1878–87.

3. Jacobsen IM, Gordon SC, Kowdley KV, et al. Sofosbuvir for hepatitis C genotype 2 or 3 in patients without treatment options. *N Engl J Med.* 2013;368(20):1867–77.
4. Fried MW, Buti M, Dore GJ, et al. Once-daily simeprevir (TMC435) with pegylated interferon and ribavirin in treatment-naïve genotype 1 hepatitis C: the randomized PILLAR study. *Hepatol.* 2013;58(6):1918–29.

CHAPTER 41 ■ HOW TO APPROACH NON-HBV/HCV HEPATITIS IN CLINICAL PRACTICE

Walid S. Ayoub, MD and Vinay Sundaram, MD, MSC

OVERVIEW

- Assessment for a patient with hepatitis starts with screening laboratory testing for viral hepatitis and metabolic liver disease as well as with abdominal imaging looking for liver masses, and radiological features of cirrhosis or vascular disease of the liver (see **Figure 41-1**).
- An abdominal ultrasound is the initial screening modality for liver masses, Budd-Chiari syndrome, and radiological features of cirrhosis and portal hypertension (nodular liver and splenomegaly).

DIFFERENTIAL DIAGNOSIS

- Viral hepatitis, metabolic disorders of the liver such as alpha-1-antitrypsin deficiency (A1AT) and Wilson disease, autoimmune hepatitis, hereditary hemochromatosis, cholestatic liver disease (primary biliary cirrhosis [PBC], primary sclerosing cholangitis [PSC]), cirrhosis, infiltrative liver disease, vascular diseases of the liver such as Budd-Chiari syndrome, drug-induced liver injuries (DILI), granulomatous diseases, thyroid disorders, celiac disease, adrenal insufficiency, liver diseases associated with pregnancy, and liver masses.
- Cytomegalovirus (CMV) and Epstein-Barr (EBV) hepatitis should be thought of, especially in young adults with persistent hepatitis. Gilbert's disease is characterized by indirect bilirubinemia and is a diagnosis of exclusion after a complete evaluation for cholestasis is performed. A liver biopsy is pursued if the workup is unrevealing with persistent abnormal liver function test (LFT).

HEREDITARY HEMOCHROMATOSIS (HFE)

- The most common genetic disorder in populations of Northern European ancestry with a prevalence of 1:220–250.
- C282Y homozygotes are the majority of HFE patients with iron overload. Fewer than 10% of homozygotes have fully expressed disease with end-organ manifestations.
- Compound heterozygotes (C282Y/H63D) have less severe iron overload and usually have normal iron studies.

```
┌─────────────────────────────┐      ┌─────────────────────────────┐
│   Elevated AST and ALT      │      │    Elevated AP or TB        │
└─────────────────────────────┘      └─────────────────────────────┘

┌─────────────────────────────┐      ┌─────────────────────────────┐
│ Review drug history         │      │ Review drug history and OCP │
│ Check for alcohol abuse     │      │ Exclude pregnancy           │
│ Assess for viral hepatitis  │      │ Check for infection         │
│ Check iron panel (ferritin, │      │ Check for use of TPN        │
│ TS)                         │      │ Assess for viral hepatitis  │
│ Abdominal ultrasound to     │      │ Check AMA (PBC screening)   │
│ assess for radiological     │      │ Check TSH                   │
│ signs of fat, cirrhosis, or │      │ Check abdominal imaging for │
│ masses                      │      │ masses, signs of biliary    │
└─────────────────────────────┘      │ obstruction (strictures with│
                                     │ PSC), or cirrhosis          │
┌─────────────────────────────┐      └─────────────────────────────┘
│ Check for AIH (IgG, ANA,    │
│ SMA)                        │      ┌─────────────────────────────┐
│ Check TSH                   │      │ Gilbert's syndrome          │
│ Assessment for celiac       │      │ (diagnosis of exclusion in  │
│ disease                     │      │ setting of indirect         │
└─────────────────────────────┘      │ hyperbilirubinemia)         │
                                     └─────────────────────────────┘
┌─────────────────────────────┐
│ Screen for Wilson disease   │
│ Assess for A1AT             │
└─────────────────────────────┘

┌─────────────────────────────┐
│ Persistent abnormal tests   │
│ for > 6 months and negative │
│ workup: consider liver      │
│ biopsy                      │
└─────────────────────────────┘
```

Figure 41-1 Approach to the patient with abnormal liver function tests.

A1AT = alpha-1 antitrypsin; AIH = autoimmune hepatitis; AMA = antimitochondrial antibody; ANA = antinuclear antibody; AP = alkaline phosphatase; OCP = oral contraceptive; PBC = primary biliary cirrhosis; PSC = primary sclerosing cholangitis; SMA = smooth muscle antibody; TB = TS = transferrin saturation; TPN = total parenteral nutrition; TSH = thyroid stimulating hormone.

PRESENTATION

Presenting symptoms include fatigue, hepatomegaly, diabetes, cardiac disease, arthropathy, skin pigmentation, and impotence.

PATHOPHYSIOLOGY

HFE mutation causes primary iron overload by increased absorption of iron from the gut.

DIAGNOSIS

- Diagnosed based on elevated serum ferritin and transferrin saturation (≥ 45%). HFE mutation analysis is usually performed afterward to confirm the diagnosis.
- The liver biopsy usually reveals a hepatic iron index of > 1.9. Patients with ferritin > 1000 μg/L are at increased risk of cirrhosis.

TREATMENT

- Treatment for HFE consists of phlebotomy with the goal to keep serum ferritin between 50 and 100 µg/L. Patients with iron overload should not take vitamin C supplements.
- Complications of HFE include cirrhosis, hepatocellular carcinoma, diabetes, skin pigmentation ("bronze diabetes"), and heart disease.
- Screening of first-degree relatives of patients with HFE-related hemochromatosis is recommended for early detection and prevention of HFE complications.

ALPHA-1 ANTITRYPSIN (A1AT) DEFICIENCY

A1AT deficiency is an autosomal-dominant disorder associated with emphysema, liver disease, and hepatocellular carcinoma.

PRESENTATION

Jaundice is the common presentation in children. Adults usually present with complications of portal hypertension (varices, splenomegaly, ascites, or coagulopathy), pruritus, or cirrhosis with liver cancer.

PATHOPHYSIOLOGY

Caused by a point mutation leading to a trapped protein in the endoplasmic reticulum of the liver cells. The mutated protein triggers a series of events leading to liver injury and predilection for liver cancer.

DIAGNOSIS

- The diagnosis is made by checking an A1AT phenotype. Patients with low serum A1AT level (less than 85 mg/dL) should have phenotypic testing to confirm the diagnosis.
- Homozygotes with PiZZ usually have positive periodic acid-Schiff (PAS) stain.

TREATMENT

There is no specific therapy for A1AT deficiency–induced liver disease. Liver transplantation is recommended for patients with cirrhosis. Smoking cessation is also recommended.

BUDD-CHIARI SYNDROME (BCS)

BCS is a vascular disorder of the liver.

PRESENTATION

- Depends on the extent and the speed of the obstructive process. Obstruction of one hepatic vein is usually asymptomatic.

- Most patients tend to be females presenting with ascites, upper abdominal pain, or upper gastrointestinal bleeding.
- Some patients have mildly elevated transaminase levels while others present with fulminant liver failure and transaminase levels over 1,000 and severe coagulopathy.

PATHOPHYSIOLOGY

- Characterized by the obstruction of the hepatic venous outflow tract in the absence of cardiac and pericardiac disease.
- Most patients have congenital or acquired risk for thrombosis such as Behçet's disease, antiphospholipid syndrome, paroxysmal nocturnal hematuria, JAK2 mutation, factor V Leiden, and myeloproliferative disease.

DIAGNOSIS

- Doppler abdominal ultrasound followed by a contrast abdominal imaging (computed tomography [CT] or magnetic resonance imaging [MRI]) usually confirms the diagnosis.
- The ascites protein content is greater than 3 g/dL with serum-ascites albumin gradient (SAAG) > 1.1 g/dL.
- If a liver biopsy is done, it reveals sinusoidal dilation.

TREATMENT

- Lifelong anticoagulation and stopping oral contraceptive are recommended.
- Recanalization of the hepatic venous outflow by expert operators has been successful in restoring the drainage of the liver. Stenting/angioplasty of short venous stenosis has been done successfully in some patients.
- Transjugular intrahepatic portosystemic shunt (TIPS) can be attempted in experienced hands. Liver transplantation is usually reserved for patients not amenable to TIPS or with fulminant liver failure.

DRUG-INDUCED LIVER INJURY (DILI)

DILI is a rare event occurring in a small percentage of patients. Acetaminophen is the most common cause of DILI in the United States.

PRESENTATION

The clinical manifestations of DILI vary widely from minor laboratory abnormalities to severe presentation with acute liver failure. Most patients present with nonspecific symptoms such as fatigue, nausea, vomiting, abdominal pain, pruritus, and jaundice.

PATHOPHYSIOLOGY

- Some drug metabolites eventually lead to apoptosis and necrosis through dysregulation of the cellular and mitochondrial machinery in

the case of DILI. DILI can produce a hepatocellular, cholestatic, or a mixed drug injury based on histology.
- Some drugs cause injury in a dose-dependent pattern, such as acetaminophen and valproic acid, while others causes idiosyncratic injury.

DIAGNOSIS

Diagnosis is usually a diagnosis of exclusion and the result of an investigational process involving a thorough investigation of the temporal relationship, clinical features, laboratory data, and current knowledge about the drug in question. In the setting of acetaminophen toxicity, the King's College Criteria is a good tool to assess the need for liver transplantation.

TREATMENT

Stopping of the offending drug usually causes reversal of the injury. Liver transplantation is needed in rare instances.

ALCOHOLIC LIVER DISEASE (ALD)

ALD is a disease of liver inflammation occurring with excessive alcohol intake—defined as greater than 30 grams daily for men and greater than 20 grams daily for women.

PRESENTATION

Can vary from abnormal liver tests without symptoms to acute alcoholic hepatitis, which can present with sudden onset of jaundice, right upper quadrant (RUQ) tenderness, and ascites.

PATHOPHYSIOLOGY

Chronic alcohol intake can cause either simple steatosis or steatohepatitis. Steatosis is fatty infiltration of the liver while steatohepatitis is an inflammatory condition characterized by presence of steatosis, infiltrate of neutrophils and lymphocytes, swelling of the hepatocytes, and Mallory bodies.

DIAGNOSIS

- Diagnosis is made based on blood tests and imaging, in combination with a history consistent with alcoholism. A blood alcohol level should be checked if there is suspicion of active drinking despite the patient stating otherwise.
- Liver function tests often demonstrate an elevated aspartate aminotransferase (AST) and alanine transaminase (ALT), with the AST to ALT ratio at 2:1 or greater. A liver ultrasound is helpful in determining the presence of steatosis or cirrhosis.
- Liver biopsy may be done if the diagnosis is unclear, and should reveal steatosis, inflammatory cell infiltrate, hepatocyte swelling, and Mallory bodies.

TREATMENT

Alcohol cessation is critical to treatment. In patients with alcoholic hepatitis, treatment with prednisone or pentoxifylline may be needed. Liver transplantation is often not an option in patients with active alcoholism.

NONALCOHOLIC FATTY LIVER DISEASE (NAFLD)

NAFLD is a disease of fatty infiltration of the liver in a patient without a history of alcoholism. Risk factors include diabetes, obesity, or metabolic syndrome.

PRESENTATION

The most common presentation is abnormal liver function tests. Patients are often asymptomatic.

PATHOPHYSIOLOGY

- Similar to ALD, NAFLD is characterized by steatosis or fatty infiltration of the liver.
- A more severe version of NAFLD is nonalcoholic steatohepatitis (NASH), a condition of steatosis and inflammation. NASH has a significantly higher risk of progressing to liver cirrhosis, as compared to simple steatosis of the liver without inflammation.

DIAGNOSIS

- Diagnosis is made based on blood tests and imaging. A history regarding alcohol intake should be performed.
- Liver function tests often demonstrate elevation of AST and ALT, with the ALT often greater than the AST. A liver ultrasound is helpful in determining the presence of steatosis or cirrhosis.
- Liver biopsy is the only method to confirm the presence of NASH. Biopsy findings demonstrate steatosis, inflammatory cell infiltrate, hepatocyte swelling, and Mallory bodies.

TREATMENT

- The primary treatment modality is weight loss. Patients are encouraged to lose weight through diet and exercise, with a goal of 1–2 pounds per week.
- Vitamin E can be considered in patients with biopsy-proven NASH.

WILSON'S DISEASE

Wilson's disease is a genetic disorder of abnormal copper deposition in the liver.

PRESENTATION

- The disease is seen most often in children of 5 years or older, though new-onset cases have been seen in adults. There is often a family history of liver or psychiatric illness.

Chapter 41: How to Approach Non-HBV/HCV Hepatitis

- Presentation can range from abnormal liver tests to fulminant liver failure. Patients may also present with neuropsychiatric symptoms including depression, seizures, or dystonia.

PATHOPHYSIOLOGY

Wilson's disease is an autosomal-dominant genetic disorder leading to loss of function of the ATP7B protein, which facilitates copper excretion into bile and allows copper to bind to ceruloplasmin.

DIAGNOSIS

- In the setting of unexplained liver disease, diagnosis is made based on three tests, of which all should be positive. These include a serum ceruloplasmin level less than 20 mg/dL, 24-hour urine copper of more than 40 mcg, and the presence of Kayser-Fleischer rings.
- If the diagnosis is indeterminate based on positivity of one or two criteria, further evaluation should be done with molecular genetic testing for Wilson's disease or a liver biopsy with measurement of dry copper weight.

TREATMENT

- Treatment is accomplished through reduction of serum copper levels. During the induction phase, a copper chelating agent such as penicillamine or trientine is used. Trientine is drug of choice because of its better side effect profile compared to penicillamine.
- Response to therapy is based on measurement of free serum copper levels and 24-hour urine copper levels. During the maintenance phase, zinc sulfate—which reduces intestinal copper absorption—can be used as monotherapy.
- Patients with fulminant liver failure should be immediately referred for liver transplant evaluation. Additionally, once a diagnosis has been established, first-degree family members should have genetic testing performed.

CHOLESTATIC LIVER DISEASE

- Cholestatic liver disease is a condition of impaired hepatic bile flow.
- The most common hepatic causes of cholestasis are primary biliary cirrhosis (PBC) and primary sclerosing cholangitis (PSC).

PRESENTATION

- Presentation involves elevation in the alkaline phosphatase level. The ALT and AST levels may also be elevated. In moderate-to-severe cholestasis, the serum bilirubin may be abnormal.
- PBC patients tend to have a positive antimitochondrial antibody (AMA). Presenting symptoms may also include fatigue, jaundice, scleral icterus, pruritus, and change in color of urine or stools.

- PBC has a female predominance and most often presents in middle-aged females. PSC has a male predominance and is associated with inflammatory bowel disease (IBD), but it can also be seen in patients without IBD.

PATHOPHYSIOLOGY

Both PBC and PSC involve immune-mediated destruction of the bile ducts. PBC tends to involve the intrahepatic bile ducts, while PSC may involve both intra- and extrahepatic bile ducts.

DIAGNOSIS

- The diagnosis of PBC is made with testing for an antimitochondrial antibody (AMA) titer and obtaining a liver ultrasound to exclude extrahepatic biliary obstruction.
- In a patient with cholestasis, normal ultrasound, and positive AMA titer, a liver biopsy is not necessary to confirm the diagnosis of PBC. The diagnosis of PSC is established with a magnetic resonance cholangiopancreaticogram (MRCP), which demonstrates stricturing of the intra- or extrahepatic ducts.
- A liver biopsy can reveal granulomas or reduced number of bile ducts in the case of PBC and "onion skinning" or bile duct proliferation in the case of PSC.

TREATMENT

- Treatment of PBC is ursodeoxycholic acid dosed at 13–15 mg per kg of patient body weight. Response to treatment is determined based on improvement in the alkaline phosphatase.
- There is no medical therapy available for PSC and ursodeoxycholic acid is not recommended. PSC patients require close monitoring for liver decompensation and development of cholangiocarcinoma. PSC patients with inflammatory bowel disease should also have colonoscopies every 1–2 years due to a high risk of colon cancer.

AUTOIMMUNE HEPATITIS (AIH)

AIH is an immune-mediated disease involving plasma cell infiltration of the liver.

PRESENTATION

- Presentation can range from elevated ALT and AST at 2–5 times the upper limit of normal without symptoms to fulminant liver failure.
- Potential symptoms include generalized abdominal pain, fatigue, nausea, or diarrhea. Patients with AIH commonly have other autoimmune disorders.

PATHOPHYSIOLOGY

The pathophysiology involves a T cell–mediated immune reaction to certain antigens on the hepatocytes, leading to liver necrosis and fibrosis.

DIAGNOSIS

- The diagnosis of autoimmune hepatitis is made with a combination of serologic testing and liver biopsy. Serologic testing indicative of AIH includes elevations in antinuclear antibody titer ($\geq 1:80$), anti-smooth muscle antibody titer ($\geq 1:80$), and immunoglobulin G (IGG) level.
- In patients with unexplained liver disease and positive testing of these studies, a liver biopsy should be considered. Histologic findings include interface hepatitis and plasma cell infiltration.

TREATMENT

- Treatment initially includes prednisone at 40–60 mg daily or a combination of prednisone and azathioprine. As serum ALT and AST levels improve, the dosage of prednisone can be tapered to as low as 5–10 mg daily.
- Maintenance therapy involves prednisone at a low dosage combined with azathioprine dosed at 50–100 mg daily. Due to high relapse rates, withdrawal should only be attempted in patients with normal ALT and AST levels, histologic evidence of no inflammation, and a minimum of 2 years of treatment.

HEPATITIS A

- Hepatitis A is endemic in developing countries. Hepatitis A is mainly transmitted by the fecal–oral route. It usually has a benign course in children but can cause significant morbidity in adults.
- Foodborne transmission occurs once an infected food handler contaminates the food during preparation of the food. Export of contaminated food from high endemic areas without sterilization is another risk factor for transmission of hepatitis A.

PRESENTATION

- In young children, acute hepatitis can be asymptomatic. In older children and adults, presentation varies from mild, short-lived, anicteric infection (flulike symptoms) to fulminant liver failure.
- Presenting symptoms include fatigue, nausea, vomiting, lack of appetite, fever > 100.4°F, and RUQ pain. As the illness progresses, patients may develop dark urine, light-colored stool, and jaundice.
- Prolonged, relapsing, and cholestatic hepatitis is a rare form of hepatitis A disease. Unlike hepatitis B and C, patients with hepatitis A do not develop chronic liver disease as a result of the acute infection. However, they develop immunity against future infection from hepatitis A.

PATHOPHYSIOLOGY

The cellular immune response leads to destruction of the infected hepatocytes and the development of symptoms and signs of disease. The humoral immune responses are the basis for diagnostic serologic assays.

DIAGNOSIS

- The diagnosis of autoimmune hepatitis is made with a combination of signs, symptoms, and blood testing.
- Hepatitis A IgM is usually present 5 days prior to symptoms development and can last for up to 6 months after infection.
- Liver biopsy is rarely pursued.

TREATMENT

- Treatment is usually supportive with rest, maintenance of good level of hydration, and avoidance of hepatotoxic substances such as acetaminophen and alcohol.
- Infected patients should not return to work or school unless the fever and jaundice have resolved.
- Majority of patients recover completely within 6 months.

REFERENCES

1. Pratt DS, Kaplan MM. Evaluation of abnormal liver-enzyme results in asymptomatic patients. *N Engl J Med.* 2000;342(17):1266–71.
2. Larson AM, ed. *Diagnosis and Management of Chronic Liver Disease.* Medical Clinics of North America, Volume 98, Issue 1 (January 2014). Philadelphia: WB Saunders Company; 2014.

CHAPTER 42 ■ APPROACH TO THE PATIENT WITH A LIVER LESION

Francisco A. Durazo, MD, FACP

OVERVIEW

- Liver lesions are frequently reported during imaging evaluation of the abdomen; most of the time they are discovered incidentally.
- A histologic prediction of the lesion is made to decide further workup and possible treatment.
- Ultimately, images may fail to yield a conclusive diagnosis, and a biopsy may be necessary. Unfortunately, liver biopsy of potentially vascular lesions may have serious consequences and may even fail to establish a diagnosis conclusively.
- On occasion, the histologic diagnosis is not made until after the lesion has been surgically resected.
- The treating physician must understand the clinical, radiologic, and pathologic characteristics of nodular liver lesions, their differential diagnosis, and a rational clinical approach to establishing a definitive diagnosis and treatment. The clinical history, physical examination, and laboratory tests are going to be crucial in making a diagnosis.
- The size of the liver mass is an important consideration in guiding the evaluation. Lesions < 1.0 cm are frequently difficult to characterize by imaging methods due to their small size, and difficult to percutaneously biopsy.
- Fine needle aspiration (FNA) biopsy is commonly used to assist in the diagnosis of a variety of liver lesions. Its overall accuracy in several series exceeds 90%. However, controversial issues surround the role of FNA in this setting. First, it is commonly nondiagnostic when used to evaluate some types of liver lesions such as hepatic adenomas and focal nodular hyperplasia. Second, it is associated with some degree of risk, including bleeding and seeding of neoplastic cells. The risk of bleeding is increased with some types of liver tumors such as hemangiomas and adenomas. Finally, its cost-effectiveness compared to nonhistologic means of diagnosis has been questioned.
- A variety of rare tumors and rare presentations of common tumors can present as a focal liver lesion. Examples include soft tissue sarcomas (such as epithelioid hemangioendothelioma, a low-grade malignant neoplasm of vascular origin), non-Hodgkin's lymphoma, and diaphragmatic cysts, which can appear to arise from the liver.

MALIGNANT LIVER TUMORS

More common than benign lesions and associated with poorer outcome

METASTATIC TUMORS

- In Western countries, metastatic liver tumors are the most common malignant hepatic neoplasm. The presence of an extrahepatic malignancy should be sought in patients with characteristic liver lesions on imaging studies.
- Ultrasound or computed tomography (CT)–guided liver biopsy or fine needle aspiration is often useful to confirm the diagnosis. However, histological confirmation is not always essential if reasonable certainty can be achieved with imaging studies or in settings in which there would be little benefit.

HEPATOCELLULAR CARCINOMA (HCC)

- A careful history should be taken to identify risk factors for chronic liver disease that could predispose the patient to hepatocellular carcinoma. Specifically, risk factors for viral hepatitis, metabolic liver diseases such as hereditary hemochromatosis, and alcohol abuse should be identified.
- Physical examination should be directed toward identifying peripheral stigmata of cirrhosis or decompensated liver disease—which should raise suspicion for HCC.

CHOLANGIOCARCINOMA

- Should be considered in patients with chronic cholestatic liver diseases who develop a discrete liver mass on standard imaging studies. These diseases include primary sclerosing cholangitis (PSC), longstanding choledochocele, and intrahepatic lithiasis, especially in those patients with parasitic diseases of the bile ducts or patients who were exposed to thorotrast for radiographic procedures.
- Endoscopic retrograde cholangiopancreatography (ERCP) with brushings of the bile ducts is often necessary to make the diagnosis, but a diagnosis is often difficult to establish. Strictures resulting from PSC are often difficult to differentiate from those due to cholangiocarcinoma.

BENIGN FOCAL LESIONS

Frequently encountered in clinical practice and include cysts, cavernous hemangiomas, focal nodular hyperplasia (FNH), hepatic adenomas (HAs), and, less commonly, abscesses

CYSTS

Hepatic cysts are the most common focal liver lesions, and their incidence increases with age. Most patients are asymptomatic except for those with very large cysts, which can produce symptoms due to a mass effect. Imaging alone can provide a specific diagnosis in most cases.

CAVERNOUS HEMANGIOMA

- It is the most common benign mesenchymal liver tumor. May present at any age or sex group but is seen most frequently in women (60–80%) between the 3rd and 5th decades of life. Its etiology is not clear but growth and initial symptoms during pregnancy or in patients receiving oral contraceptives suggest that estrogens may play a role in their development. After thrombosis or progressive fibrosis, they may appear as solid nodules or calcify.
- Usually are asymptomatic. If large, they may cause symptoms such as abdominal discomfort, pain or fullness, or compression symptoms including early satiety, anorexia, and nausea. Symptoms may also be intermittent due to thrombosis, infarcts or necrosis, pressure on adjacent structures, distension of the liver capsule, or high blood flow. Surgery may be considered an option if the patient is symptomatic. However, size alone should not be an indication for surgery given the extremely low risk of rupture.

HEPATIC ADENOMA (HA)

- It is a benign epithelial liver tumor that usually occurs in noncirrhotic liver. It is most commonly seen in premenopausal women > 30 years old. The majority have used oral contraceptives for more than 2 years prior to diagnosis. HA has also been noted in patients with type 1 glycogen storage diseases.
- > 50% of patients with HA present with symptoms of upper abdominal pain or discomfort; the tumor is noted incidentally in up to one-third of patients. It is important to establish an accurate diagnosis because these tumors have the potential to transform to HCC (although rare) or to rupture and cause life-threatening bleeding; the risk of rupture is increased during pregnancy.
- Given the risk of rupture and malignant transformation, it is recommended that HA should be resected. Pregnancy should be avoided if surgical resection is not pursued. If rupture does occur, emergency resection should be performed. Preoperative embolization may be required to achieve hemostasis prior to resection. In women with adenomas < 5 cm and oral contraceptive use, a reasonable approach would be to stop the contraceptive and to observe the lesion with serial imaging. Resection would be advised if regression does not occur.

FOCAL NODULAR HYPERPLASIA (FNH)

- A benign liver tumor that is believed to be a hyperplastic response to an anomalous artery. Like HA, FNH occurs most commonly in women in their 30s and 40s. In the majority of patients, FNH is diagnosed incidentally during imaging studies or laparotomy performed for unrelated reasons. However, pain may occur in a minority of patients. Unlike HA, the association of FNH with oral contraceptives/estrogens has not been clearly established. Pregnancy is safe in patients with small lesions because rupture is very rare. Malignant transformation probably does not occur or is exceedingly rare.
- FNH usually presents as a solitary lesion, although multiple lesions have been described. Microscopically, the lesions have fibrous septae with bile ductular proliferation, blood vessels, and inflammatory cells, which are quite readily differentiated from HA or HCC. Because FNH does *not* have malignant potential and has an extremely low risk of rupture, reassurance and prospective observation are recommended irrespective of size. Surgical resection is indicated in symptomatic patients, or when HA or HCC cannot be definitively excluded. The risks of surgical morbidity and mortality should be carefully considered, especially in patients with significant comorbid conditions.
- Differentiating FNH and HA at standard contrast-enhanced magnetic resonance imaging (MRI) can be particularly difficult if typical features are not present. The classic *T2 hyperintense scar* is absent in 20% of FNH lesions, particularly when they are small, while in HAs, intratumoral fat (leading to signal loss on the out-of-phase images) or hemorrhage (which gives rise to high signal intensity on T1-weighted imaging) is not seen in 30–40% of lesions.
- Histopathologically, FNH consists of an increased density of functional hepatocytes with abnormal blind-ending biliary ductules, which do not communicate with larger bile ducts; therefore, biliary excretion is slow compared with that of normal liver. On imaging with gadolinium-based hepatocyte-specific agents, the initial enhancement pattern in the dynamic phase is the same as with other extracellular contrast agents. That is, FNHs typically show intense homogeneous arterial enhancement with washout to isointensity on the portal venous and equilibrium phase, whereas the central scar shows slower contrast agent uptake. In the delayed phase, FNHs become hyperintense because of the high density of hepatocytes leading to retained contrast agent.
- In HA, hepatocytes are present in a cordlike pattern separated by sinusoids and lacking biliary ductules, so that normal excretion into the biliary system is impaired and bile metabolism is altered in the cells of the lesion. In the dynamic phase with gadolinium-based hepatocyte-specific agents, adenomata typically show early arterial enhancement (sometimes heterogeneous if hemorrhage is present), becoming isointense in the portal venous and equilibrium phase. At delayed phase

Chapter 42: Approach to the Patient with a Liver Lesion

imaging, HAs *do not* enhance with gadobenate dimeglumine, but variable enhancement may occur with mangafodipir trisodium and gadoxetate disodium.
- In this way, the hepatocyte-specific contrast agents can be used to diagnose FNH with a high degree of confidence. In addition, gadobenate dimeglumine may be particularly useful in discriminating HA from FNH because the former lesion does not appear to take up this agent in the hepatobiliary phase. Radiology does not always distinguish the difference between both, and an ultrasound or CT-guided biopsy is frequently nondiagnostic. When in doubt, the final diagnosis is done by excisional biopsy. In a recent study using gadobenate dimeglumine-enhanced MR, the overall accuracy for the differentiation of FNH from HA was 98.3%.

ABSCESSES

PYOGENIC ABSCESS

- The two major mechanisms for the development of liver abscesses are local spread from contiguous infections within the peritoneal cavity or hematogenous seeding of the liver. Patients generally complain of nonspecific symptoms, such as dull right upper quadrant abdominal pain, malaise, weakness, anorexia, and weight loss. They are often febrile and have rigors.
- Between 25% and 50% have hepatomegaly or splenomegaly on physical examination. A positive blood culture strongly supports the diagnosis. Laboratory findings reflect the nonspecific features of infection, such as anemia and leukocytosis. In addition, alkaline phosphatase and serum aminotransferases are often elevated.

AMEBIC ABSCESS

- Result from ingestion of cysts of *Entamoeba histolytica*, which subsequently invade the colonic mucosa and invade the mesenteric venules. These cysts eventually migrate to the liver via the portal vein and sinusoids and stimulate hepatocyte necrosis and inflammation with subsequent abscess formation. The majority of abscesses occur in the right lobe of the liver. Patients with amebic liver abscess usually present acutely with 1 to 2 weeks of fever (38.5–39.5°C) and right upper quadrant pain. Concurrent diarrhea is present in less than one-third of patients, although some patients will give a history of having had dysentery within the previous few months.
- Jaundice is uncommon. For travelers returning from an endemic area, presentation usually occurs within 8 to 20 weeks (median 12 weeks) and will be within 5 months of their return in 95% of patients, although a lag

of up to 12 years has been reported. Occasionally, patients have a more chronic presentation with months of fever, weight loss, and abdominal pain. In these patients, hepatomegaly and anemia are often associated findings. The diagnosis is usually achieved by serologic testing (ELISA) combined with imaging studies.

REFERENCES

1. Davis LP, McCarroll K. Correlative imaging of the liver and hepatobiliary system. *Semin Nucl Med.* 1994;24(3):208–18.
2. Torzilli G, Minagawa M, Takayama T, et al. Accurate preoperative evaluation of liver mass lesions without fine-needle biopsy. *Hepatol.* 1999;30(4):889–93.
3. Schwartz L, Gandras EJ, Colangelo SM, Ercolani MC, Panicek DM. Prevalence and importance of small hepatic lesions found at CT in patients with cancer. *Radiol.* 1999;210(1):71–4.
4. Tsou M, Lin YM, Lin KJ, et al. Fine needle aspiration cytodiagnosis of liver tumors. Results obtained with Riu's stain. *Acta Cytol.* 1998;42:1359–64.
5. Evans GH, Harries SA, Hobbs KE. Safety of and necessity for needle biopsy for liver tumours *Lancet.* 1987;1:620.
6. Takamori R, Wong LL, Dang C, Wong L. Needle-tract implantation from hepatocellular cancer: is needle biopsy of the liver always necessary? *Liver Transpl.* 2000;6:67–72.
7. Hobbs KE. Hepatic hemangiomas *World J Surg.* 1990;14(4):466–71.
8. Nichols FC, 3rd, van Heerden JA, Weiland LH. Benign liver tumors. *Surg Clin North Am.* 1989;69(2):297–314.
9. Grazioli L, Morana G, Kirchin MA, Schneider G. Accurate differentiation of focal nodular hyperplasia from hepatic adenoma at gadobenate dimeglumine-enhanced MR imaging: prospective study. *Radiol.* 2005;236(1):166–77.
10. Burke C, Alexander Grant L, Goh V, Griffin N. The role of hepatocyte-specific contrast agents in hepatobiliary magnetic resonance imaging *Semin Ultrasound CT MRI.* 2013;34(1):44–53.

CHAPTER 43 ■ PRIMARY SCLEROSING CHOLANGITIS

Nirupama Bonthala, MD and Saro Khemichian, MD

OVERVIEW

- Primary sclerosing cholangitis (PSC) is a chronic cholestatic disease that affects the liver and bile ducts and can progress to end-stage liver disease.
- Inflammation, fibrosis, and destruction of intra- and extrahepatic bile ducts ultimately results in biliary cirrhosis.
- Liver biopsy may demonstrate classic "onion skin" appearing fibrosis around the bile duct.
- Cholangiography will typically show "beads on string" appearance of the bile ducts.
- PSC is a progressive disease with median survival of 10 to 12 years after diagnosis without a liver transplantation.
- There is an increased associated risk of cholangiocarcinoma, gallbladder carcinoma, and colorectal cancer.

PRESENTATION

- Disease incidence is approximately 1 per 100,000 person-years. It is twice as common in men, and the average age at diagnosis is 40.
- There is a higher incidence of PSC in patients with inflammatory bowel disease (IBD), specifically ulcerative colitis (UC). Up to 90% of patients with PSC can have UC but often less than 10% of patients with UC have PSC. The severity of the IBD does not correlate with the severity of the PSC and vice versa.
- Approximately 50% of patients with PSC are asymptomatic at the time of diagnosis and are evaluated based on abnormal liver tests.
- Common symptoms include fatigue and pruritus. Fevers, chills, and right upper quadrant pain may indicate bacterial cholangitis from biliary obstruction.

- Up to half of the patients will have a normal exam. Advanced PSC can manifest on exam as jaundice, hepatomegaly, splenomegaly, and excoriations (from severe pruritus).

DIFFERENTIAL DIAGNOSIS

IgG4-associated cholangitis, PSC-autoimmune hepatitis overlap syndrome, secondary sclerosing cholangitis (caused by chronic bacterial cholangitis, choledocholithiasis, cholangiocarcinoma, recurrent pyogenic cholangitis, and ischemic cholangiopathy).

PATHOPHYSIOLOGY

The cause of PSC is unknown. First-degree relatives do have an increased risk of PSC, suggesting a genetic predisposition, but an immune reaction, ischemic injury to the bile ducts, and bacterial infections have all been proposed as possible mechanisms.

DIAGNOSIS

- Lab abnormalities typically follow a cholestatic pattern with primarily an elevation of the serum alkaline phosphatase level. Typically aspartate aminotransferase (AST) and alanine transaminase (ALT) are less than 300 IU/mL. Perinuclear antineutrophil cytoplasmic antibodies (P-ANCA) test is positive in 30–80% of patients. Increased serum IgM levels are found in up to half of patients. Antimitochondrial antibody is negative.
- While lab abnormalities can be supportive, the diagnosis is definitely made with either a magnetic resonance cholangiopancreaticogram (MRCP) or endoscopic retrograde cholangiopancreatography (ERCP) showing the characteristic multifocal strictures and segmental dilations ("beads-on-a-string"), while excluding secondary causes of sclerosing cholangitis.
- Because it is a noninvasive test with similar diagnostic accuracy to an ERCP, an MRCP is now the first test of choice for diagnosis. However, ERCP may be better for detecting early PSC and large-duct PSC and may be necessary for obtaining diagnosis in patients who cannot undergo MRCP (such as those with implanted metal devices). An ultrasound is helpful if it shows ductal abnormalities.
- A liver biopsy is helpful if it supports the diagnosis of PSC but it is rarely diagnostic and thus should not be used instead of an MRCP or ERCP. On liver biopsy the most specific finding is the so-called "onion skin" pattern of the bile ducts, which have been replaced concentrically by connective tissue. However, this is only found in less than 25% of biopsies.

Chapter 43: Primary Sclerosing Cholangitis

TREATMENT

- There are no proven medications for slowing down the progression of disease.
- Use of ursodeoxycholic acid (UDCA) is not routinely recommended, while use of high-dose regimens (> 25 mg/kg/day) is contraindicated due to increased risk of clinical deterioration.
- Patients with large bile duct strictures should be evaluated for dilation and stenting of the stricture by ERCP.
- Liver transplantation is the treatment of choice and all patients with advanced liver disease due to PSC should be referred for evaluation. Generally, patients do well after transplantation with a 5-year survival of up to 85%.
- Approximately 50% of deaths in patients with PSC are due to malignancy, thus screening is imperative. Because of the higher incidence of cholangiocarcinoma and gallbladder carcinoma, yearly imaging with ultrasounds or MRCP should be performed. A colonoscopy should also be performed every 1–2 years to evaluate for colorectal cancer.

REFERENCES

1. Chapman R, Fevery J, Kalloo A, et al. Diagnosis and management of primary sclerosing cholangitis. AASLD practice guidelines. *Hepatol* 2010;51(2):660–78.
2. Trauner M, Halilbasic E, Baghdasaryan A, et al. Primary sclerosing cholangitis: new approaches to diagnosis, surveillance and treatment. *Dig Dis*. 2012;30(Suppl 1):39–47.

CHAPTER 44 ■ PRIMARY BILIARY CIRRHOSIS

Vignan Manne, MD and Sammy Saab, MD, MPH, AGAF, FAASLD

OVERVIEW

- Primary biliary cirrhosis (PBC) is a chronic inflammatory condition that leads to the destruction of hepatic interlobular bile ducts.
- PBC is considered relatively rare. Most cases are seen in Northern European countries and the Northern United States, and with a prevalence of less than 1/2,000. The incidence and prevalence appear to be increasing worldwide.
- PBC is more commonly seen in middle-aged and elderly people and is primarily a disease of women—the ratio of women to men affected being 10:1.
- Close to 20% of PBC patients also exhibit features of other concomitant autoimmune conditions like autoimmune hepatitis (AIH), CREST syndrome, thyroiditis, and others.

PRESENTATION

- Advances in the diagnosis of PBC have lead to earlier diagnosis of the disease, and about half of patients diagnosed are asymptomatic at presentation with an incidental finding on routine lab testing of an elevated alkaline phosphatase (ALP).
- Fatigue and pruritus are the earliest presenting symptoms but can be seen in many other conditions.
- Physical examination is usually normal except late in disease in which stigmata of liver inflammation and cirrhosis can be seen such as jaundice.

DIFFERENTIAL DIAGNOSIS

AIH, primary sclerosing cholangitis (PSC), sarcoidosis, cholestatic drug reaction, biliary obstruction

PATHOPHYSIOLOGY

- The pathophysiology is still unclear, but the general consensus is that multiple genetic factors, as evidenced by high monozygotic twin

concordance, combined with environmental triggers lead to the development of disease.
- Environmental factors that are often associated with PBC include cigarette smoking and mucosal infections like urinary tract infections (UTI); other triggers still under investigation include hormonal therapy, xenobiotics, frequency of pregnancy, and cosmetics.

DIAGNOSIS (SEE FIGURE 44-1)

- American Association for the Study of Liver Diseases (AASLD) guidelines state that diagnosis is made based on three criteria: biochemical evidence of cholestasis with elevated alkaline phosphatase (ALP), presence of antimitochondrial antibodies (AMA), and histologic evidence of nonsuppurative cholangitis and destruction of small or medium-sized bile ducts on biopsy only if biopsy is deemed necessary.
- Antimitochondrial antibodies (AMA) are the hallmark of diagnosing PBC with almost 95% of patients testing positive for this marker.
- Other laboratory manifestations include hypercholesterolemia or indices of cirrhosis late in the disease course like thrombocytopenia, hypoalbuminemia, or hyperbilirubinemia.
- Imaging studies such as an abdominal ultrasound are useful to delineate extrahepatic biliary tree involvement from the intrahepatic biliary tree and are considered mandatory in patients presenting with liver abnormalities to rule out other more common causes of liver abnormalities.
- Liver biopsy is useful for histopathological staging of PBC but is usually unnecessary to diagnose and treat the disease—only being absolutely needed in the setting of an AMA-negative patient.

TREATMENT

- Ursodeoxycholic acid (UDCA) at a single or divided dose of 13–15 mg/kg/day is currently the only approved treatment for PBC and is the mainstay of treatment.
- The goal of UDCA treatment is the improvement or normalization of liver function tests (LFTs) and can usually be seen in a few weeks to several months, although some patients may take a couple years to respond.
- UDCA is a relatively safe drug with the most common side effects being gastric discomfort or weight gain.
- It should be remembered that patients taking bile acid sequestrants, such as cholestyramine, can reduce the response to UDCA because of poor absorption and should therefore take UDCA 2–4 hours before or after ingestion of the bile acid sequestrant.

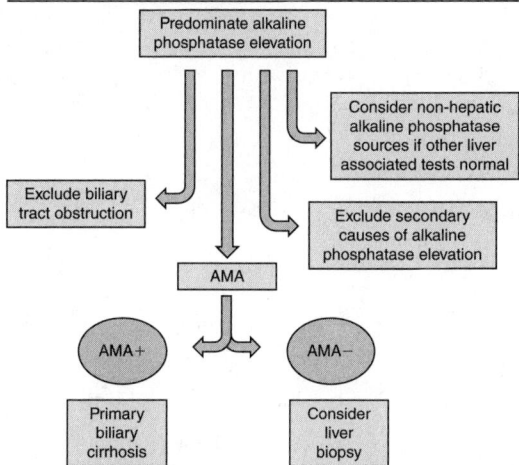

Figure 44-1 Suggested diagnostic algorithm for patients with suspected PBC.

AMA = antimitochondrial antibody; ANA = antinuclear antibody; ASMA = anti-smooth muscle antibody

- Other novel therapies are currently in development to more directly target the pathophysiology of PBC.
- Patients with incomplete or no response to UDCA and worsening disease leading to cirrhosis should be considered for liver transplantation.
- Management of symptoms of PBC (e.g., pruritus) using a variety of medications can also be considered.
- Hypercholesterolemia can also be treated with statins.

REFERENCES

1. Poupon R. Primary biliary cirrhosis: a 2010 update. *J Hepatol.* 2010;52(5):745–58.
2. Lindor KD, Gershwin ME, Poupon R, et al. Primary biliary cirrhosis. *Hepatol.* 2009;50(1):291–309.

CHAPTER 45 ■ AUTOIMMUNE HEPATITIS

Gina Choi, MD and Tram T. Tran, MD

OVERVIEW

- Autoimmune hepatitis (AIH) is a chronic, immune-mediated process of histologic injury to hepatocytes of unknown etiology.
- AIH is characterized by interface hepatitis, hypergammaglobulinemia, and autoantibodies.
- AIH is very responsive to treatment. However, if left untreated, AIH can progress rapidly to cirrhosis and the sequelae of end-stage liver disease.

PRESENTATION

- AIH has a wide clinical spectrum ranging from asymptomatic disease with abnormal liver enzymes (34–45% of cases) to acute liver failure.
- Symptoms are insidious and nonspecific, including fatigue, jaundice, nausea, abdominal pain, and arthralgias.
- Women are more affected than men (3:1 ratio).
- AIH is seen in all ages and ethnic groups.
- AIH is commonly associated with other autoimmune diseases (thyroid disease, synovitis, celiac disease, and ulcerative colitis).

DIFFERENTIAL DIAGNOSIS

Viral hepatitis (A, B, C, and E), drug-induced liver injury, alcoholic liver disease, primary biliary cirrhosis (PBC), primary sclerosing cholangitis (PSC), overlap/variant syndrome: some patients exhibit a mixed picture with features of both AIH and another disorder such as PBC and PSC. Serologies may be mixed in these overlap syndromes.

PATHOPHYSIOLOGY

- Not fully determined but thought to be due to a combination of possible environmental trigger, a failure of immune tolerance mechanisms, and genetic predisposition.

- These factors induce a T cell–mediated immune injury upon hepatocytes leading to inflammation, fibrosis, and eventually, cirrhosis.

DIAGNOSIS (SEE FIGURE 45-1)

- Predominant elevation in aspartate aminotransferase (AST) and alanine transaminase (ALT) (more than alkaline phosphatase).
- Elevated IgG > 1.5 × upper limit of normal (ULN).
- Positive autoantibodies (> 1:80): antinuclear antibody (ANA), smooth muscle antibody (SMA), anti-liver kidney microsome type 1 antibodies (LKM-1), anti-liver cytosol type 1 antibodies (LC1).
- Negative antimitochondrial antibody (AMA).
- 96% have positive ANA, SMA, or both.
- 4% have anti-LKM1 and/or anti-LC1.
- Up to 5% of patients with AIH are AMA-positive and have serological overlap with PBC but no manifestations of PBC.
- Histology: interface hepatitis, plasma cell infiltration, lobular inflammation, and bridging necrosis (granulomas are rare).
- Must exclude viral hepatitis, drug-induced liver injury, and alcohol.
- Ensure normal serum concentrations of alpha-1-antitrypsin, copper, and ceruloplasmin.

TREATMENT INDICATIONS

- The goal of treatment is to control inflammation (normalization of AST and ALT) and minimize the development of fibrosis.
- Treatment indications include: AST 10 × ULN or AST 5 × ULN + serum gammaglobulin > 2 × ULN, presence of bridging necrosis or multilobular necrosis on histology, and significant symptoms (fatigue, arthralgia, jaundice).
- Treatment is not indicated if the patient is asymptomatic with normal or near normal AST and gammaglobulin levels, if cirrhosis is present, or if the risks of treatment outweigh the benefits (psychosis, brittle diabetes, osteoporosis).

TREATMENT REGIMENS (SEE TABLE 45-1)

- Corticosteroids induce remission.
- Prednisone may be used alone or in conjunction with azathioprine (AZA).
- The dose of prednisone alone is 40–60 mg PO daily, which should be individually tapered every 1–2 weeks to maintain remission (usually down to 10 mg daily in 4 weeks).
- The preferred regimen is a combination of prednisone 30 mg plus AZA 50 mg PO daily to minimize steroid side effects.

Chapter 45: Autoimmune Hepatitis

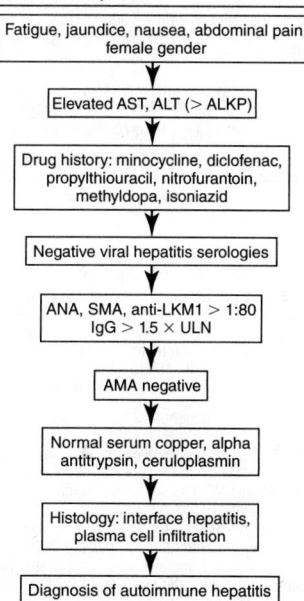

Figure 45-1 Diagnosis of autoimmune hepatitis.

AST = aspartate aminotransferase; ALT = alanine transaminase; ALKP = alkaline phosphatase; ANA = antinuclear antibody; SMA = smooth muscle antibody; LKM1 = liver kidney microsome type 1; AMA = antimitochondrial antibody; ULN = upper limit of normal

- While on AZA, monitor for leukopenia and thrombocytopenia. AZA is pregnancy category D.
- In patients without cirrhosis, budesonide 3 mg PO TID plus AZA 50 mg PO daily can also be considered. Budesonide has a significant first pass hepatic effect with fewer systemic side effects.
- As prednisone is slowly withdrawn, monitor AST and ALT every 3 weeks for flare, then every 6 months for 1 year, then yearly.
- The optimal duration of therapy is unknown. Continue treatment until AST, ALT, and gammaglobulins normalize.

Table 45-1 Treatment Regimens for Autoimmune Hepatitis

Treatment Regimen	Dose
Prednisone alone	40–60 mg PO daily Taper down to 10 mg daily in 4 weeks (depending on treatment response)
Preferred Regimen: Prednisone + Azathioprine*	30 mg PO daily + 50 mg PO daily
Budesonide + Azathioprine*	3 mg PO TID + 50 mg PO daily

*Azathioprine: Monitor for leukopenia, thrombocytopenia; pregnancy category D
PO: orally; TID: three times per day.

- Relapse rates are high and occur in 50% of patients within 6 months of treatment withdrawal and in 80% of patients who enter remission after 3 years. Long-term treatment is required for the majority of patients.
- Treatment failure is seen in 9% of patients. Salvage therapies include mycophenolate mofetil 2 g daily, cyclosporine, or tacrolimus.
- A rigorous bone maintenance regimen should be started with calcium 1–1.5 g daily and vitamin D3 400 IU daily.
- For patients with cirrhosis, surveillance for hepatocellular carcinoma is indicated.

REFERENCES

1. Strassburg CP, Manns MP. Therapy for autoimmune hepatitis. *Best Pract Res Clin Gastroenterol.* 2011;25:673–87.
2. Czaja Aj, Manns MP. Advances in the diagnosis, pathogenesis, and management of autoimmune hepatitis. *Gastroenterology.* 2010 Jul;139(1):58–72.
3. Schaefer EA, Pratt DS. Autoimmune hepatitis: current challenges in diagnosis and management of a chronic progressive liver disease. *Curr Opin Rheumatol.* 2012;24(1):84–9.
4. Manns MP, Czaja AJ, Gorham JD, et al. Diagnosis and management of autoimmune hepatitis. *Hepatol.* 2010;51(6):2193–213.
5. Manns MP, Woynarowski M, Kreisel W, et al. Budesonide induces remission more effectively than prednisone in a controlled trial of patients with autoimmune hepatitis. *Gastroenterol.* 2010;139(4):1198–206.

CHAPTER 46 ■ DRUG-INDUCED LIVER INJURY

Jeffery Kahn, MD and Hannah Do, MD

OVERVIEW

- Drug-induced liver injury (DILI) can occur after taking prescription medications, over-the-counter medications, herbals, and dietary supplements.
- The incidence is estimated to be between 1 in 10,000 and 1 in 100,000.
- It is the most common cause of acute liver failure in the United States and is frequently the reason cited when a drug is withdrawn from the market.
- More than 1,000 drugs, herbals, and supplements have been associated with the development of hepatotoxicity through a variety of mechanisms.
- The pattern of liver injury can be classified as hepatocellular (with predominantly aspartate aminotransferase/alanine transaminase [AST/ALT] elevations), cholestatic (with predominantly bilirubin and alkaline phosphatase elevation), or mixed typed.
- A high clinical index of suspicion and detailed history taking are crucial to making the diagnosis as DILI can mimic all other forms of acute and chronic liver diseases.

PRESENTATION

- The clinical presentation can vary widely and include malaise, abdominal pain, nausea, anorexia, jaundice, pruritus, rashes, arthralgias, or dark urine.
- Exposure to a drug should precede the onset of symptoms. However, the latent period after drug exposure can be highly variable.
- The combination of jaundice, encephalopathy, and elevated prothrombin time (PT) is particularly indicative of severe liver injury and has a mortality of approximately 10–50%.

DIFFERENTIAL DIAGNOSIS

Alcoholic hepatitis, viral hepatitis, shock liver, autoimmune hepatitis, non-alcoholic fatty liver disease (NAFLD), Wilson's disease, alpha-1-antitrypsin deficiency, hemochromatosis, or biliary disease—such as cholangitis

PATHOPHYSIOLOGY

- Drug-induced liver injury is a subject of ongoing research and the exact pathophysiology is still unclear.
- It is thought that most drug-induced liver injuries occur as a result of a multistep process that involves direct drug injury and subsequent activation of inflammatory pathways.
- An individual's genetic polymorphisms, inherent immunity, and environmental factors such as malnutrition, pregnancy, and alcohol use have been implicated as factors that increase susceptibility to the development of DILI.

DIAGNOSIS

- Diagnosis can be challenging, as there is no single test, including liver biopsy, that can be used to definitively diagnose DILI.
- Key element to consider is that exposure to the offending agent must precede liver injury. Underlying liver disease should be ruled out before concluding that hepatotoxicity is drug related.
- When the drug is stopped, liver injury may improve. Also, on repeated exposure to the same drug, liver injury may recur.
- A searchable database of drugs involved in DILI has been developed by National Institutes of Health (NIH): http://www.livertox.nih.gov/.

TREATMENT

- The main treatment for DILI is withdrawal of the offending agent and providing supportive care.
- In the case of acetaminophen overdose, prompt use of N-acetylcysteine is the standard of care.
- Most patients, at variable rates, will improve after cessation of the offending drug, and the improvement is not always immediate.
- Individuals with severe liver injury should be monitored closely and be seen by a transplant hepatologist.
- The injury should be reported to the Food and Drug Administration (FDA) at http://www.fda.gov/medwatch.

REFERENCES

1. Kaplowitz N, DeLeve L. *Drug-Induced Liver Disease*. 3rd ed. New York: American Press; 2013.
2. Navarro VJ, Senior JR. Drug-related hepatotoxicity. *N Engl J Med*. 2006; 354(7):731–9.

CHAPTER 47 ■ NONALCOHOLIC FATTY LIVER DISEASE

Vivian Ng, MD and Simon W. Beaven, MD, PhD

OVERVIEW

- Fat deposition (steatosis) in the liver not explained by other causes is the most common liver disorder in industrialized countries. In the United States, the prevalence of fatty liver disease ranges from 10–46%, and biopsy-based studies report a prevalence of nonalcoholic steatohepatitis (NASH) of 1–17%. Systematic reviews suggest nonalcoholic fatty liver disease (NAFLD) prevalence in adults is probably 25–33%, while NASH prevalence is 2–5%. Thus, the natural history remains poorly understood and the influence of genetics remains to be delineated.
- NAFLD is divided into nonalcoholic fatty liver (NAFL), simple steatosis, and NASH, which is steatosis with hepatic inflammation. Liver function tests cannot differentiate the two.
- Long-standing NAFLD can progress to cirrhosis and may impart a risk for cancer (even without cirrhosis).
- NAFLD is strongly associated with the metabolic syndrome: obesity, insulin resistance/diabetes, dyslipidemia, systemic hypertension, atherosclerotic disease. Also suspect in young women with polycystic ovarian syndrome (PCOS).

PATHOPHYSIOLOGY

- Multifactorial, but likely that hepatic insulin resistance is the key feature driving hepatic steatosis to become NASH. The obese state, with inflammatory cytokines from obese adipose tissue and macrophages, also contribute, but there are lean patients with NASH. Muscle insulin resistance, central nervous system (CNS) alterations (sleep/circadian rhythm disturbances), and pancreatic function also likely play roles. Reactive oxygen species (ROS), endoplasmic reticulum (ER) stress, and unfolded protein response are important too.
- Only a minority (15–25%) will develop progressive NASH and cirrhosis. Genetic factors are important in determining disease risk, but there is no clinical utility at this time to test for any specific gene mutations or polymorphisms.
- Aberrations in the circadian rhythm can lead to metabolic dysfunction: disruption of the circadian clock causes animals to develop hyperlipidemia, hyperglycemia, hypoinsulinemia, and hepatic steatosis.

- The intestinal microflora has a critical role in normal physiology and pathologic development of NAFLD/NASH, likely through lipid flux to the liver and inflammatory signaling (Toll-like receptor signaling, TLR4/9).

PRESENTATION

- Most patients with NAFLD are asymptomatic, although some patients with NASH may complain of fatigue, malaise, and intermittent right upper abdominal discomfort or aching.
- Patients are typically diagnosed with NAFLD later in adult life (age 40 to 50 or later). Pediatric NAFLD is poorly understood.
- Patients are more likely to come to attention when laboratory tests reveal elevated liver aminotransferases or when hepatic steatosis is detected incidentally on abdominal imaging. Alanine aminotransferase (ALT) elevations of 2–3 × upper limit of normal (ULN) are typical.

DIAGNOSIS (SEE FIGURE 47-1)

- Diagnosis requires the finding of hepatic steatosis by imaging or biopsy in appropriate clinical setting.
- *Need to exclude significant alcohol use,* certain medications (e.g., steroids, tamoxifen, amiodarone, highly active antiretroviral therapy [HAART] therapy), pancreaticobiliary diversion or bypass, total parenteral nutrition (TPN), and, rarely, inborn errors of metabolism.
- NAFLD patients usually have mild or moderate elevations of aspartate aminotransferase (AST) and alanine aminotransferase (ALT), at 2–5 × the upper limit of normal (ULN). Usually, the AST:ALT ratio $< \times 1$.
- The degree of aminotransferase elevation does not predict the degree of hepatic inflammation or fibrosis. The alkaline phosphatase may be elevated to 2–3 × ULN. Serum albumin and bilirubin levels are typically within the normal range, unless cirrhosis has developed. Gamma-glutamyl transpeptidase (GGT) is a better predictor of alcohol use than fatty liver—do not recommend using.
- Full workup for chronic liver disease includes assessment of viral hepatitis serologies, iron studies, autoimmune markers (antinuclear antibodies [ANAs], antimitochondrial antibodies [AMAs], anti-smooth muscle antibodies [ASMAs]), and thyroid function. Other tests to consider, on an individual basis, could include ceruloplasmin (Wilson's disease), endomysial antibody (celiac disease), or alpha-1-antitrypsin. Patients with NAFLD or significant alcohol use often have an elevated serum ferritin concentration or transferrin saturation from secondary iron overload.
- Ultrasound, computed tomography (CT), and magnetic resonance imaging (MRI) are imaging modalities that can detect hepatic steatosis.

Chapter 47: Nonalcoholic Fatty Liver Disease

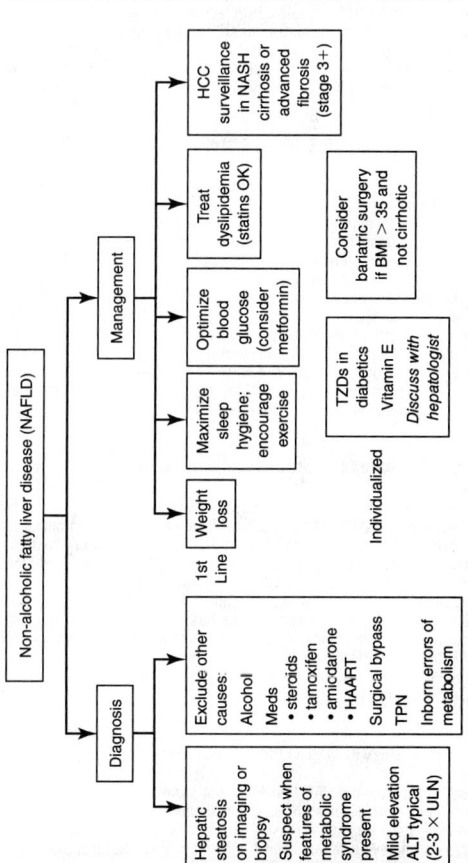

Figure 47-1 Diagnostic and treatment algorithm for nonalcoholic fatty liver disease.

ALT = alanine aminotransferase; BMI = body mass index; HAART = highly active antiretroviral therapy; HCC = hepatocellular carcinoma; NASH = nonalcoholic steatohepatitis; TPN = total parenteral nutrition; TZDs = Thiazolidinediones; ULN = upper limit of normal

Ultrasonography often reveals a hyperechoic texture or a "bright liver" because of diffuse fatty infiltration. CT and MRI can identify steatosis but are not sufficiently sensitive to detect inflammation or fibrosis.
- Hepatic elastography at experienced centers may be better predictor of fibrosis, but obesity limits its sensitivity.

ROLE OF LIVER BIOPSY

- Liver biopsy is the gold standard for diagnosing NAFLD (NAFL or NASH) for histological confirmation.
- Presumptive diagnosis can often be made based upon the patient's history, laboratory tests, and imaging findings.
- A biopsy may be useful in establishing advanced fibrosis or cirrhosis, and this should trigger hepatocellular carcinoma (HCC) surveillance.
- Histologic scoring of NAFLD should use the NAFLD Activity Score (NAS), a validated measure that diagnoses NASH reliably from liver biopsy. The NAS is the sum of the individual biopsy scores for steatosis (0 to 3), lobular inflammation (0 to 2), hepatocellular ballooning (0 to 2). NAS of 1–2 corresponds to NAFL, 3–4 corresponds to borderline NASH, and a score of 5–8 corresponds to NASH. Note that fibrosis (measure of disease chronicity) is scored separately (0–4).

NATURAL HISTORY AND CANCER RISKS

- NAFLD may eventually develop cirrhosis as steatosis progresses to inflammation/NASH with fibrosis. Having simple steatosis on biopsy is reassuring, but those with NASH are at risk (~30–40%) for progression.
- Older age, diabetes mellitus, body mass index (BMI) $\geq \times 28$, and high visceral adiposity index are predictors for fibrosis progression.
- Hepatocyte ballooning, Mallory's hyaline, lobular inflammation, and fibrosis on biopsy are histologic risk factors.
- Hepatocellular carcinoma (HCC) is associated with cirrhosis due to NAFLD. HCC surveillance is recommended for patients with NASH-related cirrhosis and should be strongly considered in patients with advanced fibrosis too (stage 3+).

TREATMENT (SEE FIGURE 47-1)

- Current treatment of NAFLD includes optimizing blood glucose control in patients with diabetes or insulin resistance, treating dyslipidemia, reducing body weight, increasing physical activity, normalizing sleep hygiene, improving dietary habits, and stopping alcohol use.

- Weight loss improves liver enzymes, histological activity, and insulin levels; reasonable goal is to lose 0.5–1 kg/week.
- Metformin lowers blood glucose by decreasing hepatic gluconeogenesis, stimulating glucose uptake by muscle, and increasing fatty acid oxidation in adipose tissue. While metformin does not improve liver fibrosis, it is effective in diabetes, may delay the onset of diabetes from prediabetes, and is useful in polycystic ovarian syndrome (PCOS).
- Thiazolidinediones (TZDs) are peroxisome proliferator-activated receptor gamma (PPARG) agonists primarily targeting adipocytes and macrophages to improve insulin action. TZDs also improve liver histologic parameters in patients with NASH. Long-term use of TZDs may be complicated by weight gain, edema, heart failure, and bone metabolic changes. Use of TZDs in nondiabetics cannot be recommended at this time.
- Bariatric surgery should be strongly considered for patients with BMI > x 35, especially if diabetes is present. Histologic and clinical outcomes from bariatric surgery far outstrip any pharmacologic intervention.
- Treatment of dyslipidemia lowers risks of cardiovascular disease and stroke, and may be beneficial in NAFLD. Statin therapy has been shown to be safe in patients with NAFLD.
- Many therapies have been studied for NAFLD. Caffeine consumption may be associated with a lower risk of disease progression in patients with NAFLD. Vitamin E is thought to decrease oxidative stress, and may have benefit in patients with NASH without diabetes, but observational studies have also shown a possible increase in all-cause mortality with high-dose vitamin E supplementation (> x 400 IU/day). Omega-3 fatty acids have been suggested to benefit patients with NAFLD or NASH. Phentermine (amphetamine-related), topiramate (anti-epileptic), and lorcaserin (5-HT$_{2c}$ agonist) all have mild weight-loss effects but have high potential for side effects and dependency.

REFERENCES

1. Schuppan D, Schattenberg JM. Non-alcoholic steatohepatitis: pathogenesis and novel therapeutic approaches. *J Gastroenterol Hepatol*. 2013;28 (Suppl 1):68–76.
2. Sanyal AJ, Chalasani N, Kowdley KV, et al. Pioglitazone, vitamin E, or placebo for nonalcoholic steatohepatitis. *N Engl J Med*. 2010; 362(18):1675–85.
3. Schauer PR, Kashyap SR, Wolski K, et al. Bariatric surgery versus intensive medical therapy in obese patients with diabetes. *N Engl J Med*. 2012;366(17):1567–76.

CHAPTER 48 ■ INHERITED METABOLIC LIVER DISEASES

Nikhil Agarwal, MD and Mohamed El-Kabany, MD

OVERVIEW

- Inherited metabolic liver diseases should be considered as a cause of abnormal liver tests in adult patients.
- Wilson's disease, alpha-1-antitrypsin deficiency, and hereditary hemochromatosis are the leading causes of inherited metabolic liver disease in adults.
- In an adult with acute or subacute liver failure with a positive family history and extrahepatic manifestations, think inherited metabolic liver disease!

WILSON'S DISEASE

PRESENTATION

- Acute liver failure or chronic hepatitis and cirrhosis typically in children or adults < age 35 (although patients have been diagnosed in their 70s). Expect to see this in unexplained liver disease or in autoimmune liver disease that does not respond to steroids.
- Neurologic or psychiatric disease may be present.
- Kayser-Fleischer rings may be present.
- Low ceruloplasmin, hemolytic anemia, and low alkaline phosphatase are often found in laboratory analysis.

DIFFERENTIAL DIAGNOSIS

Viral hepatitis, alcohol abuse, autoimmune hepatitis, drug-induced liver injury, hereditary hemochromatosis, alpha-1-antitrypsin deficiency

PATHOPHYSIOLOGY

An inherited genetic abnormality leads to impaired cellular copper transport. Over time, accumulation of copper in the liver (and other organs) leads to progressive injury and eventually cirrhosis.

DIAGNOSIS

- Wilson's disease should be considered in children and adults with unexplained hepatic, neurologic, or psychiatric disease.

- Low serum ceruloplasmin levels < 20 mg/dL, the presence of Kayser-Fleischer rings, and an elevated 24-hr urine copper (> 100 mcg) can provide the diagnosis for Wilson's disease about half the time.
- Liver biopsy with copper concentration (> 250 mcg) may be needed to confirm the diagnosis.
- Genetic testing should be performed in first-degree relatives of affected patients.

TREATMENT

- Pharmacologic treatment consists of orally administered agents aimed at removing tissue copper and preventing reaccumulation.
- Chelating agents, such as d-penicillamine or trientine are used to help remove tissue copper.
- Chelators or zinc salts are used to prevent reaccumulation.
- A low-copper diet is rarely recommended to patients.
- Patients with acute liver failure or decompensated cirrhosis should be referred for liver transplantation.

ALPHA-1-ANTITRYPSIN DEFICIENCY

PRESENTATION

- Many phenotypes are present with bimodal peaks in neonates, infants, and adults.
- Chronic obstructive pulmonary disease with chronic hepatitis or cirrhosis is the typical presentation in an adult.
- Lung disease presents at an earlier age than smoking-related emphysema, and manifests in the base of the lung with a panacinar pathology as opposed to smokers who have a predominately apical lung disease with a centrilobular pathology.

DIFFERENTIAL DIAGNOSIS

Viral hepatitis, alcohol abuse, autoimmune hepatitis, drug-induced liver injury, hereditary hemochromatosis, Wilson's disease

PATHOPHYSIOLOGY

An inherited genetic abnormality in the protease inhibitor alpha-1 antitrypsin leads to an accumulation of proteins in the hepatocytes, which leads to chronic injury and eventually fibrosis

DIAGNOSIS

- Diagnosis is usually made with a low serum alpha-1-antitrypsin level in combination with a severe deficient phenotype by isoelectric focusing.

- Genotype analysis can identify the most common deficient alleles and confirm the diagnosis.
- Liver biopsy with light microscopy reveals cytoplasmic diastase-resistant, periodic acid-Schiff positive globules.

TREATMENT

- Liver transplantation is the only option for advanced liver disease.
- Liver transplantation should be pursued before lung decomposition precludes transplantation.

HEREDITARY HEMOCHROMATOSIS (HH)

PRESENTATION

- Caused by an inherited defect in iron metabolism, which leads to progressive iron overload in many organ tissues—including liver, heart, and pancreas.
- Liver disease may present in combination with skin hyperpigmentation, arthralgia, diabetes mellitus, and heart disease.
- Classic triad of cirrhosis, diabetes mellitus, and skin hyperpigmentation ("bronze diabetes") is rare and is usually a manifestation of late disease.

DIFFERENTIAL DIAGNOSIS

Viral hepatitis, alcohol abuse, autoimmune hepatitis, drug-induced liver injury, Wilson's disease, alpha-1-antitrypsin deficiency

PATHOPHYSIOLOGY

- An inherited defect in the normal HFE gene leads to increased absorption of iron and progressive iron accumulation into organ tissues.
- After many years of excess iron deposition, cellular injury and organ damage occur leading to liver disease, arthralgia, diabetes mellitus, heart disease, etc.

DIAGNOSIS

- In target individuals (abnormal liver tests, family history, or symptoms of HH) iron studies should be obtained.
- A transferrin saturation of > 45% or a serum ferritin of > 200 mcg warrants further genotype analysis.
- A C282Y homozygote or C282Y/H63D heterozygote may not need further workup to confirm the diagnosis.
- Liver biopsy may be necessary in heterozygotes or compound heterozygotes to confirm the disease.

TREATMENT

- Initial treatment should be to perform phlebotomy of one unit of blood (500 mL) weekly or twice weekly as tolerated.
- Once hematocrit levels decrease by 20% of starting value, or ferritin levels reach < 50 mcg/mL, phlebotomy should be switched to maintenance.
- Maintenance phlebotomy should be performed every 2–3 months to achieve a ferritin level of 25–50 mcg.
- Vitamin C supplements and alcohol should be avoided.

REFERENCES

1. European Association for Study of Liver (EASL). EASL Clinical Practice Guidelines: Wilson's disease. *J Hepatol.* 2012;56(3):671–85.
2. Fairbanks KD, Tavil AS. Liver disease in alpha-1 antitrypsin deficiency: a review. *Am J Gastroenterol.* 2008;103(8):2136–41.
3. Tavil AS, American Association for the Study of Liver Diseases, American College of Gastroenterology, American Gastroenterological Association. Diagnosis and management of hemochromatosis. *Hepatol.* 2001;33(5):1321–8.

CHAPTER 49 ■ ASCITES

Gina Choi, MD and Bruce Allen Runyon, MD

OVERVIEW

- Cirrhosis is the most common cause of ascites in the United States.
- Ascites is the most common of the three major complications of cirrhosis (the other two being hepatic encephalopathy and variceal hemorrhage).
- Ascites is the most common complication of cirrhosis that leads to hospital admission.
- Ascites has a 1-year mortality of 15% and a 5-year mortality of 44%.

PRESENTATION

- Symptoms include abdominal pain, discomfort, weight gain, and shortness of breath.
- Physical exam findings include increased abdominal girth and the presence of shifting dullness (about 1.5 L of fluid required for positive test).

DIFFERENTIAL DIAGNOSIS (SEE TABLE 49-1)

- 85% have liver disease, 15% have another cause.
- The differential diagnosis includes malignancy, heart failure, renal disease, thyroid disease, tuberculosis, and combinations of causes for fluid retention, such as cirrhosis, heart failure, and chronic kidney disease.

PATHOPHYSIOLOGY

Portal hypertension leads to arterial vasodilation and a decreased effective arterial volume, followed by renal sodium and water retention, which leads to overflow of fluid into the peritoneal cavity. This is mediated by elevated levels of vasoconstrictors that are compensating for the vasodilatory effect of nitric oxide.

DIAGNOSIS

- Detailed history inquiring about risk factors for liver disease (ascites may be the first sign of cirrhosis).

Table 49-1 Differential Diagnosis of Ascites

Differential diagnosis of ascites
Cirrhosis
Alcoholic hepatitis
Heart failure (check BNP: median 6100 pg/mL in heart failure, 166 pg/mL in cirrhosis)
Cancer (peritoneal carcinomatosis, liver metastases)
Pancreatitis
Nephrotic syndrome
Tuberculous peritonitis (recent immigration from endemic area, immunocompromised)
Acute liver failure
Budd-Chiari syndrome
Sinusoidal obstruction syndrome
Postoperative lymphatic leak
Myxedema

BNP = pro-brain natriuretic peptide

- Paracentesis with ascitic fluid analysis must be performed.
- Send ascitic fluid cell count and differential, total protein, albumin (and serum albumin) to calculate serum ascites albumin gradient (SAAG).
- SAAG ≥ 1.1 g/dL is consistent with portal hypertension (responds to salt restriction and diuretics).
- SAAG ≤ 1.1 g/dL is not consistent with portal hypertension (does not respond to salt restriction and diuretics except in nephrotic syndrome).
- If infection is suspected (fever, abdominal pain, unexplained encephalopathy, acidosis, azotemia, hypotension, hypothermia), send ascitic fluid for culture in blood culture bottles, Gram, glucose, lactate dehydrogenase (LDH), and amylase.
- Polymorphonuclear leukocytes (PMNs) > 250 cells/mm^3 is consistent with spontaneous bacterial peritonitis (SBP).

TREATMENT (SEE FIGURE 49-1 AND TABLE 49-2)

FIRST-LINE MANAGEMENT

- First-line management of ascites due to cirrhosis includes: abstinence from alcohol when present (ascites may resolve or become more responsive to medical therapy), sodium-restricted diet (2 g/day), and once daily dosing (to maximize compliance) of dual diuretics with spironolactone 100 mg (maximum dose 400 mg) and furosemide 40 mg (maximum dose 160 mg) with monitoring of urine Na, urine K, and daily weights (once edema has resolved, 0.5 kg is a reasonable daily maximum weight loss).

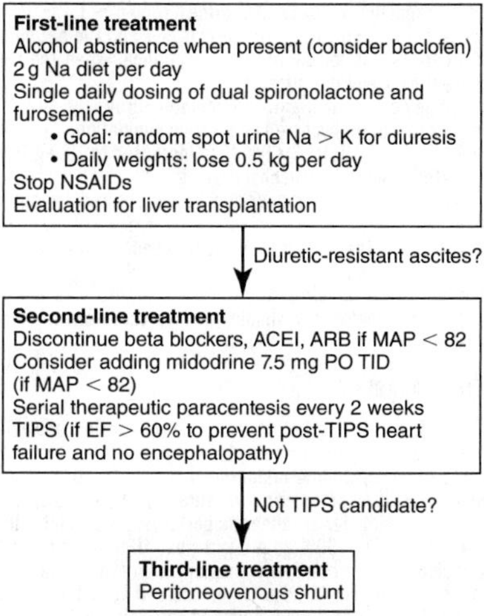

Chapter 49: Ascites

First-line treatment
Alcohol abstinence when present (consider baclofen)
2 g Na diet per day
Single daily dosing of dual spironolactone and furosemide
- Goal: random spot urine Na > K for diuresis
- Daily weights: lose 0.5 kg per day

Stop NSAIDs
Evaluation for liver transplantation

↓ Diuretic-resistant ascites?

Second-line treatment
Discontinue beta blockers, ACEI, ARB if MAP < 82
Consider adding midodrine 7.5 mg PO TID (if MAP < 82)
Serial therapeutic paracentesis every 2 weeks
TIPS (if EF > 60% to prevent post-TIPS heart failure and no encephalopathy)

↓ Not TIPS candidate?

Third-line treatment
Peritoneovenous shunt

Figure 49-1 Treatment regimen for the management of ascites due to cirrhosis.

Na = sodium; K = potassium; kg = kilogram; ACEI = angiotensin-converting enzyme inhibitors; ARB = angiotensin receptor blockers; MAP = mean arterial pressure; TIPS = transjugular intrahepatic portosystemic shunt

Table 49-2 Treatment of Ascites

Ascitic Condition	Antibiotic of Choice
SBP	Cefotaxime 2 g IV Q8H × 5 days
SBP prophylaxis (Indications: prior history of SBP, ascitic total protein < 1.5 g/dL, Cr > 1.2, BUN > 25, Na < 130, TB > 3, Child's Pugh score > 9)	Norfloxacin 400 mg PO daily Trimethoprim/sulfamethasoxazole one DS tablet PO daily
Cirrhosis + GI bleed	Ceftriaxone 1 g IV Q24H × 7 days Norfloxacin 400 mg PO BID × 7 days

SBP = spontaneous bacterial peritonitis; Cr = creatinine; BUN = blood urea nitrogen; Na = sodium; TB = total bilirubin; DS = double strength

- When the random spot urine Na to urine K ratio is > 1, the patient should be losing fluid weight. When the ratio is > 1 and the patient is not losing weight, assess for dietary noncompliance. When the ratio is < 1, increase the dose of diuretics.
- Discontinue nonsteroidal anti-inflammatory drugs (NSAIDs).
- Consider referral for liver transplantation evaluation.
- Baclofen 5 mg PO TID for 3 days, then increased to 10 mg TID (or higher as tolerated) can reduce alcohol craving.
- Amiloride (10–40 mg per day) can be substituted for spironolactone if intolerant.
- Hold diuretics in the setting of active GI bleed, hepatic encephalopathy, or renal dysfunction.
- Serum Na < 120 mmol/L, serum Cr > 2 mg/dL, and uncontrolled or recurrent encephalopathy should lead to cessation of diuretics and re-evaluation.

SECOND-LINE MANAGEMENT

- Includes: discontinuing beta blockers, angiotensin-converting enzyme inhibitors, and angiotensin receptor blockers if mean arterial pressure is < 82. Consider adding midodrine 7.5 mg PO TID to increase blood pressure (BP) if mean arterial pressure < 82, serial therapeutic paracenteses, transjugular intrahepatic portosystemic shunt (TIPS) (if ejection fraction [EF] > 60% to prevent post-TIPS heart failure and if no encephalopathy), and/or liver transplantation evaluation.
- Recommend albumin infusion when more than 5 L of ascitic fluid is removed (6–8 g of albumin per liter of fluid removed).

THIRD-LINE MANAGEMENT

- Includes peritoneovenous shunt.
- Do not advise bed rest, fluid restriction, vaptans (vasopressin receptor antagonists) for hyponatremia, and intravenous diuretics.

SPONTANEOUS BACTERIAL PERITONITIS

- *SBP treatment* includes cefotaxime 2 g IV every 8 hours for 5 days.
- *SBP prophylaxis* is recommended for patients with prior history of SBP, low-protein ascites (< 1.5 g/dL), Cr > 1.2, BUN > 25, Na < 130, TB > 3, and Child's Pugh score > 9 with norfloxacin 400 mg PO daily, ciprofloxacin 750 mg PO weekly, or one trimethoprim/sulfamethoxazole double-strength tablet PO for 5 days per week.

REFERENCES

1. Runyon BA. Introduction to the revised American Association for the Study of Liver Diseases Practice Guideline management of adult patients with ascites due to cirrhosis 2012. *Hepatol.* 2013;57(4):1651–3.
2. Runyon BA. Management of adult patients with ascites due to cirrhosis: update 2012. *American Association for the Study of Liver Diseases (AASLD) Practice Guidelines.* Available at: http://www.aasld.org/practiceguidelines/Pages/default.aspx. Accessed February 2013.

CHAPTER 50 ■ HEPATIC ENCEPHALOPATHY

Justin A. Reynolds, MD

OVERVIEW

- Hepatic encephalopathy (HE) represents a spectrum of reversible neuropsychiatric abnormalities ranging from subtle alterations in mental status to deep coma.
- HE is most often seen in patients with advanced liver disease, but may also be seen in acute liver failure or in patients with portosystemic bypass shunts.

PRESENTATION

- The cognitive, psychiatric, and neuromuscular deficits that accompany HE vary across a spectrum of severity. Other causes of mental status change should be excluded.
- Cognitive findings include subtle features like difficulty with computation, shortened attention span, loss of time or place, and gross disorientation.
- Psychiatric findings include irritability, decreased inhibitions, inappropriate behavior, apathy, paranoia, or anger.
- Neuromuscular findings include tremor, incoordination, asterixis, slurred speech, ataxia, nystagmus, rigidity, and coma.
- Physical exam findings may include ataxia, bradykinesia, slurred speech, hyperactive deep tendon reflexes, nystagmus, and asterixis. Asterixis is a commonly recognized sign on exam and describes a flapping motion of the hands when the wrists are dorsiflexed and arms fully extended.

PATHOPHYSIOLOGY

- HE is thought to be multifactorial, although the exact mechanism is unclear. Ammonia likely plays a key role, although other endotoxins and cytokines may contribute as well.
- Ammonia accumulates via many mechanisms in cirrhotic patients: increased gut flora production, impaired hepatic clearance or portosystemic shunting, decreased glutamine synthesis, reduced renal excretion, etc.

- Inflammatory cytokines or endotoxins may also accumulate due to concurrent infection or alterations in the gut–endothelial barrier. All of these, plus ammonia, may serve to alter the permeability of the blood–brain barrier and permit neurological changes.
- Cerebral edema and increased intracranial pressure have been observed in acute hyperammonemia (such as that seen in acute liver failure from acetaminophen toxicity), but more low-grade cerebral edema may contribute to encephalopathy in cirrhotic patients.
- Many potential precipitants of hepatic encephalopathy have been identified: infection (e.g., urinary tract, spontaneous bacterial peritonitis, pneumonia), gastrointestinal (GI) bleeding, acute kidney injury, electrolyte disturbances (e.g., hypokalemia, hyponatremia), dehydration and/or excessive diuresis, medications (especially sedatives, hypnotics, or opiates), shunts (e.g., splenorenal shunt, transhepatic portocaval shunt).

DIAGNOSIS

- The diagnosis is primarily made on clinical grounds.
- Lab abnormalities are not specific, although elevations in plasma ammonia may be seen. Venous ammonia samples lack adequate specificity, but arterial ammonia levels can be helpful if properly collected.
- Plasma ammonia may be elevated in a variety of conditions, and can be influenced by many factors (e.g., use of a tourniquet, whether sample was placed on ice), thus limiting the usefulness of the test.
- The severity of HE has traditionally been graded according to clinical manifestations:
  - Grade 1: disordered sleep, change in behavior, occasional asterixis, mild lack of awareness
  - Grade 2: irritability, moderate confusion, slurred speech, lethargy
  - Grade 3: incoherent speech, marked confusion, somnolence
  - Grade 4: coma (unresponsive to verbal or noxious stimuli), decorticate or decerebrate posturing

TREATMENT

- Many episodes of acute hepatic encephalopathy are triggered by a specific event such as infection or a GI bleed. Searching for a precipitant and appropriately directed treatment is of paramount importance.
- Lactulose, a synthetic disaccharide, is the mainstay of treatment for overt encephalopathy. It is converted to short-chain fatty acids by colonic bacteria, which lowers colonic pH, traps ammonia within the colon (by forming NH_4 from NH_3), thus reducing plasma ammonia levels.

- Lactulose induces an osmotic diarrhea, and the dosage is typically titrated to achieve 2 to 3 bowel movements daily. Other common side effects include bloating, flatulence, and abdominal cramping.
- Lactulose may be given as a syrup formulation to be taken orally, or as a powder that is reconstituted in water. Lactulose enemas may also be given in patients who cannot receive medications by mouth.
- Rifaximin, a minimally absorbed oral antibiotic, causes alteration in gut flora and can reduce the nitrogenous load within the intestine, thus reducing plasma ammonia. It is generally given in addition to lactulose therapy.
- Zinc is a frequently used adjunct for overt encephalopathy, particularly in patients who have breakthrough episodes despite lactulose and rifaximin. This is based on an observation that zinc deficiency is common in cirrhotics with encephalopathy. Several small case series also indicate a potential role, although larger studies are lacking.
- Protein restriction was once thought to help reduce the nitrogenous load within the gut. However, it has fallen out of favor due to concern for exacerbating malnutrition that is often seen in late-stage cirrhotics.
- Outside of the United States, L-ornithine-L-aspartate (LOLA) is frequently prescribed for the treatment of hepatic encephalopathy and is thought to lower plasma ammonia levels by increasing its metabolism to glutamine. Sodium benzoate has also been used for HE with some reported success. Further studies are needed to document their efficacy.

REFERENCES

1. Khungar V, Poordad F. Hepatic encephalopathy. *Clin Liver Dis.* 2012;16:301–20.

CHAPTER 51 ■ HEPATORENAL SYNDROME

Gina Choi, MD and Bruce Allen Runyon, MD

OVERVIEW

- Hepatorenal syndrome (HRS) is one of many possible causes of acute kidney injury in the setting of acute, subacute, and chronic liver disease.
- HRS represents the end stage of continued reduction in renal perfusion due to worsening liver disease.
- Two types of HRS have been described: type 1 (which is more rapidly progressive and serious) and type 2, based on the timing of decline in kidney function.
- HRS is a diagnosis of exclusion and portends a poor prognosis.

PRESENTATION

- HRS should be suspected in acute, subacute (severe alcoholic hepatitis), and chronic liver disease (cirrhosis with portal hypertension).
- The onset is usually insidious but can be triggered by an acute insult, including bacterial infection or gastrointestinal hemorrhage.
- Clinical signs include a progressive rise in serum creatinine (Cr), normal urine sediment, no or minimal proteinuria (< 500 mg per day), low urine Na (< 10 meq/L), and terminal oliguria.
- Type 1 HRS is more serious and develops in less than 2 weeks.
- Type 2 HRS is less severe than type 1 and occurs in patients with ascites resistant to diuretics.
- Diuretics do not cause HRS.

DIFFERENTIAL DIAGNOSIS

The differential diagnosis includes other potential etiologies of acute kidney injury including excessive or rapid diuresis, renal hypoperfusion (due to beta blockers, angiotensin-converting enzyme inhibitors or angiotensin receptor blockers), shock, nephrotoxic drugs (nonsteroidal anti-inflammatory drugs [NSAIDs], aminoglycosides, contrast agents), parenchymal renal disease (glomerulonephritis, vasculitis), and postrenal obstruction seen on ultrasound.

PATHOPHYSIOLOGY

- Portal hypertension causes arterial vasodilation (mediated by nitric oxide) in the splanchnic circulation.
- In response, there is a progressive fall in systemic vascular resistance, despite intense renal vasoconstriction, which is mediated by the renin-angiotensin system. A fall in cardiac output triggers the onset of HRS.

DIAGNOSIS

- The diagnosis of HRS includes excluding other potential etiologies of acute kidney injury in the setting of certain clinical criteria.
- There is no single diagnostic test, however, urinary neutrophil gelatinase-associated lipocalin (NGAL) is under investigation to aid in the diagnosis: levels of 20 ng/mL re seen in prerenal azotemia, 50 ng/mL in chronic kidney disease, 105 ng/mL in HRS, and 325 ng/mL in acute kidney injury.
- The criteria for diagnosis in a consensus statement include: cirrhosis with ascites, serum Cr > 1.5 mg/dL, no improvement of serum Cr (decrease to a level ≤ 1.5 mg/dL) after 2 days of diuretic withdrawal and volume expansion with albumin 1 g/kg of body weight per day (maximum of 100 g/day), absence of shock, no current or recent treatment with nephrotoxic drugs, absence of parenchymal kidney disease (proteinuria > 500 mg/day, microhematuria > 50 red blood cells (RBCs) per high power field, abnormal renal ultrasound).
- Type 1 is characterized by a rapid, progressive reduction in renal function, defined by a doubling of the initial serum Cr to a level > 2.5 mg/dL or a 50% reduction of the initial 24-hour Cr clearance to a level lower than 20 mL per minute during a period of less than 2 weeks.
- Type 2 does not have a rapidly progressive course, is less severe than type 1, and is seen in patients with diuretic-resistant ascites.

TREATMENT (SEE FIGURE 51-1)

- Discontinue all diuretics, beta blockers, angiotensin-converting enzyme inhibitors, angiotensin receptor blockers, and nephrotoxic medications.
- In patients admitted to the ICU, recommend norepinephrine 0.5–3 mg/hr continuous intravenous (IV) infusion plus albumin 1 g/kg IV bolus per day (100 g daily maximum) × 2 days with the goal of raising the mean arterial pressure by 10–15 mmHg.
- In patients not admitted to the ICU, recommend midodrine 7.5 mg PO three times per day (maximum dose 15 mg PO three times per day),

Chapter 51: Hepatorenal Syndrome

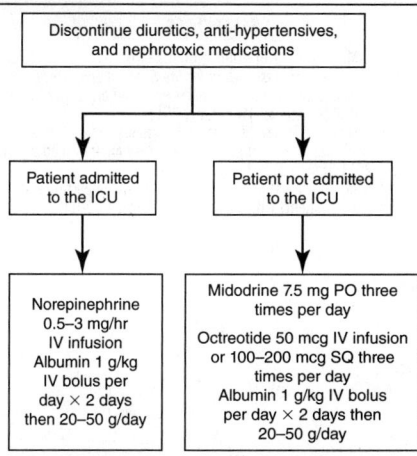

Figure 51-1 Treatment of hepatorenal syndrome. The goal with norepinephrine, midodrine, and octreotide is to increase mean arterial perfusion by 10–15 mmHg. Recommend medical treatment trial for 2 weeks. ICU = intensive care unit.

octreotide 50 mcg continuous IV infusion (or 100–200 mcg SQ three times per day), plus albumin 1 g/kg IV bolus per day (100 g daily maximum) × 2 days, followed by 20–50 g/day until midodrine and octreotide therapy is discontinued. The goal is to increase the mean arterial pressure by 10–15 mmHg.
- HRS is considered refractory if there is no response to medical therapy after 2 weeks of treatment.
- Transjugular intrahepatic portosystemic stent shunt (TIPS) may be considered in highly selected patients (usually with type 2 HRS) who fail medical therapy and have no contraindications to the procedure. It is optimal to decrease the Cr as low as possible (preferably ~2 mg/dL) prior to TIPS with the therapy detailed above and in Figure 51-1. However, there are risks associated with the procedure. Intravenous contrast can further worsen an already high pre-TIPS Cr and renal function.
- Patients who are appropriate transplant candidates with cirrhosis, ascites, and HRS should be referred for liver transplant evaluation with dialysis as a bridge to transplantation.

REFERENCES

1. Runyon BA. Management of adult patients with ascites due to cirrhosis: update 2012. *American Association for the Study of Liver Diseases (AASLD) Practice Guidelines.* Available at: http://www.aasld.org/practiceguidelines/Pages/default.aspx. Accessed February 2013.
2. Salerno F, Cazzaniga M, Merli M, et al. Diagnosis, treatment and survival of patients with hepatorenal syndrome: a survey on daily medical practice. *J Hepatol.* 2011;55(6):1241–8.
3. Martín-Llahí M, Guevara M, Torre A, et al. Prognostic importance of the cause of renal failure in patients with cirrhosis. *Gastroenterol.* 2011;140(2):488–96.

CHAPTER 52 ■ LIVER DISORDERS DURING PREGNANCY

Justin A. Reynolds, MD

OVERVIEW

- Liver disease in pregnancy is uncommon, but when present, requires prompt and accurate diagnosis due to the risk of morbidity and mortality to the mother and her fetus.
- Experienced healthcare providers will recognize the normal physiological and laboratory changes that occur during pregnancy. Fortunately, there are very few changes that occur in expectant mothers' standard liver tests aside from a third trimester rise in serum alkaline phosphatase (much of which is placental in origin). Thus, any alteration in liver transaminases, total bilirubin, or gamma-glutamyl transpeptidase (GGT) is abnormal and requires evaluation.
- Many chronic liver diseases can exist prior to pregnancy such as chronic viral hepatitis, primary sclerosing cholangitis, Wilson's disease, or autoimmune hepatitis. Others may be coincidental with pregnancy such as gallstone disease, acute viral hepatitis, and Budd-Chiari syndrome. The focus of this chapter will be on those liver diseases that are unique to pregnancy.

HYPEREMESIS GRAVIDARUM

- Hyperemesis gravidarum (HG) can occur in up to 0.3% of all pregnancies and is characterized by intractable nausea and vomiting within the first trimester—often with associated lab abnormalities, dehydration, and need for intravenous fluids.
- No uniform diagnostic criteria exist for HG although some informal criteria include weight loss exceeding 3 kg or 5% of prepregnancy weight, ketonuria, electrolyte disturbances, and orthostatic hypotension.
- Abnormal liver tests may be seen in up to 50% of women with HG. In those affected, liver transaminases can range up to a 20-fold elevation with occasional jaundice.
- Risk factors for HG are not clearly defined but may include multiple gestation pregnancy, genetic, psychological, or psychiatric factors.
- Differential diagnosis includes acute viral hepatitis, cholecystitis, choledocholithiasis, molar pregnancy, and diabetic ketoacidosis.

- Diagnosis is clinical and the remainder of the differential diagnosis must be excluded. Liver biopsy is generally unnecessary and, if performed, typically appears normal.
- Treatment includes hospitalization with intravenous hydration, correction of any electrolyte disturbances, supportive measures including antiemetics, and nutritional support.

INTRAHEPATIC CHOLESTASIS OF PREGNANCY

- Incidence in a given population is highly variable likely reflecting geographic and ethnic variations that predispose to intrahepatic cholestasis of pregnancy (ICP).
- ICP is characterized by significant pruritus and elevated serum bile acids, with onset typically late second trimester or early third trimester. ICP tends to recur in pregnancy.
- Pruritus can be extreme and is generalized but often predominates on the palms and soles and worsens at night. Jaundice occurs in a minority of cases, and abnormal liver transaminases are commonly seen up to 20-fold elevation. Prompt resolution of all symptoms and biochemical abnormalities is typical postpartum.
- Pathogenesis is multifactorial but includes genetic and hormonal factors as likely contributors to ICP. Exogenous factors like diet and geography may also play a role.
- Elevation in serum bile acid concentrations (cholic acid and chenodeoxycholic acid) and the presence of pruritus are important for diagnosis. Diarrhea may also occur due to steatorrhea.
- Maternal risk in ICP is negligible aside from bothersome symptoms and the risk of recurrence in future pregnancies.
- Management of ICP includes symptomatic therapy for the mother with ursodiol (15 mg/kg per day), which lowers serum bile acid levels without risk to the fetus. Fat-soluble vitamins may also be given in cases of significant steatorrhea. Cholestyramine and dexamethasone have been examined but are less effective.
- Risks to the fetus are more significant in ICP and include prematurity, placental insufficiency, sudden fetal death, and increased risk of neonatal respiratory distress. These risks predominate in the final 2–4 weeks of pregnancy and referral to a high-risk obstetrician and early delivery is often advised.

HELLP SYNDROME

- HELLP is an acronym referring to a syndrome that occurs in 10–20% of patients with preeclampsia (0.2%–0.6% of pregnancies overall) and includes hemolysis (H), elevated liver enzymes (EL), and low platelet counts (LP).

Chapter 52: Liver Disorders During Pregnancy

- HELLP syndrome is a microangiopathic hemolytic anemia associated with endothelial damage, platelet activation and consumption, and a risk of bleeding and disseminated intravascular coagulation (DIC).
- The pathogenesis of the HELLP syndrome is unclear but maternal risk is elevated with a family or personal history of HELLP.
- Clinical features include abdominal pain or tenderness, nausea, vomiting, malaise, hypertension, and proteinuria. Onset is typically between 28 and 36 weeks of gestation, but up to 25% may have onset in the early postpartum period.
- There is no consensus regarding diagnosis via laboratory criteria, but the following features are necessary: (1) hemolysis as documented by peripheral smear and elevated lactate dehydrogenase (LDH); (2) hepatic dysfunction with elevated LDH and aspartate transaminase (AST); and (3) thrombocytopenia with platelets less than 150,000 cells/mm^3.
- Differential diagnosis includes acute fatty liver of pregnancy (AFLP), antiphospholipid syndrome, hemolytic uremic syndrome (HUS), and thrombotic thrombocytopenic purpura (TTP). Rapid diagnosis is critical due to maternal and fetal risk and the need for urgent delivery.
- Major maternal and fetal risks include DIC, abruptio placenta, renal failure, acute respiratory distress syndrome (ARDS), hepatic subcapsular hematomas, hepatic infarction, and hepatic rupture or liver failure.
- Management includes prompt diagnosis, maternal stabilization, assessment of fetal status and lung maturity, and early delivery. AFLP must be excluded due to its overlap with HELLP syndrome, and its heightened risks of mortality and liver failure.
- Liver rupture is a much-feared (but rare) complication of HELLP, typically preceded by an intraparenchymal bleed that progresses to a subcapsular hematoma and rupture. Survival depends on rapid diagnosis and aggressive care via surgery and/or hepatic arterial embolization.

ACUTE FATTY LIVER OF PREGNANCY

- Acute fatty liver of pregnancy (AFLP) is a severe illness occurring almost exclusively in the third trimester, characterized by microvesicular fatty infiltration of hepatocytes potentially leading to acute liver failure. This is arguably the most critical liver disease in pregnancy because of risk to mother and fetus.
- AFLP is rare, occurring in between 1 in 10,000 and 1 in 20,000 deliveries. It appears to be more common with multiple gestations, and is always present before delivery although sometimes is misdiagnosed as HELLP or preeclampsia before the onset of jaundice or encephalopathy.
- Many cases of AFLP involve abnormalities in hepatic mitochondrial fatty acid oxidation, specifically in the long-chain 3-hydroxyacyl-CoA dehydrogenase (LCHAD) enzyme. All infants born to mothers with AFLP ought be tested for LCHAD deficiency or other disorders of fatty acid oxidation.

- Clinical features include nausea, vomiting, headaches, and abdominal pain in most patients. In more severe cases, women may have hypoglycemia, jaundice, ascites, hepatic encephalopathy, and coagulopathy as well.
- Approximately 50% of women with AFLP have features of preeclampsia and there are shared features with HELLP syndrome as well.
- In AFLP, liver transaminases can range up to 1000 U/L, but are typically between 200 and 500 U/L, and bilirubin is usually below 5 mg/dL except in severe cases. Other features include leukocytosis, thrombocytopenia, coagulopathy, renal dysfunction, and hypoglycemia.
- Liver biopsy is definitive and shows microvesicular steatosis predominantly in zone 3. However, performing a liver biopsy in pregnancy should only be done with great caution and be reserved for cases of doubt or where management will be impacted.
- Treatment is emergent delivery and supportive care for the mother. Maternal stabilization often requires correction of coagulopathy and continuous intravenous fluids with dextrose to prevent hypoglycemia.
- Liver transaminases and encephalopathy typically improve within several days of delivery. In women with progressive liver dysfunction, transfer to a liver transplant center is indicated.
- Complications of postpartum bleeding and other infections are common. Pulmonary edema may also develop in the mother due to low plasma oncotic pressure. Rarely, liver transplant is necessary due to fulminant liver failure.

REFERENCE

1. Hay, JE. Liver disease in pregnancy. *Hepatol.* 2008;47(3):1067–76.

CHAPTER 53 ■ HEPATOCELLULAR CARCINOMA

Mariela Macias, MD and Saeed Sadeghi, MD

OVERVIEW

- Hepatocellular carcinoma (HCC) accounts for 90% of primary liver tumors with the other 10% consisting mainly of biliary carcinomas. It is the third leading cause of cancer-related deaths worldwide, and the sixth most common malignancy in the world.
- Main risk factors for HCC are any disorder that leads to cirrhosis such as chronic viral infections with hepatitis B (HBV) or C (HCV), alcohol abuse, hereditary conditions (such as alpha-1-antitrypsin deficiency or hemochromatosis), and in the United States, nonalcoholic steatohepatitis (NASH).
- Factors associated with protection include: statin use, coffee consumption (> 2 cups/day), treatment of viral hepatitis infections, intake of lean meats and omega fatty acids.
- While the vast majority of HCCs are adenocarcinoma, the fibrolamellar type of HCC occurs more commonly in younger individuals in the second or third decade of life—without gender predilection or underlying cirrhosis.

PRESENTATION

- Majority of patients with HCC are asymptomatic, however, there should be a high degree of suspicion for HCC when a compensated cirrhotic patient suddenly becomes decompensated.
- Some nonspecific symptoms are related to mass effect from increasing tumor size including early satiety, abdominal pain/bloating, palpable mass, and bruit over liver from hypervascularity of mass.
- Less commonly, HCC may present with paraneoplastic syndromes such as hypoglycemia due to tumor's glucose consumption, hypercalcemia due to bone involvement or parathyroid hormone-related peptide release, and elevated hematocrit due to tumor erythropoietin production.

DIFFERENTIAL DIAGNOSIS

In cirrhotic patients, includes regenerating nodule from underlying cirrhosis, dysplastic nodule, and HCC. In both cirrhotic and noncirrhotic patients, the differential can also include hepatic hemangioma, focal nodular hyperplasia, cholangiocarcinoma, metastasis from solid tumors, lymphoma, or fibrolamellar HCC.

PATHOPHYSIOLOGY

- Underlying cirrhosis with its constant hepatocyte destruction and repair gives rise to multiple mutations in tumor suppressor genes such as TP53 and pro-oncogenic mutations in beta-catenin and c-MET. This, along with chronic inflammation from viral infection (hepatitis B or C) can lead to development of HCC.
- Fibrolamellar HCC is thought to arise from progenitor hepatocyte cells that share immunohistochemical-staining pattern of both HCC and cholangiocarcinomas. Fibrolamellar HCC has more chromosomal stability with fewer mutations and transforming growth factor beta may drive its pathogenesis. Fibrolamellar HCC also has high expression of epidermal growth factor receptor (EGFR), which may be a potential therapeutic target.

DIAGNOSIS

- HCC can be diagnosed by imaging alone based on the American Association for the Study of Liver Diseases (AALSLD) guidelines. Any mass greater than 1 cm in size that demonstrates hypervascularity on arterial phase and delayed washout on venous phase, on either quadriphasic computed tomography (CT) or dynamic magnetic resonance imaging (MRI), fulfills the criteria for HCC diagnosis.
- If there is uncertainty with the first imaging modality (i.e., CT), an MRI can be used to confirm diagnosis. Liver biopsy can be utilized to diagnose suspicious lesions that do not fulfill diagnostic criteria for HCC.
- Screening is recommended in patients with cirrhosis, and HBV infection even in absence of cirrhosis, using abdominal ultrasound every 6 months +/− alpha-fetoprotein (AFP) tumor marker based on AALSLD guidelines.

TREATMENT (SEE TABLE 53-1)

- Treatment is guided by tumor stage and underlying liver function of the patient. The Barcelona Clinic Liver Cancer (BCLC) staging and treatment guideline is a useful validated modality that links patient and tumor characteristics with the appropriate treatment.
- Curative strategies, which include liver resection and liver transplantation, are associated with 5-year survival exceeding 70% when done

Chapter 53: Hepatocellular Carcinoma

Table 53-1 Barcelona Clinic Liver Cancer (BCLC) Staging and Treatment Guideline

BCLC Stage	PS/Child-Pugh	Incidence	Tumor Characteristics	Liver function	Treatments	~5 year Survival
Stage 0	0/A	~5% (Stage 0–A)	< 2 cm	Normal PH and bilirubin	Curative Treatments (LR, LT > AT)	~70%
Stage A	0/A–B	As Above	Single < 5 cm or 3 nodules < 3 cm	Elevated PH +/– normal bilirubin	Curative (LT/AT)	~50%
Stage B	0/A–B	~20–30%	Large multinodular	No portal invasion +/– normal bilirubin	TACE/TAE	~20%
Stage C	1–2/A–B	~30%	Vascular invasion/ advanced	Portal invasion	Sorafenib	~7%
Stage D	> 2/C	5–15%	Any	+PH/abnormal bilirubin	Palliative care	0%

PH = portal hypertension; LR = liver resection; LT = Liver transplantation; AT = Ablative Therapies; TA(C)E = Transarterial (chemo)embolization

- by high-volume centers. Liver resection is generally limited to patients who are noncirrhotic and have small tumors. In cirrhotic patients with evidence of portal hypertension, liver transplantation is the best modality for cure.
- In the United States, liver transplant outcomes are significantly improved when patients are within the Milan transplantation criteria (solitary lesion < 5 cm or three nodules < 3 cm and no vascular invasion). Another validated set of criteria, the University of California San Francisco (UCSF) criteria, is becoming accepted as well given that it has less restrictive size criteria (solitary lesion of < 6.5 cm or three nodules with sum diameter total of 8 cm and with largest tumor ≤ 4.5 cm and no vascular invasion) without compromising survival benefit.
- Ablative therapies (AT) such as transarterial chemoembolizations (TACE) with chemotherapy or radiofrequency ablation can be used as bridging modalities to control the disease until a liver donor is available.
- In patients with locally advanced tumors without portal vein thrombosis not meeting the above criteria, AT with TACE or radioactive microspheres such as yttrium-90 have been utilized to control the disease. However, it is unclear if they confer a survival advantage for the patient. Two small studies have shown a benefit for survival for TACE and recently small retrospective cohort studies have shown a trend toward improved overall survival using yttrium-90 radioembolization.
- Patients with Child-Pugh score A/B who have advanced tumors with portal vein thrombosis or metastatic disease can be treated with sorafenib, a small-molecule multitargeted tyrosine kinase inhibitor against RAF, vascular endothelial growth factor receptors, and platelet-derived growth factors. Sorafenib is the only therapeutic intervention to date in this patient population that has been associated with a survival advantage of 2.8 months. Results from clinical trials to evaluate the benefit of sorafenib in post-resection and post-transplant settings are currently pending.

REFERENCES

1. Vivarelli M, Montalti R, Risaliti A. Multimodal treatment of hepatocellular carcinoma on cirrhosis: an update. *World J Gastroenterol.* 2013;19(42):7316–26.
2. Michael NM, Skye CM, Omar H, Timothy MP. A systematic review: treatment and prognosis of patients with fibrolamellar hepatocellular carcinoma. *J Am Coll Surg.* 2012;215:820–30.
3. Van Meer S, De Man RA, Siersema PD, van Erpecum KJ. Surveillance for hepatocellular carcinoma in chronic liver disease: evidence and controversies. *World J Gastroenterol.* 2013;19(40):6744–56.
4. Lin S, Hoffman K, Schemmer P. Treatment of hepatocellular carcinoma: a systematic review. *Liver Cancer.* 2012;1(3-4):144–58.

CHAPTER 54 ■ FULMINANT HEPATIC FAILURE

John Baber, MD and Vatche G. Agopian, MD

OVERVIEW

- Fulminant hepatic failure (FHF), also known as acute liver failure (ALF), is defined as severe acute liver injury with encephalopathy and impaired synthetic function (international normalized ratio [INR] > 1.5) in a patient without cirrhosis or preexisting liver disease developing within 26 weeks of the onset of illness.
- Acetaminophen toxicity is the leading cause of FHF in the United States and Europe.
- Etiology is the primary determinant of outcome, and early recognition and transfer to a liver transplant center is essential for effective treatment.

PRESENTATION

- Nonspecific symptoms (malaise, nausea, vomiting) typically precede overt signs of jaundice and encephalopathy.
- Hepatocellular dysfunction leads to coagulopathy, hypoglycemia, and lactic acidosis.
- Hypotension, hypoventilation, tachycardia, and renal failure can develop as late-stage sequelae.
- Rapid onset of encephalopathy confers a high likelihood of cerebral edema.

PATHOPHYSIOLOGY AND ETIOLOGIES

- Viral hepatitis accounts for 12% of FHF in the United States, most commonly hepatitis B (HBV) and hepatitis A. Hepatitis D superinfection in an HBV-positive individual and hepatitis E are also culprits. Herpes simplex virus (HSV), varicella zoster virus (VZV), cytomegalovirus, Epstein-Barr virus, adenoviruses, parvovirus B-19, and dengue fever may cause FHF in immunocompromised patients.
- Hepatotoxins: acetaminophen toxicity is dose-dependent and is the leading cause of FHF in the United States, accounting for approximately 42% of cases. Idiosyncratic drug reactions (11%) are dose-independent, and commonly include nonsteroidal anti-inflammatory drugs (NSAIDs), antimicrobials, antiepileptic medications, herbal supplements, and illicit

drugs. Mushroom poisoning (*Amantia phalloides*) is rare, but it portends a poor prognosis without liver transplantation (30% mortality).
- Pregnancy-related complications due to fatty liver, eclampsia, or HELLP syndrome (*h*emolysis, *e*levated *l*iver tests, *l*ow *p*latelets) can cause FHF.
- Shock liver (low cardiac output, systemic hypotension), Budd-Chiari syndrome (hepatic venous outflow obstruction), sinusoidal obstruction from bone marrow transplantation, and liver infiltration by malignancies such as lymphoma may result in FHF.
- Acute exacerbation of underlying liver disease in Wilson's disease and autoimmune hepatitis can present as FHF.

DIAGNOSIS

- History of chronic liver disease, alcohol intake, illicit drug use, tattoos, medications including supplements, travel history, immunization history, and family history should be elicited.
- Physical examination should evaluate for signs of chronic liver disease (hepatosplenomegaly, spider angiomas, ascites, palmar erythema, caput medusae).
- Neurological exam detects the presence of hepatic encephalopathy (HE). Patients with Grade I HE (mild confusion) demonstrate mild asterixis, while pronounced asterixis is present in Grade II (lethargy, moderate confusion) and Grade III (stuporous, incoherent speech, sleeping but arousable) HE. Decorticate or decerebrate posturing may be seen in Grade IV HE (coma, unresponsive to pain).
- Cerebral edema is rare in patients with Grade I/II HE but is seen in 25–35% of patients with Grade III and 65–75% of patients with Grade IV HE.
- Laboratory evaluation includes a complete blood count, comprehensive metabolic panel, INR, arterial blood gas and lactate, plasma ammonia, aerobic and anaerobic blood cultures, serum Factor V and VII levels, viral hepatitis serologies, hepatitis C polymerase chain reaction (HCV PCR), HSV PCR, VZV PCR, serum acetaminophen level, toxicology screen, urine pregnancy test, autoimmune markers, total serum immunoglobulins, serum ceruloplasmin, and serum amylase and lipase.
- Studies: chest X-ray, electrocardiogram (EKG), and liver ultrasound with Doppler studies of the hepatic vasculature should be performed routinely. If there is a concern for cerebral edema, a noncontrast computed tomography (CT) scan of the head should be performed. Liver biopsy can be performed if the etiology of FHF remains unclear.

TREATMENT

- Any patient with suspected FHF merits immediate ICU admission in a liver transplant center for close monitoring, as significant hepatocyte

death can produce systemic inflammatory response syndrome (SIRS) and multiorgan dysfunction, in addition to encephalopathy and coagulopathy.
- Balanced fluid administration to maintain perfusion but avoid exacerbation of cerebral edema is essential—as is early nutritional support.
- Reducing ammonia levels with enteral lactulose and antibiotics targeting urease-producing gut bacteria (neomycin, rifaximin) may lower plasma ammonia and ameliorate the development of HE and cerebral edema.
- Patients with Grade III/IV encephalopathy merit immediate intubation and mechanical ventilation. Sedation, minimization of stimulation, and elevating the head of bed at 30 degrees reduces the risk of intracranial hypertension.
- Coagulopathy is a defining feature of FHF, although correction of the INR is not advisable in the absence of bleeding, as this obscures INR trends that are helpful in monitoring disease progression.
- Etiology-specific therapy includes intravenous N-acetylcysteine for acetaminophen toxicity, antiviral therapy for HBV, immediate gastric lavage with activated charcoal for mushroom poisoning, acyclovir for suspected HSV, restoration of hepatic drainage in Budd-Chiari syndrome, and delivery of the fetus in pregnancy-related FHF. The utility of intravenous (IV) corticosteroids in acute autoimmune hepatitis is debated. Plasma exchange may lower the serum copper and halt hemolysis, but it is unlikely to avert the need for liver transplantation in fulminant Wilson's disease.
- Liver transplantation is the definitive therapy for patients with progressive liver dysfunction and cerebral edema who do not respond to supportive treatment.

REFERENCES

1. Lee WM, Stravitz RT, Larson AM. Introduction to the revised American Association for the Study of Liver Diseases Position Paper on acute liver failure 2011. *Hepatol.* 2012;55(3):965–7.
2. Stravitz RT, Kramer DJ. Management of acute liver failure. *Nat Rev Gastroenterol Hepatol.* 2009;6(9):542–53.

CHAPTER 55 ■ LIVER TRANSPLANTATION

John Baber, MD and Vatche G. Agopian, MD

OVERVIEW

- Liver transplantation (LT) is the definitive lifesaving therapy for irreversible hepatic failure of any etiology—acute or chronic.
- The Model for End-Stage Liver Disease (MELD) score is an accurate predictor of 3-month mortality due to liver failure, and it has become the standard for deceased-donor organ allocation in the United States since 2002.

INDICATIONS FOR LIVER TRANSPLANTATION

- Hepatitis C virus (HCV): with 20% of HCV-infected patients progressing to cirrhosis at 20 years, HCV is the most common indication for LT in the United States, accounting for 33% of all adult transplants. Reinfection of the allograft is universal in recipients with detectable viral loads at the time of LT, and is the leading cause of graft loss in these patients.
- Alcoholic liver disease (ALD): ALD accounts for 10–12% of LT in the United States. Recipients with ALD must demonstrate sobriety for a minimum of 6 months prior to LT, although the risk of recidivism approaches 33% after transplantation.
- Nonalcoholic steatohepatitis (NASH): with the epidemics in obesity, diabetes, and metabolic syndrome, NASH is now the third leading indication (10%) for LT in the United States and poised to become the leading indication in the next several decades. NASH likely accounts for the majority of patients previously categorized as having cryptogenic cirrhosis, although this association is difficult to confirm because steatosis/steatohepatitis frequently disappears with the progression of cirrhosis and hence is not observed on explant pathology.
- Hepatitis B virus (HBV): chronic HBV accounts for 5% of LTs. The introduction of high-dose intravenous hepatitis B immunoglobulin and antiviral therapy has significantly reduced the rate of recurrent HBV in the allograft and allowed for transplantation with excellent long-term survival.
- Cholestatic liver disease: chronic cholestasis leading to liver failure results most commonly from primary biliary cirrhosis (PBC), primary sclerosing cholangitis (PSC), and secondary biliary cirrhosis. Altogether they account for approximately 10% of all LTs, with excellent long-term survival.

- Fulminant hepatic failure (FHF): FHF occurs infrequently (~2000 cases/year) in the United States, with acetaminophen toxicity accounting for 40% of cases, and acute viral hepatitis, idiosyncratic drug reactions, hepatotoxins, autoimmune hepatitis, Wilson's disease, herbal supplements, and pregnancy-related complications accounting for the remainder. Prompt recognition and early referral to a transplant center is essential to identify those patients who will likely require LT (cerebral edema, severe acidosis, renal failure).
- Metabolic disorders: accounting for less than 5% of all LTs, these rare disorders lead to chronic liver disease in adulthood and include Wilson's disease, genetic hemochromatosis, and alpha-1-antitrypsin deficiency.
- Malignancy: well selected patients with hepatocellular carcinoma (HCC), cholangiocarcinoma, metastatic neuroendocrine tumors, and hepatoblastoma and hemangioendothelioma may all benefit from LT. Of these, HCC represents the majority (93%) and now accounts for approximately 20% of all LTs in the United States.
- Pediatric indications for LT most commonly include cholestatic liver disease (most commonly extrahepatic biliary atresia: 40%), hepatic malignancy (most commonly hepatoblastoma), and metabolic disorders (alpha-1-antitrypsin, urea cycle enzyme deficiencies, glycogen storage disease, Wilson's disease, cystic fibrosis, and primary hyperoxaluria).

PERIOPERATIVE COMPLICATIONS

- Infection: leading cause of mortality following LT within the first 3 months due to highest levels of immunosuppression. Offending organisms most commonly include bacterial, fungal, and viral infections.
- Graft nonfunction: primary nonfunction (within 7 days) and delayed nonfunction (> 7 days) complicate 5–8% of all LTs and lead to retransplantation and mortality.
- Hepatic artery thrombosis (HAT): HAT complicates 3.9% of adult and 8.5% of pediatric LT, and leads to graft loss, biliary strictures, intrahepatic abscesses. Early revascularization may avert the development of biliary complications, after which retransplantation becomes necessary. Observation is appropriate for asymptomatic HAT.
- Portal vein thrombosis (PVT): PVT complicates 2.1% of adult and 6.3% of pediatric LT, commonly leading to portal hypertension and graft failure.
- Biliary complications: anastomotic leaks, intra-/extrahepatic strictures, intrahepatic biliary abscesses, and bile duct stones complicate 16–30% of all LTs. Risk factors include excessive duct dissection, hepatic artery thrombosis/stenosis, prolonged ischemia, donation after cardiac death (DCD) donors, ABO mismatch transplantation, and sclerosing cholangitis. Minimally invasive endoscopic or percutaneous transhepatic interventions are diagnostic and therapeutic.

- Rejection: acute rejection occurs in 20–60% of LT recipients, most commonly within the first year. Usually suspected based on the development of hepatic biochemical test abnormalities, diagnosis is confirmed histologically and it is readily treated by bolus corticosteroids.

FOLLOW UP

- Early follow up is provided by transplant physicians with weekly comprehensive laboratory testing (complete blood count [CBC], chemistry, renal and hepatic panels, and immunosuppressive drug levels) with transition to primary care after 3 months.
- Long-term consequences of calcineurin and glucocorticoid immunosuppression include the development of hypertension (65–70%), de novo diabetes mellitus (5–30%), obesity (20%), hypercholesterolemia (16–43%), hypertriglyceridemia (40–47%), chronic kidney disease (20% at 5 years), bone loss, and de novo malignancy—most commonly skin cancer (0.9–3.2%) and post-transplant lymphoproliferative disease (0.9–2.6%).
- Excellent 20-year long-term graft (43%) and patient (52%) survival can be achieved with LT—a durable gold-standard therapy for patients with irreversible liver failure.

REFERENCES

1. Agopian VG, Petrowsky H, Kaldas FM, et al. The evolution of live transplantation during 3 decades: analysis of 5347 consecutive liver transplants at a single center. *Ann Surg.* 2013;258(3):409–21.
2. Zarrinpar A, Busuttil RW. Liver transplantation: past, present, and future. *Nat Rev Gastroenterol Hepatol.* 2013;10(7):434–40.

CHAPTER 56 ■ ALCOHOLIC HEPATITIS

Christopher V. Almario, MD and Mohamed El-Kabany, MD

OVERVIEW

- Alcoholic hepatitis (AH) is an acute form of alcohol-induced liver injury.
- AH is often seen in patients who have consumed large quantities of alcohol over an extended period of time.
- The spectrum of AH severity ranges from mild to severe. Patients with severe AH may have 50% mortality in the first 28 days of hospitalization.

PRESENTATION

- Patients with AH present with a wide spectrum of severity and symptoms.
- Symptoms are often nonspecific and include fever, anorexia, weight loss, abdominal pain, distension, nausea and vomiting, or encephalopathy.
- Physical exam can reveal jaundice, ascites, hepatomegaly, spider angiomas, asterixis, or encephalopathy.

DIFFERENTIAL DIAGNOSIS

Drug-induced liver injury, acute viral hepatitis, nonalcoholic steatohepatitis, ischemic hepatitis, Wilson's disease, autoimmune hepatitis, toxin-induced hepatitis, alpha-1-antitrypsin deficiency, and Budd-Chiari syndrome.

PATHOPHYSIOLOGY

Pathogenesis is not clearly established, but possible contributing factors include metabolism of alcohol to toxic products, oxidative stress, and cytokines.

DIAGNOSIS

- Diagnosis of AH requires a high index of clinical suspicion and is generally made through alcohol intake history and supported by physical exam and lab tests.

- Typically, labs reveal an aspartate aminotransferase/alanine transaminase (AST/ALT) ratio of > 2:1. AST is generally < 500 IU/mL and ALT < 200 IU/mL.
- Anemia, leukocytosis, and elevated bilirubin are common, but nonspecific.
- If diagnosis is in doubt, liver biopsy can be considered.

TREATMENT

After evaluation and treatment of withdrawal symptoms (see **Figure 56-1**).

- All patients with AH should remain abstinent from alcohol and undergo nutritional assessment and intervention.
- Patients with severe AH should also be treated with either prednisolone or pentoxifylline. Pentoxifylline is preferred because it is safer and less expensive.
- Severe AH is suggested by Maddrey's Discriminant Function ≥ 32, Model for End-Stage Liver Disease > 18. Discriminant Function = $4.6 \times$ (patient's prothrombin time − control prothrombin time) + total bilirubin.
- If corticosteroids are initiated, Lille score should be calculated after 1 week on therapy. Patients with a Lille score > 0.45 at 1 week should discontinue corticosteroids. Score can be calculated at: http://www.lillemodel.com.

REFERENCES

1. Choi G, Runyon BA. Alcoholic hepatitis: a clinician's guide. *Clin Liver Dis.* 2012;16:371–85.
2. Sohail U, Satapathy SK. Diagnosis and management of alcoholic hepatitis. *Clin Liver Dis.* 2012;16:717–36.

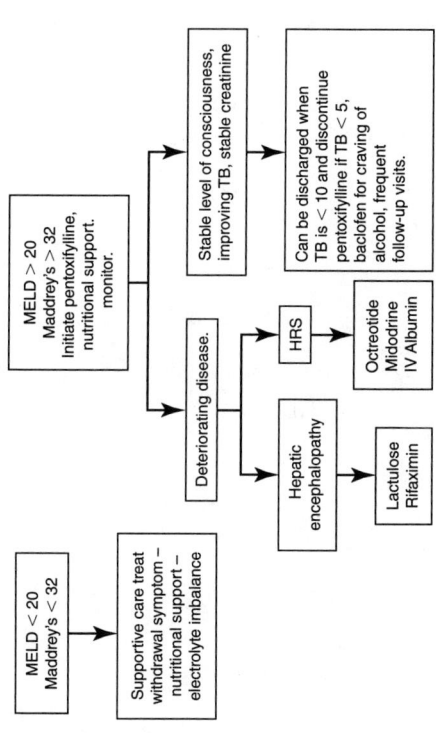

HRS = hepatorenal syndrome; TB = total bilirubin; MELD = Model for End-Stage Liver Disease

Figure 56-1 Management of alcoholic Hepatitis.

PART IV NUTRITION

CHAPTER 57 ■ NUTRITIONAL SUPPORT WITH ENTERAL FEEDING

Michael J. Albertson, MD

OVERVIEW

- The goal of enteral feeding is to supply nutritional support to meet the needs of patients who are not able to eat.
- In acute critical illness, catabolism increases in relation to anabolism and metabolic needs may not be met without supplementation. Nutritional support is necessary to inhibit the breakdown of muscle proteins into amino acids.
- Studies have shown that adequate nutritional support may alter the outcome of critical illness.

INDICATIONS

- Critically ill patients who cannot maintain nutritional support.
- Patients with neurologic deficits that prevent swallowing (such as in stroke or Parkinson's disease).
- Patients with obstruction due to esophageal cancer.
- Prophylactically, before radiation therapy for esophageal cancer. It is not unusual to develop transient edema as a result of radiation therapy that may result in temporary inability to maintain oral nutrition. A gastrostomy tube (G-tube) can be placed in anticipation of problems and removed later on.
- Patients with projected long-term intensive care unit (ICU) care on ventilatory assistance who cannot eat.

CONTRAINDICATIONS TO THE START OF ENTERAL FEEDING

- Patients who are or who have been hemodynamically unstable
- Low intravascular volume that has not been corrected
- Bowel obstruction
- Severe ileus
- Major upper gastrointestinal (GI) bleed
- Intractable nausea/vomiting or diarrhea
- Gastrointestinal ischemia
- High-output fistulae

VALUE OF ENTERAL NUTRITION

- May decrease the incidence of infection in critically ill patients—possibly due to preservation of gut immune function and decrease in inflammation.
- May prevent the onset of "stress ulceration" in the gastric mucosa.
- Provides calories, protein, electrolytes, vitamins, minerals, and trace elements.

PRE- OR POST-PYLORIC FEEDING

- Gastric feeding is usually via nasogastric tube into the stomach. In some cases the feeding tube is placed post-pylorus. Studies have not shown a beneficial effect of post-pyloric placement in preventing aspiration. Post-pyloric placement of a feeding tube can be difficult and requires expertise in endoscopic placement. Enteral feeding is usually successful with intragastric placement of a feeding tube via the nares. Position of the tube must be documented radiographically before any feeding is started.
- After the tube is placed, the head of the bed should be elevated to between 30 and 45 degrees to prevent aspiration.
- Early initiation of enteral feeding, within 48 hours, appears to be beneficial.

NUTRITIONAL REQUIREMENTS

DOSING WEIGHT

- For patients with a body mass index (BMI) between 18.5 kg/m^2 and 29.9 kg/m^2, use the actual weight for determination of caloric needs. For patients with a BMI > 30 kg/m^2, adjust the caloric needs downward.
- Calorie goal of 25–30 kcal/kg per day (1800–2100 kcal/day).
- Protein requirement depends on severity of illness.
- 0.8–1.2 g/kg/day is a goal. Critically ill patients may require 1.2–1.5 g/kg/day, and burn patients may require up to 2.0 g/kg/day.

COMPOSITION OF NUTRITIONAL SUPPORT

■ Carbohydrate/Fat

- Standard enteral nutrition delivers 49–53% of calories as carbohydrate and 29–30% of calories as fat.
- Vitamins and trace elements are critical additives to enteral nutritional support and have been shown to decrease mortality rates.

FORMULATIONS

- In patients not requiring fluid restriction:
  - Isotonic to serum
  - 1 kcl/mL
  - Lactose-free
  - Nonhydrolyzed protein content of 40 g/1000 mL
  - Nonprotein calorie to nitrogen ratio of 150
  - Mixture of simple and complex carbohydrates
  - Long-chain fatty acids
  - Vitamins, minerals, and trace elements
- A registered dietitian in the ICU can calculate the caloric needs of your patient and give advice about the most appropriate current formulation available in the hospital.
- Patients on fluid restriction may need a more concentrated formulation to avoid fluid overload and supply necessary nutritional support. The solutions available are usually hyperosmolar and supply 1.2–2.0 kcal/mL.

INEFFECTIVE FORMULATIONS AND ADDITIVES

Many studies have evaluated different formulations for patients with renal and hepatic insufficiency but have not been shown to be more effective than standard formulas. Various combinations of carbohydrate/fat/protein ratios with addition of amino acids have been investigated. They include:

- Low-carbohydrate/high-fat enteral nutrition, low-protein supplements in renal patients, peptide-based enteral nutrition, omega-3 fatty acids, arginine and ornithine, prebiotics, probiotics, and fiber

CONTINUOUS VERSUS BOLUS FEEDING

- No difference in outcome.
- Starting with a lower volume, 10–20 mL/hr, causes less adverse effects (nausea, vomiting, and diarrhea) than starting with higher volumes. The rate can be raised incrementally to a steady state of 40 mL/hr to reach a calorie goal of 18–25 kcal/kg/day.

COMPLICATIONS

ASPIRATION

- Can be ameliorated by raising the head of the bed to 45 degrees. Aspiration risk is low and most pneumonias are caused by aspirated nasopharyngeal secretions. Checking residuals is often encouraged but does not necessarily prevent aspiration. Various hospital protocols call

for stopping or slowing the rate of enteral feeding if residuals are high but this may prevent adequate daily calorie intake.
- Motility agents: not effective unless the patient suffers from gastroparesis.

DIARRHEA

Occurs in 15–18% of patients on enteral nutrition. The mechanism is unknown but may be due to decreased transit time or fluctuations in the gut microbiota. Check for concomitant use of antibiotics or proton pump inhibitors (PPIs). Additives mixed with sorbitol can also be the cause.

METABOLIC

Fluid and electrolytes should be monitored frequently to prevent complications associated with elevations or decreases in potassium, magnesium, and phosphorus (see Refeeding Syndrome).

FLUID AND WATER

Most patients will require supplemental free water unless there is a problem with fluid overload.

CONSTIPATION

- Patients may need a laxative with long-term enteral nutrition.
- Bulking agents are not recommended.

REFEEDING SYNDROME

- During refeeding, increased blood glucose results in increased insulin production, which stimulates glycogen, fat, and protein synthesis. This requires phosphate, magnesium, and thiamine. There is net absorption of K^+ into the cells along with Mg^{++} and phosphate. This results in a serum decrease in already depleted levels of phosphate, Mg^{++}, and K^+.
- Cardiac complications such as arrhythmia and congestive heart failure can occur—as can seizures. Impaired diaphragmatic contractility due to weakness or low phosphate can result in dyspnea. Liver tests can be elevated. Muscular involvement can include myalgias, weakness, tetany, and in rare cases, rhabdomyolysis.

REFERENCES

1. Gramlich L, Kichian K, Pinilla J, et al. Does enteral nutrition compared to parenteral nutrition result in better outcomes in critically ill adult patients? A systematic review of the literature. *Nutrition*. 2004;20(10):843–8.
2. Koretz RL, Avenell A, Lipman TO, et al. Does enteral nutrition affect clinical outcome? A systematic review of randomized trials. *Am J Gastroenterol*. 2007;102:412–29.

3. Montejo JC, Minambres E, Bordeje L et al. Gastric residual volume during enteral nutrition in ICU patients: the REGANE study. *Intensive Care Med.* 2010;36(8):1386–93.
4. Mehanna HM, Moledina J, Travis J. Refeeding syndrome: what is it, and how to prevent and treat it. *Brit Med J.* 2008;336(7659):1495–98.

CHAPTER 58 ■ PARENTERAL NUTRITIONAL SUPPORT

Jorge H. Vargas, MD

OVERVIEW

- Intravenous alimentation is used when the oral or enteral routes are not functional or possible (intestinal failure). Although not physiologic, it constitutes an effective therapy.
- The nutrients are delivered into the systemic circulation and not through the portal system (as with normal enteral feeding)—this route has metabolic implications and alterations in the circadian rhythms of hunger and satiety.
- This infusion of macro- and micronutrients intravenously for prolonged periods of time allows for the correction of nutritional deficits and may also maintain and ensure normal growth.
- It has thus become an essential tool in the improvement of the prognosis and outcomes of numerous medical and surgical conditions.

INDICATIONS

Both adults and children share a series of categories of indications to provide intravenous calories and nutrients, and the length of the indication may be quite variable.

INTESTINAL FAILURE

■ Congenital anomalies

- Structural or developmental anomalies of the intestine
  - Microvillus inclusion disease
  - Tufting enteropathy
  - Intestinal atresia resulting in short bowel syndrome
  - Congenital short gut
- Developmental anomalies of the intrinsic nervous system of the gastrointestinal (GI) tract (visceral neuropathies)
  - Aganglionosis
- Developmental anomalies of the intestinal smooth muscle (visceral myopathies)
- Intestinal lymphangiectasia

Acquired or postnatal

- Necrotizing enterocolitis
- Mid-gut volvulus on anomalies of intestinal rotation
- Radiation enteritis
- Thromboembolic episodes of mesenteric vessels
  - Trauma
- Internal hernias, volvulus as complications of abdominal surgeries
  - Postbariatric surgery
- Inflammatory bowel disease
  - Crohn's disease
    - Recurrent resections
    - Obstruction
    - Fistulae
- Collagen vascular disease
  - Scleroderma
- Autoimmune enteropathy

CALCULATING NUTRITIONAL NEEDS AND FORMULATIONS

The calculation of nutritional requirements varies according to age, degree of development, clinical situation, and specific therapeutic goals and should be individualized. Keep in mind that carbohydrates (dextrose) and fat emulsions are the main sources of energy. Nitrogen for protein synthesis is supplied as crystalline amino acids.

- Protein requirements: 1–2.5 g/kg day.
- Lipid requirements: 25–40% of non protein calories or 2–3 g/kg/day.
- Carbohydrates (glucose): 60–75% of non protein calories or 50% of total calories.
- A detailed fluid balance of the individual is then important to calculate needs.
- Electrolytes, micronutrients, minerals, and vitamins may also be individualized.
- Special types of amino acids may be required in situations of chronic liver disease; the carbohydrate content may be tailored to tolerance and insulin response, and the lipid infusions can also be tailored according to tolerance and ability to clear.

HOW TO DETERMINE THE COMPOSITION OF PARENTERAL NUTRITION

Determine the energy requirements of the individual patient.

- May use indirect calorimetry, calculation by Harris-Benedict equation, or use standardized tables.

Chapter 58: Parenteral Nutritional Support

- Children
  - 100 kcal/kg/day for first 10 kg, 50 kcal/kg/day added for weight between 10 and 20 kg, and 25 kcal/kg/day for weight between 20 and 30 kg. Above 30 kg may use adult parameters.
- Adults
  - Baseline needs: 25–30 kcal/kg/day
  - Additional injury/stress: 35–40 kcal/kg/day
  - Severe stress/injury: 40–55 kcal/kg/day

These calculations can be based on ideal body weight (IBW), weight × height, or current weight, plus additional percentage of calories for "catch-up growth" in cases of severe malnutrition or weight loss.

VASCULAR ACCESS

Provided at different ages, patient size, and clinical setting by a variety of devices.

- Peripheral angiographic catheter (angio-cath).
- Larger, deeper, and longer catheters that can be placed percutaneously (peripherally inserted central catheter, or PICC) by specialized phlebotomists or interventional radiologist and surgeons.
  - Tunneled catheters with single or multiple lumens.
  - "Port" type of catheters, with no external access, which are not really designed for daily use.
  - The materials and designs of the catheters do not seem to really influence outcomes, including infectious episodes. The choice between a peripheral vein versus a central one will depend on several factors including the age of the patient, the degree of malnutrition or severity of the compromise of this function, the osmolarity of the solutions to cover the delivery of adequate energy, and mainly the duration of the need for nutritional support.
- The "central" position of these lines ensures a rapid flow and thus the ability to administer large osmotic loads.
- Tunneled lines perhaps allow better mobility and freedom of patient activities, particularly when they are young, but do not seem to have better outcomes in terms of incidence of infections or contamination when compared to other types. They may offer a lower risk of being pulled out or displaced.
- Once the lines are in place, the patient or caregiver needs to learn to handle the aseptic technique of caring for the line and the site as well connecting the solutions at home and setting up the infusion pump.

THE INFUSIONS

Once the decision is made to provide nutritional support intravenously and having calculated the fluid, carbohydrates, protein, fat, electrolytes, vitamins, micronutrients, and general nutritional needs of the patient, the solutions can and should be infused in a "cycled" manner, when their need is prolonged or "long-term."

- "Compressing" the administration of the solutions:
  o Overnight and for 8–12 hours: allows time off any pumps and equipment, for patients to return, at least in part, to a more normal life, and for children to have time for activities, development, or school.
- Variations in fluid and electrolytes
  o Maintain strict fluid balances.
    – Measurable and "insensible" losses to maintain homeostasis
  o May also be calculated to cover only nutritional needs.
    – Then adding balance of losses separately
      - These solutions may be given in "parallel" or after parenteral nutrition has been delivered and may be given at faster rates (e.g., NS [normal saline], ½ NS c KCl [potassium chloride], LR [lactated Ringer's], etc.)

MONITORING AND FOLLOW UP

The frequency of the analytical determinations and follow up will depend on the clinical situation and the duration of the nutritional support. Besides closely monitoring the patient's weight and other anthropometrics, the patients are seen periodically with an emphasis on checking for and preventing complications from the nutritional therapy, such as:

- Patency and flow through the line
- Hemodynamics: fluid retention
- Metabolic problems:
  o Hyperglycemia: thirst, polyuria
  o Hypoglycemia: jitteriness, pallor, diaphoresis
- Vascular problems: thrombosis, phlebitis

Lab work should include complete blood counts, comprehensive metabolic panel to assess for electrolyte and acid-base balance, triglycerides and cholesterol, liver and renal function, and protein status (total protein and albumin). Protein assessment should include evaluation of protein synthesis by measuring a faster metabolized protein like prealbumin, and, periodically, a micronutrient assessment including iron (Fe), zinc (Zn), selenium (Se), and perhaps copper (Cu) levels.

Chapter 58: Parenteral Nutritional Support

COMPLICATIONS

Can be minimized with an adequate use of the indications, a well balanced mixture of nutrients, and close vigilance to the patient's response.

MECHANICAL COMPLICATIONS

Technical problems at insertion of the catheters or lines used to deliver the solutions.

- Pneumothorax, vascular lacerations, cardiac perforations and tamponades, air embolism, or nerve injury.
- Lines can rupture, dislodge, migrate, and occlude, and the latter can be the result of either clotting, deposition, or precipitation of chemicals in the solution or medications infused.
  - Repair under aseptic technique via repositioning or a total replacement.
  - Thrombosis of the line
    - Infusion of blood or blood products
    - Lack of adequate line care
    - Lack of infusion of anticoagulants after use
    - Involvement of the line in a diffuse thromboembolic episode of the vein that harbors the catheter

METABOLIC COMPLICATIONS

Related to the over-infusion or deficits of metabolic components of the solutions.

- Carbohydrates, proteins, and fats
  - Hyperglycemia
    - Glycosuria, water, and electrolyte loss
  - Hypoglycemia
    - Inadequate taper or sudden discontinuation of solution
  - "Refeeding syndrome"
  - Protein
    - Elevation of blood urea nitrogen (BUN)
    - Encephalopathy in context of liver disease
  - Fats
    - Hypertriglyceridemia
    - Fat overload syndrome (> 4 g/kg of fat/day, > 60% of total calories as fat)
- Excess of fluid and sodium
  - Water retention, edema, respiratory difficulty, excess weight gain
- Excess of additives used
- Deficiencies of components that are normally absorbed through the intestinal route and are part of our daily diets
  - Fe, Zn, Se, Cu, and P (phosphorus), as well as vitamins A, B1, B12, E, folates, etc.

INFECTIOUS COMPLICATIONS

- Local, cutaneous entry-site infections
- Line infections
  - Poor or lapse in the aseptic technique in the handling
  - Bacterial migration from the intestinal lumen, bypassing the reticuloendothelial system of the liver
    - Bacterial and fungal elements and may constitute an indication for removal of the line as the only effective therapy. In general, however, most of the infections can be successfully treated with antibiotics, keeping the lines in place—particularly in those patients with indications for long-term need of nutritional support.

OTHER CATEGORIES

- Liver disease, although transient and reversible, particularly in the young patient, still constitutes a major source of worry as it has major consequences in the morbidity and mortality of those patients, limiting the ability to tolerate feedings and thus limiting the development of adaptation to conditions like short bowel syndrome. May lead to irreversible end-stage liver disease and need for transplantation at a young age. The etiology of the liver disease is still not completely understood but several major factors have been identified as contributors, such as recurrent Gram-negative infections and the lack of infusion of certain types of fats as omega-3 fatty acids.
- Bone disease is also another complication despite the fact that aluminum was taken away from the solutions when amino acids were directly produced and synthesized. It appears that the balance of Ca (calcium) and PO_4 (phosphate) in serum and excretions, despite better control of vitamin D levels, may be a factor for this disorder—again seems to be more severe in developing children.
- Thromboembolic
  - Physical characteristic of the nutritional solutions (high osmolarity), used with certain chronicity, are responsible for the initiation of thrombotic or vascular complications—hence the potential indication to consider the administration of antiplatelet aggregation products or anticoagulants to the nutritional solutions as well.

REFERENCES

1. Koletzko B, Goulet O, Hunt J, et al. Guidelines on Paediatric Parenteral Nutrition of the European Society of Paediatric Gastroenterology, Hepatology and Nutrition (ESPGHAN) and the European Society for Clinical Nutrition and Metabolism (ESPEN), Supported by the European Society of Paediatric Research (ESPR). *J Pediatr Gastroenterol Nutr.* 2005;41(Suppl 2):81–4.

2. Koshevar M, Guenter P, Holcombe B, et al. ASPEN statement on parenteral nutrition standardization. *J Parent Enteral Nutr.* 2007;31:441–8.
3. Ayers P, Adams S, Boullata J, et al. A.s.p.e.N. Parenteral nutrition safety consensus recommendations. *J Parenter Enteral Nutr.* 2014;38(3):296–333.

CHAPTER 59 ■ DIETARY MODIFICATIONS FOR GASTROINTESTINAL SYMPTOMS

Nancee Jaffe, MS, RD

OVERVIEW

- Many gastrointestinal (GI) disorders warrant dietary intervention, including celiac disease/gluten sensitivity, chronic constipation and/or diarrhea, colorectal cancer, food allergies/intolerance (lactose intolerance, fructose malabsorption), gas and bloating, gastroparesis, inflammatory bowel diseases (IBD), irritable bowel syndrome (IBS), gastroesophageal reflux disease (GERD), small bowel syndrome/ostomies, and small intestine bacterial overgrowth.
- Most commonly seen GI complaints that involve nutritional intervention are gas/bloating, gastroesophageal reflux disease, diarrhea, and constipation.

GAS/BLOATING

Intestinal gas comes mainly from two sources: air we ingest orally and gas naturally produced in the body as certain foods are broken down and digested by colonic bacteria.

DIETARY CHANGES

- *Reduce intake of raffinose/stachyose*: sugars found in such foods as beans, mushrooms, cabbage, Brussels sprouts, broccoli, and asparagus. Products like Beano® help break down these sugars.
- *Reduce intake of lactose*: a sugar found in dairy products such as milk and ice cream.
- *Reduce intake of fructose*: a sugar found in certain fruits and vegetables such as apples, watermelon, pears, onions, and garlic, as well as sweeteners like high fructose corn syrup.
- *Reduce intake of sugar alcohols (sorbitol, mannitol, xylitol, maltitol)*: a sugar found naturally in fruits such as prunes, apples, and peaches. Also used as a sweetener in sugar-free processed foods such as gums, mints, and diabetic products.
- *Prescribe the low FODMAP (fermentable oligosaccharides, disaccharides, monosaccharides and polyols) diet*: a diet that eliminates specific sugars from the diet that can contribute to gas and bloating. This diet is indicated for irritable bowel syndrome and small intestine bacterial overgrowth patients. Recommended patients work with a skilled registered

dietitian as the diet is difficult to follow without proper instruction and guidance. See **Table 59-1**.

Swallowing excess air happens when one chews gum, smokes, uses a straw, drinks or eats too quickly, and/or experiences chronic or severe stress and anxiety.

GERD

- Symptoms are often precipitated or exacerbated by dietary intake.
- Symptoms include: heartburn, acid taste in mouth, burping, chronic cough, trouble swallowing, recurrent sore throat, and/or hoarseness.

DIETARY CHANGES

Elimination of classic trigger foods can reduce symptoms:

- Citrus fruits (oranges, lemons, limes, grapefruit)
- Caffeine (chocolate, tea, coffee, soda, energy drinks)
- Alcohol
- Fried, greasy, oily, or fatty foods
- Garlic and onions
- Mint, peppermint, or spearmint
- Spicy foods
- Tomato-based food products (sauces, ketchup, salsa)
- Carbonated beverages

LIFESTYLE MODIFICATIONS

- Raise the head of the bed by 4–6 inches or use a wedge pillow.
- Eat small, frequent meals instead of large meals.
- Save beverages for between meals instead of drinking at a meal.
- Stay upright for at least an hour after eating.
- Avoid eating 2–3 hours before going to sleep.
- Wear loose fitting clothing around the abdomen and chest.
- Lose weight if overweight or obese.
- Stop smoking.

DIARRHEA

Diarrhea is generally defined as having three or more loose, watery stools per day.

DIETARY INTERVENTIONS

To help minimize stool output:

- BRAT diet: banana, rice (white not brown), applesauce, and toast (white not whole grain)

Table 59-1 High FODMAP Foods

Fructose	Lactose	Fructans	Galactans	Polyols
FRUITS: apples, boysenberry, cherries, mango, peaches, pears, figs, raspberries, watermelon **VEGETABLES**: artichoke, asparagus, sugar snap peas **SWEETENERS**: agave, honey, high fructose corn syrup **ALCOHOL**: rum	Custards, ice cream, milk (any fat content or format), soft cheeses (ricotta, cottage), yogurt	**FRUIT**: nectarines, raspberries, watermelon **VEGETABLES**: asparagus, beets, broccoli, Brussels sprouts, cabbage, garlic, kale, onions, radicchio, scallions, shallots, snow peas **GRAINS**: barley, bulgar, couscous, rye, wheat **SWEETENERS**: chicory root, inulin	**VEGETABLES**: asparagus, broccoli, Brussels sprouts, cabbage, cauliflower **LEGUMES/NUTS/SEEDS**: beans: butter, chickpea, lima, soy; cashews, lentils, pistachios, split peas, tempeh **SWEETENERS**: chicory root, inulin	**FRUITS**: apples, apricots, avocado, blackberries, nectarines, peaches, pears, plums, prunes, watermelon **VEGETABLES**: broccoli, cauliflower, fennel, green bell peppers, mushrooms, pumpkin, snow peas, sweet corn **SWEETENERS**: isomalt, mannitol, maltitol, sorbitol, xylitol (sugar-free products such as gum, mints, cough drops, medications)

Sources:
1. Catsos P. *IBS: Free at Last!: Change Your Carbs, Change Your Life with the FODMAP Elimination Diet*. 2nd ed. Portland, ME: Pond Cove Press; 2012.
2. Muir JG. HPLC separation of carbohydrates in vegetables and fruits. *J Agric Food Chem*. 2009;57(2):554–65.
3. Scarlata K. FODMAPs. *Well Balanced Food Life Travel*. Available at: http://blog.katescarlata.com/category/fodmaps/. Accessed August 2014.
4. Monash University. *The Monash University Low FODMAP diet*. Available at: http://www.med.monash.edu/cecs/gastro/fodmap/. Accessed August 2014.

- Other foods that might decrease stool output are:
  - White potatoes (no skin)
  - White pasta
  - Saltine crackers
  - Well cooked carrots
  - Baked, poached, or roasted chicken without skin or fat
- Until diarrhea subsides, avoid:
  - Caffeine (chocolate, tea, coffee, soda, energy drinks)
  - Fried, greasy, oily, or fatty foods
  - Dairy products
  - Foods high in insoluble fiber
  - Foods high in simple sugars such as juices
  - Sugar alcohols (sorbitol, maltitol, mannitol, xylitol)
  - Alcohol
- Oral rehydration solutions (ORS) should be considered in cases of chronic diarrhea to avoid dehydration. They have specific amounts of fluid, sodium, and carbohydrates.
  - Recommended ORS recipes:
    - 1 liter G2 + ½ teaspoon salt
    - 2 cups Gatorade + 2 cups water + ½ teaspoon salt
    - 1 liter Pedialyte + ¼ teaspoon salt

CONSTIPATION

Constipation is defined as producing less than three bowel movements per week and can include dry, hard, or pellet-like stools that require straining.

DIETARY INTERVENTIONS

To help maximize stool output in functional constipation patients:

- Increase insoluble fiber to help stool pass quickly; if stool is hard or dry, add psyllium husk to help soften stool first before introducing insoluble fiber.
- Limit foods that have little or no fiber, such as dairy products and animal proteins.
- Drink fluids and avoid dehydration. The Institute of Medicine recommends women drink approximately 2.7 liters of fluid each day and men approximately 3.7 liters of fluid daily.
- Hot liquids, especially in the morning, may help encourage a bowel movement. Prune juice mixed with warm water works well for some patients.

REFERENCES

1. U.S. Department of Health and Human Services, National Institutes of Health (NIH) Publication. *Constipation*. No. 07–2754. Bethesda, MD: Author; July 2007. Print.

2. U.S. Department of Health and Human Services, National Institutes of Health (NIH) Publication. *Diarrhea*. No. 11–2749. Bethesda, MD: Author; January 2011. Print.
3. U.S. Department of Health and Human Services, National Institutes of Health (NIH) Publication. *Gas*. No. 08–883. Bethesda, MD: Author; January 2008. Print.
4. U.S. Department of Health and Human Services, National Institutes of Health (NIH) Publication. *GERD*. No. 07–0882. Bethesda, MD: Author; May 2007.
5. Rees Parrish, C. *A Patient's Guide to Managing a Short Bowel*. Bedminster, NJ: NPS Pharmaceuticals; 2011.
6. Institutes of Medicine, *Dietary Reference Intakes: Water, Potassium, Sodium, Chloride, and Sulfate*. Washington, DC: The National Academies; 2004.
7. Dennis M. *Calming Inflammation and Healing the Gut*. Santa Barbara, CA: Casa de Maria; February 2013.
8. Rhoda K, Wolff J. "Diet for Diarrhea: Going Beyond the BRAT Diet." ADA Food and Nutrition Conference and Exposition. American Dietetic Association. San Diego Convention Center San Diego; 27 Sept. 2011. Lecture.
9. Krames StayWell, *Lifestyle Changes for Controlling GERD*. Yardley, PA: Author; 2000–2013.

PART V ENDOSCOPY GUIDELINES

CHAPTER 60 ■ ENDOSCOPY GUIDELINES

Stephen Kim, MD and Eric Esrailian, MD, MPH

OVERVIEW

Endoscopic procedures have various indications, but the indications for urgent procedures are limited. We summarize published guidelines for antibiotic prophylaxis and the management of antithrombotic agents around the time of endoscopy.

INDICATIONS FOR URGENT ENDOSCOPY

- Although endoscopy is typically performed for a variety of indications, there are only a few reasons to perform gastrointestinal endoscopy on an urgent basis.
- The following are the indications for urgent endoscopy, as it relates to each type of endoscopic procedure:
  - Esophagogastroduodenoscopy (EGD)
    - Active or recent upper gastrointestinal bleeding
    - Foreign body removal
    - Assessment of injury after caustic ingestion
  - Colonoscopy/flexible sigmoidoscopy
    - Active or recent lower gastrointestinal bleeding
    - Foreign body removal
    - Decompression of sigmoid volvulus or acute megacolon
  - Endoscopic retrograde cholangiopancreatography (ERCP)
    - Acute cholangitis due to bile duct obstruction
  - Endoscopic ultrasound (EUS)
    - None; no urgent indications for performing EUS

ANTIBIOTIC PROPHYLAXIS IN ENDOSCOPY

- From an infection standpoint, gastrointestinal endoscopy is generally considered to be safe and carries a lower risk of transient bacteremia than routine daily activities such as brushing and flossing teeth.
- However, bacteremia can occur after endoscopy due to bacterial translocation of microbial flora from mucosal trauma related to the procedure.

- The prophylactic use of antibiotics is recommended for endoscopic procedures that are thought to carry a higher risk of developing iatrogenic infectious complications.
- Antibiotic prophylaxis is indicated for the following procedures and patient conditions:
  1. Percutaneous endoscopic gastrostomy (PEG) tube placement
     - Cefazolin 1 g IV × 1 (or equivalent) given 30 minutes prior to procedure
  2. Cirrhosis with acute gastrointestinal bleeding
     - Ceftriaxone 1 g IV daily × 7 days (or equivalent) with first dose given prior to procedure
  3. Acute cholangitis due to bile duct obstruction
     - Coverage for enteric Gram-negative organisms and enterococci
  4. Bile duct obstruction in the absence of cholangitis with anticipated incomplete drainage at ERCP (hilar stricture, primary sclerosing cholangitis, etc.)
     - Coverage for enteric Gram-negative organisms and enterococci
  5. EUS with fine-needle aspiration (FNA) of cystic lesions
     - Fluoroquinolone given before the procedure and continued for 3 days
  6. Drainage of sterile pancreatic fluid collections
     - Fluoroquinolone given before the procedure and continued for 3 days
- Antibiotic prophylaxis is *not recommended* for the following procedures and patient conditions:
  - Any cardiac condition including prosthetic valves
  - Bile duct obstruction in the absence of cholangitis with complete drainage
  - EUS with FNA of solid lesions
  - Synthetic vascular grafts, cardiovascular devices, prosthetic joints

ANTITHROMBOTIC AGENTS IN ENDOSCOPY

- Antithrombotic medications include antiplatelet agents (aspirin, nonsteroidal anti-inflammatory drugs [NSAIDs]), thienopyridines (clopidogrel, ticlopidine), and anticoagulants (warfarin, heparin, direct thrombin, and factor Xa inhibitors).
- When performing endoscopy on patients taking antithrombotics, the bleeding risk of the endoscopic procedure and the thromboembolic risk of interrupting antithrombotic therapy should be considered.
- Endoscopic procedures are divided into low and high risk of bleeding (see **Table 60-1**).
- Similarly, cardiovascular conditions are separated into low and high risk of causing a thromboembolic event (see **Table 60-2**).

Chapter 60: Endoscopy Guidelines

Table 60-1 Endoscopic Procedures Listed by Risk of Bleeding

Low Risk	High Risk
Diagnostic endoscopy with biopsy	Polypectomy
ERCP without sphincterotomy	ERCP with sphincterotomy
EUS without FNA	EUS with FNA
Capsule endoscopy	PEG placement
Enteral stent placement	Pneumatic or bougie dilation
	Treatment of varices
	Tumor ablation
	Balloon-assisted enteroscopy
	Cystogastrostomy

Table 60-2 Patient Conditions Listed by Risk of Thromboembolic Event

Low Risk	High Risk
Atrial fibrillation • uncomplicated • paroxysmal	Atrial fibrillation associated with: • valvular heart disease • prosthetic valves • active congestive heart failure • ejection fraction < 35% • history of thromboembolic event • hypertension • diabetes mellitus • age > 75
Mechanical aortic valve	Mechanical mitral valve
Bioprosthetic valve	Any mechanical valve and previous thromboembolic event
Deep vein thrombosis	Recent (< 1 year) coronary stent placement
	Acute coronary syndrome
	Non stented percutaneous coronary intervention after myocardial infarction

- Endoscopic procedures with a low risk of bleeding can be performed safely while continuing patients on antithrombotic therapies.
  - Nevertheless, consider discontinuing anticoagulation in patients with a low risk of thromboembolic events in the peri-endoscopic period.
- Endoscopic procedures with a high risk of bleeding require closer management:
  - Antiplatelet agents (aspirin, NSAIDs) can be continued.

- Thienopyridines (clopidogrel) should be discontinued for at least 7–10 days prior to the procedure when possible. If the thromboembolic risk is high, aspirin monotherapy can be started or continued. Elective procedures should be postponed.
  - Anticoagulants should be discontinued prior to the procedure when possible. If the thromboembolic risk is high, consider bridging therapy with a shorter acting anticoagulant. For patients on temporary anticoagulation, elective procedures should be postponed until antithrombotic therapy has been completed.
- No optimal timing of restarting antithrombotics has been established. The decision to restart antithrombotics should be individualized on a case-by-case basis.

REFERENCES

1. ASGE (American Society for Gastrointestinal Endoscopy) Standards of Practice Committee. Antibiotic prophylaxis for GI endoscopy. *Gastrointest Endosc.* 2008;67(6):791–8.
2. ASGE Standards of Practice Committee. Appropriate use of GI endoscopy. *Gastrointest Endosc.* 2012;75(6):1127–31.
3. ASGE Standards of Practice Committee. Management of antithrombotic agents for endoscopic procedures. *Gastrointest Endosc.* 2009;70(6):1060–70.

INDEX

Note: Page numbers followed by f or t indicate material in figures or tables respectively.

A

abdomen/pelvis
  with contrast, routine CT, 47–48
  MRI, 50–51
  with noncontrast CT, 49
abdominal computerized tomography (CT) scan, 8
abdominal pain, 87
  aggravating/alleviating factors of, 7
  associated symptoms of, 7
  conditions of, 4
  evaluation of, 4
  historical elements of, 7
  imaging of, 8, 48f
  key concepts of, 3
  laboratory testing of, 8
  pain symptoms, characterization of, 5–7
  pathophysiology of, 3–4
  physical findings of, 7–8
abdominal radiograph, 51
abdominal ultrasound, 49, 136
ablative therapies (AT), 270
abnormal blind-ending biliary ductules, 222
abnormal liver tests, 192f
  abbreviations, 195–196
  approach to patient with, 209, 210f
  causes of injury, 193–195
  initial approach, 193
  liver panel tests, 191, 192f
  patterns of injury, 193
abscesses, 223–224
acalculous cholecystitis, 141
acetaminophen, 212
acetaminophen toxicity, 213, 271

ACG guidelines. See American College of Gastroenterology guidelines
achalasia, 11
activated charcoal, 44
acute bloody diarrhea, 27
acute cholecystitis, 140t
acute diarrhea, 29, 30
acute diverticulitis, 153
acute fatty liver of pregnancy (AFLP), 19, 265–266
acute gastroenteritis, management algorithm for, 159f
acute infection, HBV, 197–198
acute invasive, diarrhea, 27
acute liver failure (ALF). See fulminant hepatic failure (FHF)
acute mesenteric ischemia (AMI), 4, 102–103
acute painless lower GI bleeding, diagnostic algorithm for adults, 115f
acute pancreatitis, 135
  inflammatory process of, 136
acute pouchitis, 176, 178
acute processes, 19
acute watery diarrhea, 27
adenocarcinoma, 117
adenoma detection rate (ADR), 162
adenomas, 162
adenomatous polyps, 161
adenovirus, 158
adequate perfusion, 101
AFLP. See acute fatty liver of pregnancy
AGA. See American Gastroenterological Association

aggravating/alleviating factors, abdominal pain, 7
AH. See alcoholic hepatitis
AIH. See autoimmune hepatitis
alanine aminotransferase, 191
alanine transaminase (ALT), 234
alcohol use, 135
alcoholic hepatitis (AH)
  diagnosis, 279–280
  differential diagnosis, 279
  gastropaedica, 279
  management, 280, 281f
  pathophysiology, 279
  presentation, 279
  treatment, 280
alcoholic liver disease (ALD), 213–214, 275
alkaline phosphatase, 191
alosetron, 91
alpha-1-antitrypsin (A1AT) deficiency, 211, 246–247
ALT. See alanine transaminase
AMA. See antimitochondrial antibodies
ambulatory intraesophageal pH testing, 56
amebic abscess, 223–224
American Association for the Study of Liver Diseases (AASLD) guidelines, 230
American College of Gastroenterology (ACG) guidelines, 66
American Gastroenterological Association (AGA), 20, 60

311

Index

American Gastroenterological Association (AGA) (*Cont.*)
  surveillance guidelines for average-risk individuals, 161t
AMI. *See* acute mesenteric ischemia
ammonia, 255
amylase, 136
anal fissures, 70
  diagnosis, 71
  differential diagnosis, 71
  pathophysiology, 71
  presentation, 70–71
  treatment, 71
anorectal biofeedback for sphincter retraining, 26
antibiotics, 158
anticoagulants, 310
antidepressants, 91
antidiarrheal therapy, 91, 180
antiemetics, 137
antimitochondrial antibodies (AMA), 215, 216, 230
antispasmodic agents, 91
arthritis, 73
ascending cholangitis, 140t, 141t
ascites
  diagnosis, 249–250
  differential diagnosis, 249, 250t
  pathophysiology, 249
  presentation, 249
  treatment, 250–252, 251f, 251t
aspartate aminotransferase (AST), 191, 234
asterixis, 255
astrovirus, 158
asymptomatic cholelithiasis, 140t, 141t
AT. *See* ablative therapies
autodigestion, 136
autoimmune hepatitis (AIH), 216–217
  diagnosis, 234, 235f

B

baclofen, 56
bacterial gastroenteritis, 18
bacteriology, 65
balloon-occluded retrograde transvenous obliteration (BRTO), 111
Barcelona Clinic Liver Cancer (BCLC), staging and treatment guideline, 268, 269t
bariatric surgery, 243
Barrett's esophagus (BE)
  diagnosis, 60
  management/treatment, 60–63, 61f
  pathophysiology, 59–60
  presentation, 59
BCS. *See* Budd-Chiari syndrome
BE. *See* Barrett's esophagus
benign anorectal disorders, 69–72
  anal fissures, 70–71
  condyloma, 71–72
  hemorrhoids, 69–70
benign focal lesions, 220–223
benign liver tumor, 222
benzamides, 22
biliary disease, 97
biliary dyskinesia, 141
bloating, 299–300
blood supply, 101
  anatomy, 102
blood transfusion, 114
bloody diarrhea, 7
BMI. *See* body mass index
boceprevir, 205
body mass index (BMI), 286
bolus feeding *vs.* continuous feeding, 287
bone disease, 296
borderline resectable tumors, 130
bowel obstruction
  differential diagnosis, 233
  pathophysiology, 233–234
  presentation, 233
  treatment, 234–236, 236f

BRTO. *See* balloon-occluded retrograde transvenous obliteration
Budd-Chiari syndrome (BCS), 211–212, 273
bulk laxative, 25t
button batteries, 34

C

CA 19-9, 128
Campylobacter jejuni, 158
Candida (monilial) esophagitis, 95
carbolic acid, 42
caustic ingestions
  acute workup, 42
  caustic substances, 41–42, 41t
  clinical presentation, 42
  endoscopy, 43
  long-term sequelae, 45
  treatment, 43–44
cavernous hemangioma, 221
CD. *See* celiac disease; Crohn's disease
CDI. *See* Clostridium difficile infection
celiac artery pathology, 105
celiac disease (CD)
  diagnosis, 78–80, 79f
  differential diagnosis, 78
  pathophysiology, 78
  presentation, 77
  treatment, 80
cell culture cytotoxicity assay, 185
cellular immune response, 217
central nervous system (CNS), causes, 18
cerebral cortex, 17
chemotherapy, 270
chloride channel agonist, 25t

diagnosis, 150
differential diagnosis, 149
gastropaedica, 149
pathophysiology, 150
presentation, 149
treatment, 151